BACTERIAL MENINGITIS

BACTERIAL MENINGITIS

Allan R. Tunkel, M.D., Ph.D.

Professor & Vice Chair for Education, Department of Medicine
Director, Internal Medicine Residency Program
MCP Hahnemann University
Philadelphia, Pennsylvania

Contribution by

W. Michael Scheld, M.D.

Wyeth-Ayerst Professor of Infectious Diseases
Professor, Department of Internal Medicine
University of Virginia School of Medicine
and
Attending Physician, Department of Internal Medicine
University of Virginia Health System
Charlottesville, Virginia

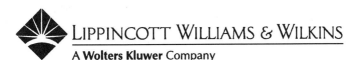

LIPPINCOTT WILLIAMS & WILKINS
A **Wolters Kluwer** Company
Philadelphia • Baltimore • New York • London
Buenos Aires • Hong Kong • Sydney • Tokyo

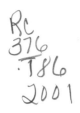
Acquisitions Editor: Jonathan W. Pine, Jr.
Developmental Editor: Selina M. Bush
Production Editor: John C. Vassiliou
Manufacturing Manager: Benjamin Rivera
Cover Designer: Karen Quigley
Compositor: Techbooks
Printer: Edwards Brothers

© **2001 by LIPPINCOTT WILLIAMS & WILKINS**
530 Walnut Street
Philadelphia, PA 19106 USA
LWW.com

Library of Congress Cataloging-in-Publication Data
Tunkel, Allan R.
   Bacterial meningitis / Allan R. Tunkel.
      p. ; cm.
   Includes bibliographical references and index.
   ISBN 0-7817-1102-9
   1. Meningitis.   I. Title.
   [DNLM: 1. Meningitis, Bacterial. WL 200 T926b 2001]
   RC376 .T86 2001
   616.8′2 — dc21   2001016444

10 9 8 7 6 5 4 3 2 1

To my wife, Randy, for her love, encouragement, and understanding;
To my children, Lindsay and Emily, for their hugs and
kisses at the end of a hard day;
and
To my Mom and Dad, for a lifetime of support and guidance.

Contents

Foreword

Few diagnoses are as frightening to the patient, his family, his clinician, and the community as the diagnosis of "bacterial meningitis." Bacterial meningitis is a disease that frequently strikes at the healthy of all ages, it can occur in epidemic outbreaks, it can be caused by a myriad of pathogens, and it carries a high rate of mortality and of neurologic sequelae. Consequently, an intense world-wide diagnostic and therapeutic focus has been directed at bacterial meningitis for two centuries. Furthermore, as medicine has become more technologically based, an extraordinary spurt of research data has been generated that addresses the host/pathogen interactions in the evolution of the disease. Therapeutic options are complex and under constant reevaluation as a consequence of the continuing emergence of organisms resistant to conventional therapy.

Dr. Allan R. Tunkel began his infectious disease career at the University of Virginia, working with Dr. W. Michael Scheld, investigating the pathogenesis of bacterial meningitis in the rat model. His initial bench-side focus subsequently shifted to the clinical. He has published extensively on the topic and is currently recognized nationally and internationally as an outstanding clinician and educator in the diagnosis and management of bacterial meningitis. He has now single-handedly (or almost, he leaves one chapter to his mentor) undertaken an ambitious summary and analysis of what is known about bacterial meningitis. In nine chapters, using clear, comprehensible language and tables, extensive annotation, and a sprinkling of illustrative clinical photographs, this superb teacher explores a subject that fascinates him. *Bacterial Meningitis* is a solid compendium and intermeshing of the clinical and the investigational. *In vitro* and animal data clarify the pathogenesis. Epidemiologic sections address the international relevance of the disease and the impact of the regional emergence of resistant organisms. Clinical chapters not only examine the typical presentations of meningitis but also explore outliers based on age, pathogen, and comorbidity. The diagnostic sections analyze the currently available diagnostic modalities and offer clear recommendations as to specificity and sensitivity. Discussions of therapy integrate animal data with individual clinical studies and with meta-analyses, where appropriate, to assess the efficacy of antibiotics and adjunctive therapy. This volume is also an excellent reference source for central nervous system drug penetration and activity. Areas of uncertainty and those requiring further work are clearly delineated for the reader. The references are sweeping and up-to-date.

So in summary, this book is a single source of everything current you want to know about bacterial meningitis. I hope you're not afraid to read and ask.

Oksana M. Korzeniowski, M.D.
Professor, Department of Medicine
Division of Infectious Diseases
MCP Hahnemann University
Philadelphia, Pennsylvania

Preface

Bacterial meningitis has been recognized for centuries and continues to be a condition that carries a significant morbidity and mortality. The last century has witnessed profound advances in the approach to the patient with bacterial meningitis, including improvements in diagnostic technologies, development of antimicrobial agents, and vaccination. This last advance has led to a significant decrease in the incidence of meningitis caused by specific bacterial pathogens.

In this single-author work (with the exception of the first chapter, contributed by my mentor, Mike Scheld), I have attempted to produce a well-organized overview of bacterial meningitis; to my knowledge, this is the only book dedicated specifically to this disorder. In the ten chapters that follow, the reader will understand the history of meningitis; the current state of knowledge related to epidemiology, etiology, pathogenesis, pathophysiology, clinical features, diagnosis, therapy, and prevention; important considerations in differential diagnosis; and the expected future trends into the 21st century. I present evidence for specific recommendations in the sections on diagnosis, therapy, and prevention, as well as indicate areas of controversy that will require more research to resolve these clinical challenges.

This book is not meant to be an exhaustive review of every facet of bacterial meningitis, but rather a practical, clinically-oriented approach to this disorder. Pathogenesis and pathophysiology are reviewed to help the reader understand how basic science knowledge has contributed to the approach to diagnosis and management. *Bacterial Meningitis* is intended for residents in training, primary care practitioners, emergency medicine physicians, critical care specialists, neurologists, and clinical infectious diseases specialists. It is my hope that the information in this book will help to improve the management and outcome of patients with this devastating disease.

BACTERIAL MENINGITIS

1

A Brief History

W. Michael Scheld

Headache roameth over the desert, blowing like the wind,
Flashing like lightning, it is loosed above and below;
It cutteth off like a reed, him who feareth not his god;
Like a stalk of henna it slitteth his thews.
It wasteth the flesh of him who hath no protecting goddess,
Flashing like a heavenly star, it cometh like the dew;
It standeth hostile against the wayfarer, scorching him like the day.
This man it hath struck and
Like one with heart disease he staggereth,
Like one bereft of reason he is broken,
Like that which hath been cast into the fire he is shrivelled,
Like a wild ass...his eyes are full of cloud,
On himself he feedeth, bound in death;
Headache whose course like the dread windstorm none knoweth,
None knoweth its full time or its bond.

—Mesopotamian incantation, 4000 to 3000 BC

Although bacterial meningitis has been recognized for millennia, the morbidity and mortality associated with this condition remain unacceptably high at the dawn of the twenty-first century, despite advances in diagnosis and antimicrobial therapy (1,2). In addition, the disorder remains common (3), especially in developing countries and, in particular, the "meningitis belt" of sub-Saharan Africa, the modern desert of prevalent headache recounted in the 5,000-year-old incantation that opens this chapter. The most recent significant advance in the management of meningitis and related invasive disease, the introduction of effective immunization against *Haemophilus influenzae* type b (4) is the greatest achievement in pediatric infectious diseases in this generation. New conjugate vaccines for the prevention of invasive disease caused by the other two major meningeal pathogens, *Streptococcus pneumoniae* (5) and *Neisseria meningitidis,* offer considerable hope for the control of this disorder in the near future. This brief chapter outlines some of the major historical milestones in our understanding and management of this frightening disease as a prelude to this marvelous single-author work. The chapter is divided into sections describing historical land-marks in the elucidation of anatomic structures central to an understanding of the pathogenesis and pathophysiology of central nervous system infections, description of the clinical syndrome focusing on epidemic meningococcal meningitis, the intro-duction of diagnostic tests, and the various attempts at management, emphasizing the early triumphs of the current antimicrobial era.

ANATOMIC CONSIDERATIONS

The diagnosis of bacterial meningitis still requires analysis of the cerebrospinal fluid (CSF). The diagnostic method for sampling the CSF was not available until the late nineteenth century but provided the opportunity for the rapid development of various diagnostic tests in the succeeding decades (see later). However, a history of studies of the CSF requires some attention to the historical descriptions of the meninges and the ventricles, as these are the anatomic constraints through which the CSF flows.

Hippocratic writers (430 to 350 BC) referred to the falx cerebri, and Hippocrates himself described the association of headache and tinnitus with inflammation of the brain, including recognition of the high mortality. Greek physicians also, in treatises on head wounds, described the meninges and various aspects of brain anatomy, including delineation of thick and thin layers (i.e., the dura and pia mater) (6). In descriptions of trepanning, an ancient practice, Greek physicians recognized the importance of the membrane known as the dura mater and stated specifically that it should never be wounded. However, landmark descriptions of the ventricular system awaited the great advances, fostered by the performance of autopsies and anatomic dissection, of the physicians of the Alexandrian school (7,8). The two best known of these physicians, Erasistratus (c. 260 BC) and Herophilus of Chalcedon (c. 300 BC), provided extensive descriptions of the meninges and central nervous system anatomy, including delineation of the lateral, third, and fourth ventricles. Centuries later, Claudius Galen of Pergamum (129 to 199 AD) offered a detailed account of the ventricular system based on dissections of the ox brain. As in almost everything else medical, the field languished until the great contributions of Andreas Vesalius (1514 to 1564). Although Leonardo da Vinci had produced a wax cast of the human ventricular system in about 1504, this work was unknown and did not influence medical thought at the time. Further description of the ventricular system was produced by Giulio Aranzi (1530 to 1589). In 1587, he provided a clear depiction of the choroid plexus and the temporal horns of the lateral ventricles. He described the passage from the third to the fourth ventricles as an "aqueduct," and this conduit was later named after François De Le Boë Sylvius (1614 to 1672) (8,9).

The first recognition of CSF is attributed to Galen's account in the second century of a clear fluid residue in the ventricles of the living brain, a description based on animal studies. The fluid was viewed as a vaporous humor; Galen believed it was produced by the brain and provided energy for the entire body. This belief was an extension of earlier concepts of "vitalism," a central tenet of Greek medical thought. According to this ancient view, the heart produced the vital spirit, which was the vaporous life determinant (and often referred to as the psychic "pneuma"), which was distributed peripherally to every organ in the body (8,10). It was not until 1692 that another scientific reference to CSF was published by Antonio Valsalva (1666 to 1723), when he drained the clear fluid from the lumbar sac of a dog and compared it with samples of synovial fluid. A clear and complete description of the CSF was provided by Domenico Cotugno (1736 to 1822) in 1764. He was the first to recognize the continuity between the cerebral and spinal fluids; thus his observations should be recognized as the initial contribution to modern CSF physiology (11). This particular conclusion remained in obscurity for some 60 years until rediscovered by François Magendie (1783 to 1855). Magendie stressed the normal presence of CSF in the brain and ventricles (in 1825 and 1827); prior to these seminal observations (12), any CSF found around the brain or within the ventricles at autopsy was regarded as an abnormal response to the presence of disease.

In 1854, J. Faivre suggested that the CSF was produced by the choroid plexus. In the following year, Hubert von Luschka (1820 to 1875) described the lateral recesses of the fourth ventricle through which the CSF flows into the subarachnoid space that bears his name. Definitive demonstrations of CSF formation, flow, and absorption were made in 1876 by Ernest Key (1832 to 1901) and Gustav Retzius (1842 to 1919) (8). These contributions to an understanding of the anatomy of the ventricular system, the meninges, and the CSF provided a framework that permitted the introduction of the lumbar puncture for CSF analysis, the first ancillary investigation to be introduced into the practice of neurology.

CLINICAL DESCRIPTIONS

As stated earlier, Hippocrates realized the potential for important intracranial consequences of otitic infection, but clear clinical descriptions of bacterial meningitis, particularly the epidemic variety, were not provided until the nineteenth century (13). In 460 BC, Hippocrates commented on a syndrome of purulent otitic fever associated with cerebral symptoms as follows: "We need to pay attention in acute ear pain accompanied by fever because the patient can become delirious and, in a short time, die." However, this description has been attributed to a case of brain abscess in association with otitis (14), and Hippocrates himself may have believed that the intracranial infection was primary and that involvement of the ear was secondary, being a conduit for drainage of focal suppuration of the brain.

While it has been claimed that early authors such as Galen and Rhazes also recognized meningitis, this is debatable. Thomas Willis (1621 to 1675), an English physician, was probably the first to describe an outbreak of bacterial meningitis (15); his description dates from 1661. However, the first clear account of the disease in modern times is usually credited to Vieusseux, a Swiss physician who described an outbreak of epidemic meningitis in Geneva and its environs in March 1805 (13,15–17). This outbreak began on the left bank of Lake Geneva in the suburb of Eaux-Vives and then became widespread throughout the city. Thirty-three deaths were reported. This epidemic of "malignant purpuric fever" was the first clear clinical description of meningococcemia with meningitis; Vieusseux noted the symptoms of violent headache, vomiting, stiffness of the spine, and livid patches on the skin in several cases. The pathologic findings were described in the French literature within a year by Matthey, a local pathologist who found pus at the base of the brain, congestion of meningeal vessels, and a hemorrhagic gelatinous exudate over the surface of the brain (15).

The first American account of epidemic meningococcemia and meningitis appeared in a letter to the editor of the *Medical and Agricultural Register* for the years 1806 and 1807 (vol. 1, no. 5, by L. Danielson and E. Mann of Medfield, MA, in May 1806) (18). The contents were later recorded in the communications of the Massachusetts Medical Society (vol. 2, page 36) (19). They reported nine cases, all fatal, with onset between March 8th and 31st of 1806; the rapid progression and violent nature of the disease was clearly evident from these early reports. For example, Danielson and Mann wrote in their initial letter the following:

> Without any apparent previous predisposition, the patient is suddenly taken with violent pain in the head and stomach, succeeded by cold chills, and followed by nausea and puking; ...respirations short and laborious; tongue a little white toward the root, and moist; velocity of the blood increased with a very sensible diminution of momentum...the eyes have a wild vacant stare...the heat of the skin soon becomes much increased...these symptoms are accompanied by a peculiar fearfulness...and continue from six to nine hours, when coma (suppression of sense and voluntary motion) commences...the extremities become cold; livid, spots resembling petechiae (purple spots which appear in the last stages of certain fevers) appear under the skin, on the face, neck, and extremities; pulse small, irregular, and unequal; spasms occur at intervals, which increase in violence and frequency in proportion as the force of the circulation decreases; at this time, the eyes appear glassy, and the size of the pupil varies suddenly...these symptoms seem to mark the second period of the disease, and continue from three to five hours. The third and last stage is distinguished by a total loss of pulsation at the wrists; livid appearances become more general; spasms more violent; coma more profound; death! The patient has in general continued in the last stage from six to twelve hours.... Evacuation of the bowels, administration of bark and wine were ineffectual.... Induction of emesis as well as bleeding were employed in some of the cases to no effect (18,19).

Danielson and Mann also described the pathologic findings in five cases, with an excerpt as follows:

> The first examination was made on a boy, ten years old, seven hours after death, whose case was strongly marked, terminating in twenty-two hours. On removing the cranium and dividing the dura mater, there was discharged, by estimation, half an ounce of serous fluid. The dura and pia mater in several places adhere together, and both to the substance of the brain. The veins of the brain were uncommonly turgid, with a fluid similar to that which was discharged from between its membranes, and the substance of the brain itself remarkably soft, offering scarcely any resistance to the finger when thrust into it: the cerebellum also was found in the same state...The lungs were rather darker than usual; otherwise all the viscera (bowels, etc.), both of the thorax and abdomen, were in a healthy state.

It is interesting that Danielson and Mann described "nothing peculiarly morbid" in three of their five cases examined at post mortem except a remarkable turgidity of the veins and sinuses of the brain (18,19). These cases may have represented overwhelming fulminant meningococcemia in the absence of meningitis.

Many of these early descriptions were collated in a comprehensive treatise by Elisha North (1771 to 1843) of Connecticut in 1811 (20). He described a "great surprising and sudden loss of strength" as well as the appearance of the extremities: "in the cold stage, appear of a purplish or livid color." He also recognized that meningococcemia was not always associated with petechial eruption at onset, as follows: "Sometimes delirium is among the first symptoms; sometimes coma; and many times petechia. This symptom does not occur so often as the name which the disease has obtained would lead one to expect; these vary in size, and in color, from a bright red to a dark purple" (20,21). Although recognizing that petechiae marked the worst form of the disease, he stressed, based on observations by a colleague, Dr. Strong, that "spotted fever" may be a misnomer, since comatose patients clearly died in the absence of a skin eruption, an early delineation of meningococcemia from meningitis without this characteristic finding. North also recognized the development of peripheral gangrene in some cases and presaged later clinical descriptions on the involvement of larger blood vessels and of "purpura fulminans."

In the early nineteenth century, as in the present day, this disease could present dramatically in a fulminant form, as alluded to earlier. The epidemic nature of meningococcemia with or without meningitis was terrifying to physicians and laypersons alike. For example, Dr. Samuel Woodward, of Torrington, Connecticut, wrote the following in *The American Mercury,* Hartford, in 1807:

> The violent symptoms were great lassitude, with universal pains in the muscle; chills; heats, if any, were of short duration; unusual prostration of strength; delirium, with severe pain in the head, vomiting, with undescribable anxiety of stomach; eyes red and watery, and rolled-up, and the head drawn back with spasms; pulse quick, weak, and irregular; petechiae and vibices all over the body, and a cadaverous countenance and smell; death often closed the scene in ten or fifteen hours after the first attack...the body near the fatal period, and soon after, became spotted as an adder... (13).

Similarly, the following was written by the Reverend Festus Foster of Petersham, Massachusetts, as a letter to the editor of *The Worchester Spy,* dated March 6, 1810:

> I hasten to give you a sketch of the spotted fever in this place. It made its first appearance about the beginning of January last; but the instances were few and distant from each other, until last week. Although it had proved fatal in most instances, seven only had died belonging to this town previous to the 25th of February. Since that time, the disorder has come upon us like a flood of mighty waters. We have buried eight persons within the last eight days. About twelve or fifteen new cases appeared on Thursday last; many of them very sudden and violent. This was the most melancholy and alarming day ever witnessed in this place. Seven or eight physicians were continually engaged in the neighborhood north of the meeting house, and I believe not one half hour passed in the forenoon without presenting a new case. Pale fear and extreme anxiety were visible in every countenance... (13).

Spotted fevers have been recognized for millennia. Descriptions of typhus, typhoid, disseminated syphilitic eruptions, smallpox, and so on, were well known to physicians of the early nineteenth century. It is inconceivable that this fulminant form of meningococcemia had been previously unrecognized, especially given the excellent clinical descriptions of rashes in the literature from this period. One must speculate that the virulence of meningococci for humans somehow changed in the early nineteenth century (13).

Throughout the nineteenth century, explosive epidemics of bacterial meningitis were described from North America, Europe, and even the Fiji Islands. The predilection of the disease for the military was an early observation; in fact, Baron Laurey in 1807 described "méningite de congélation" in a soldier in Napoleon's army (22). The sudden onset of meningococcal disease, its extremely high mortality, the contagious nature and ability of the disease to spread rapidly within a given family or cluster, and the lack of any specific treatment are well outlined in the introduction to the masterful monograph on meningococcal disease by Keith Cartwright (15). Although these early descriptions of meningococcemia and meningitis clearly described cardinal symptoms and signs such as fever, alterations in consciousness, and skin eruptions, specific meningeal signs and neck stiffness were not emphasized by Vieusseux or by Danielson and Mann (23). Hippocrates may have been speaking of meningitis when he taught in the fifth century BC "if, during fever, the neck shall have been suddenly twisted, the deglutition be rendered difficult without any tumor, it is a fatal sign" (23,24). The first description of neck stiffness in meningitis, however, can perhaps be attributed to Andreas Vesalius, mentioned earlier, for his pioneering anatomic work, *De Humani Corporas Fabrica*. In 1559, he was called to attend to King Henri II of France, who had sustained a head wound while in a tournament. After Vesalius inserted a cloth between the king's teeth and pulled it out vigorously, the king screamed in agony. The reaction by Vesalius was to immediately pronounce the patient beyond cure, uttering, "Chiornium vulnus," meaning, "wound of the centaurs." Later medical commentators have suggested that the patient had meningitis secondary to trauma, and that this crude head flexion maneuver by Vesalius elicited this sign of meningeal irritation (23,25).

Another early reference to meningeal irritation can be found in the visionary engraving by William Blake (1757 to 1827) depicting the trials of Job in an opisthotonic posture with the devil perched on his knees. Although the inspiration for this engraving is unknown and may have reflected Blake's own life experiences, he may have been interpreting Job's words, "my skin is black upon me, and my bones are burned with heat" in the context of meningeal irritation, a description not inconsistent with meningococcemia (23). Finally, following the early accounts of suspected meningitis in New England, Nathan Strong's "Inaugural Dissertation on the Disease Termed Petechial Spotted Fever," submitted in 1810 to the Medical Society of Connecticut for his medical degree, states the following: "the extensor muscles of the head and neck were, in almost every case, affected with tonic spasm" (26).

In addition to these early descriptions, several signs of meningeal irritation were subsequently described and have been considered by clinicians as useful adjuncts in the early examination of a patient with suspected meningitis. Vladimir Mihailovich Kernig described the sign that now bears his name in 1882 (27). He was apparently well aware of neck stiffness as a sign of meningeal irritation prior to his description of the sign, for he states, "One finds, as is well-known, in the majority of cases of tuberculous and epidemic cerebrospinal meningitis, the classical more or less intense neck and back rigidity." The maneuver as originally described by Kernig was performed with the patient in a sitting position with the hips flexed 90° to the trunk, whereas students now interpret Kernig's sign upon hip flexion in the supine position (23). Jozef Brudzinski, a Polish physician who eventually became dean of the University of Warsaw, described at least five different physical signs of meningeal irritation (23). The nape of the neck sign is best known and was described in 1909 (23,28). Upon flexion of the neck by the examiner, hip and knee flexion is produced. His early report states that this neck sign was present in 96% of cases of meningitis, whereas Kernig's sign was present in only 57%. Brudzinski also described several other meningeal signs, including contralateral reflexes and a reciprocal contralateral sign of meningeal irritation, which are less well appreciated by modern students of medicine (23). Opisthotonus is not common in patients with bacterial meningitis outside of the neonatal period, although it is a regular feature of advanced tetanus. Some patients with meningitis may spontaneously assume the tripod position (also called Amoss sign or Hoyne sign). Recently, an additional maneuver in assessing for meningitis has been described by Japanese investigators as "jolt accentuation of headache." By asking the patient to turn his or her head horizontally at a frequency of 2 or 3 rotations per second, worsening of a baseline headache represents a positive sign, with a sensitivity of 97% and a specificity of 60% in the original study (29). Analysis in the interim has suggested that in patients with fever and headache, a lack of jolt accentuation of headache on physical examination essentially excludes meningitis from consideration (30).

Finally, in addition to the classic descriptions of patients with bacterial meningitis in the medical literature as enumerated earlier, it should be recognized that this syndrome has been the subject of detailed depictions in great literature authored by physicians and laypersons alike. One such example occurs in the beautiful but devastating short story "Danse Pseudomacabre," by William Carlos Williams, a physician, but one of the great poets of the twentieth century (31), as follows:

> It is a baby. There is a light at the end of a broken corridor. A man in a pointed beard leads the way. Strong foreign accent. Holland Dutch. We walk through the corridor to the back of the house. The kitchen. In the kitchen turn to the right. Someone is sitting back of the bedroom door. A nose, an eye emerge, sniffing and staring, a wrinkled nose, a cavernous eye. Turn again to the right through another door and walk toward the front of the house. We are in a sickroom. A bed has been backed against the corridor entry making this detour necessary.
>
> Oh, here you are doctor. British. The nurse I suppose.
>
> The baby is in a smother of sheets and crumpled blankets, its head on a pillow. The child's left eye closed, its right partly opened. It emits a soft whining cry continuously at every breath. It can't be more than a few weeks old.
>
> Do you think it is unconscious, doctor?
>
> Yes.
>
> Will it live? It is the mother. A great tender-eyed blonde. Great full breasts. A soft gentle-minded woman of no mean beauty. A blue cotton house wrapper, shoulder to ankle.

If it lives it will be an idiot perhaps. Or it will be paralysed—or both. It is better for it to die.

There it goes now! The whining has stopped. The lips are blue. The mouth puckers as for some diabolic kiss. It twitches, twitches faster and faster, up and down. The body slowly grows rigid and begins to fold itself like a flower folding again. The left eye opens slowly, the eyeball is turned so that the pupil is lost in the angle of the nose. The right eye remains open and fixed staring forward. Meningitis. Acute. The arms are slowly raised more and more from the sides as if in the deliberate attitude before a mad dance, hands clenched, wrists flexed. The arms now lie upon each other crossed at the wrists. The knees are drawn up as if the child were squatting. The body holds this posture, the child's belly rumbling with a huge contortion. Breath has stopped. The body is stiff, blue. Slowly it relaxes, the whimpering cry begins again. The left eye falls closed.

It began with that eye. It was a lovely baby. Normal in every way. Breast fed. I have not taken it anywhere. It is only six weeks old. How can he get it?

The pointed beard approaches. It is infection, is it not, doctor?

Yes.

But I took him nowhere. How could he get it?

He must have gotten it from someone who carries it, maybe from one of you.

Will he die?

Yes, I think so.

MICROBIAL ETIOLOGY AND APPROACH TO DIAGNOSIS

Following Robert Koch's pioneering discovery of the cause of anthrax in 1876, the last two decades of the nineteenth century witnessed an explosion of new knowledge on the microbial etiology of disease. As bacteriology evolved from an art into a science, the first report of meningococcal isolation was attributed to Anton Weichselbaum in 1887 (15,32). He observed gram-negative diplococci in the CSF of a young patient who had died in Vienna of sporadic meningitis and isolated the organism (which he called *Diplococcus intracellularus meningitidis*) from the meningeal exudate of six of eight patients. As he isolated a pneumococcus from the other two cases, he was therefore cautious in his interpretation of these findings (32). All three of the major meningeal pathogens (*Neisseria meningitidis, Streptococcus pneumoniae,* and *Haemophilus influenzae*) were first isolated and described in a 10-year period at the close of the nineteenth century.

The development and perfection of the technique of lumbar puncture by Heinrich Quinke (1842 to 1922) in 1891 (33) facilitated the formal examination of CSF and the diagnosis of meningitis. Quinke was searching for a safe and simple method to remove CSF from children with hydrocephalus. Although Quinke described bacteria in the fluid in pathological circumstances, it took nearly 20 years before the first comprehensive description of the chemical composition of CSF was published by William Mestrezat (1883 to 1928) in 1911 (34). The earliest example of the diagnostic value of CSF analysis by biochemical methods was published in 1893 by Ludwig Lichthein (1845 to 1928) when he observed that CSF glucose concentrations were low in the presence of bacterial and tuberculous meningitis. This observation led to the measurement of CSF glucose in the initial diagnostic approach to patients with suspected meningitis over the past century. The other major abnormalities in the CSF found in patients with bacterial meningitis (i.e., the CSF neutrophilic pleocytosis and elevated protein concentration) were well described in the early years of the twentieth century (reviewed in 8,13). Interpretation of the CSF glucose concentration in relation to plasma values was introduced as early as 1925 by George Goodwin and Harold Shelley. Advances during the twentieth century on these critical analyses were largely methodological in nature, including enzymatic glucose-oxidase and hexokinase methods for determination of CSF glucose and colorimetric methods for determination of CSF protein that supplanted early turbidimetric procedures in the early 1950s. The low CSF pH in bacterial meningitis cases was noted as early as 1911, but the contribution of elevated lactate concentrations was first described in 1924 by K. Nishimura (35). While CSF lactate concentrations are not routinely measured in patients with suspected bacterial meningitis, the height of the CSF lactate correlates directly with prognosis and may be useful in differentiating bacterial meningitis from an abnormal CSF following neurosurgery, based on the neurosurgical procedure itself.

Following the documentation of the primary CSF abnormalities observed in cases of bacterial meningitis in the early years of the twentieth century, including CSF pleocytosis, elevated protein, and depressed glucose concentrations, many other diagnostic aids were described in the clinical literature, including detection of bacterial antigens by various techniques, and the polymerase chain reaction for direct identification of microbial DNA in clinical specimens. These advances, as well as their limitations, are amply outlined in the pages that follow. Recent contributions to the literature include a suggestion that determination of serum C-reactive protein and procalcitonin may be useful in identification of patients with bacterial meningitis when compared with viral syndromes (36). These new, inexpensive, and rapid techniques show great promise in the delineation of bacterial from viral meningitis when more established techniques yield equivocal results.

HISTORICAL LANDMARKS IN THE THERAPY OF MENINGITIS

Although dependent on multiple factors, particularly the implicated pathogen and patient age, bacterial meningitis prior to the introduction of specific antisera was a highly lethal disease (mortality 70% to 100%). Soon after the description of the lumbar puncture, CSF drainage was introduced for the treatment of meningitis. During the early decades of the twentieth century, various modifications of CSF drainage were employed, including irrigation of the subarachnoid space with Ringer's lactate solution or chemical agents (e.g., gentian violet, mercurochrome, and optochin), air injections through the lumbar needle with exit via the cisterna magna, continuous drainage of the CSF, and even bilateral injection of an iodine-containing solution into the carotid arteries (reviewed in ref. 37). In addition to substantial toxicity, all these procedures lacked clinical efficacy.

At the turn of the twentieth century in the United States, meningococci ranked second only to *Mycobacterium tuberculosis* as a cause of meningitis and sporadic, explosive outbreaks continued to occur. Following devastating epidemics of meningococcal meningitis in New York in 1904 to 1905 and in eastern Germany in 1905 to

1907, investigators in Germany and the United States were working almost simultaneously on the development of antimeningococcal antisera. This line of investigation was based on studies in animals (15), which documented formation of agglutinating antibodies and partial protection in guinea pigs with the prior injection of an immune horse serum before meningococcal challenge. This led to human trials of antisera, first given subcutaneously with subsequent doses administered by the intraspinal route. In one initial series, 12 of 17 treated patients survived, excellent results when compared with the mortality of 70% to 80%, which was routine at the time. Working in the midst of these explosive outbreaks of meningococcal meningitis (e.g., more than 5,000 deaths in 6,755 cases in New York City in 1904 to 1905), Simon Flexner and James Jobling of the Rockefeller Institute in New York began an elegant series of experiments that eventually demonstrated the protective effect of antimeningococcal antiserum in humans. They raised the serum in horses by injection with heat-killed whole organisms and proved efficacy in experimental animals, including primates. After a series of studies by various routes of administration, it was recognized that intraspinal, intracisternal, or intraventricular injection was necessary for maximal protective benefit. Since meningococcal meningitis was so prevalent at this time, intrathecal injection of 20 to 30 mL of antiserum for disease in adults was administered after the first lumbar puncture yielded cloudy fluid; therapy was then continued daily for about 4 days. This practice was the first important advance in the treatment of meningococcal meningitis. The survival rate increased from 10% to 30% in untreated patients to approximately 70% in 1,224 cases treated with antimeningococcal serum in 1913 (37,38). Multiple complications of this novel and highly effective therapy were noted in up to 50% of patients, including fever, skin eruptions, arthritis, and digestive complaints. "Serum sickness" was born. Secondary or fatal meningitis induced by the introduction of extraneous bacteria was rare, but recorded. These results were upheld in a series of studies reported between 1915 and 1922. During World War I, 2,466 military personnel were admitted to hospitals in the United States with meningococcal meningitis; 67% survived with antisera treatment (reviewed in ref. 37).

    Thus direct inoculation of antimeningococcal antisera became the mainstay of therapy for meningococcal meningitis until the availability of antibacterial agents in the 1930s. During this time, massive epidemics of this disease occurred in the civilian populations of Detroit, Milwaukee, and Indianapolis in 1928–1929. Because of the large number of infant cases, the overall mortality remained extremely high at approximately 50%, despite the administration of antimeningococcal antiserum therapy; the mortality rate in infants was 84% in Detroit, and 72% in adults older than 40 years of age (15,37). In the early 1930s, Ferry demonstrated the production of exotoxins in filtrates of meningococci and produced antitoxins for testing in humans. Although some favorable responses were initially obtained, the intravenous or intrathecal antitoxin administration schedules eventually were proven of no adjunctive value over standard therapy with antimeningococcal antiserum (or later, with sulfonamides) and this treatment was abandoned (37). Perhaps this is illustrative of the current status of the treatment of sepsis and septic shock caused by meningococci with antiendotoxin modalities in the current antimicrobial era.

Therefore in the late 1930s, meningococcal meningitis remained a common disease capable of explosive and often highly fatal outbreaks with a high mortality rate in the range of 70% to 80% unless antisera was judiciously employed. Despite these encouraging results, the mortality remained in the range of 30% to 40% before the introduction of the sulfonamides.

Sulfanilamide was first synthesized in 1908, but many decades passed before the antibacterial properties of this class of drugs were recognized. The first experiments documenting these effects were performed in 1932, in the last month before Hitler's ascension to power. In 1933, Domack, while working on aniline dyes at Bayer AG in Leverkusen in western Germany, discovered the antibacterial activity of sulfachrysoidine (Prontosil), which led to experiments in laboratory animals and the first clinical report detailing the experience with the use of these compounds in human infections, as published in the landmark study that appeared in *Deutsche Medizinische Wochenschrift* on February 15, 1935. The first patient treated with a sulfonamide in this country was a 10-year-old girl with *Haemophilus influenzae* meningitis and epiglottitis at the Columbia University Medical Center in 1935. This was followed by documentation of the therapeutic efficacy of sulfanilamide in group A β-hemolytic streptococcal infections, including erysipelas, septicemia, infected abortions, and pelvic peritonitis. One event that brought the sulfonamides to the attention of the American public was the treatment of Franklin Delano Roosevelt, Jr. (the president's son) at the Massachusetts General Hospital in November, 1936. His prompt recovery from a streptococcal sore throat with the use of a German experimental drug (Prontolyn) was reported widely in the press (e.g., *New York Times,* December 17, 1936). Since another president's son, Calvin Coolidge Jr., had died of streptococcal septicemia 12 years earlier, sulfonamides soon became available to American physicians. Early work documented that the administration of sulfonamides prevented septicemia, meningitis, and death after the intraperitoneal injection of meningococci in mice. Furthermore, some experimental evidence suggested that sulfonamides attained therapeutic concentrations in the CSF.

These studies suggested a role for sulfanilamide in the treatment of meningitis and led to a report by Schwentker and colleagues in the April 24, 1937 issue of the *Journal of the American Medical Association.* Schwentker et al. (39) described the results of treatment of 11 cases of meningococcal disease (10 patients with meningitis and one patient with only meningococcemia) with sulfanilamide. As positive cultures were obtained in all but one case, the diagnosis could not be questioned. Sulfanilamide was administered simultaneously by both the subcutaneous and intrathecal routes. Despite modest dosages, the response to treatment was good, and only one patient died, for a mortality of 9%. The one death resulted from pneumonia and, since the CSF and blood cultures were sterile at the time of death, may have represented a superinfection. Although a shortcoming of the article, there was no mention of the use of concomitant meningococcal antisera or antitoxin therapy, leading to the assumption that sulfanilamide was administered alone (37). The drug was well tolerated and there were no local or systemic reactions to the intrathecal injections. Appropriately cautious in their conclusions, the authors suggested that (a) their small series required larger numbers of patients, (b) sulfonamide was more effective than repeated subarachnoid drainage based on retrospective experience, and (c) sulfonamides might replace, or serve as an adjunct to, antimeningococcal serum therapy. The study by Schwentker and colleagues was the first demonstration of cure of meningococcal meningitis by a synthetic chemotherapeutic agent. Within the year, other investigators quickly confirmed these results. Furthermore, during the next decade, these studies were followed by other reports documenting the efficacy of this approach.

The sulfonamides not only cured meningitis caused by *Neisseria meningitidis* with a low frequency of adverse events, they also ushered in the modern scientific era of medicine. Lewis Thomas, in a beautifully written memoir, *The Youngest Science: Notes of a Medicine Watcher,* describes the major diseases confronting him on the wards of the Boston City Hospital during his internship, including syphilis, delirium tremens, pneumococcal pneumonia, tuberculosis, and rheumatic fever. Only a few drugs with any therapeutic benefit (morphine, insulin, quinine, digitalis, and liver extract) were available to him, and only the administration of specific antipneumococcal or antimeningococcal antisera could occasionally reverse the course of an otherwise lethal disease. As an intern in 1937, Thomas observed the dramatic effect of sulfonamide therapy on the course of pneumococcal and streptococcal septicemia as follows (40):

> For most of the infectious diseases on the wards of Boston City Hospital in 1937, there was nothing to be done beyond bedrest and good nursing care. Then came the explosive news of sulfanilamide, and the start of the real revolution in medicine. I remember the astonishment when the first cases of pneumococcal and streptococcal septicemia were treated in Boston in 1937. The phenomenon was almost beyond belief. Here were moribund patients, who would surely have died without treatment, improving in their appearance within a matter of hours of being given the medicine, and feeling entirely well within the next day or so. The professionals most deeply affected by these extraordinary events were, I think, the interns. The older physicians were equally surprised, but took the news in stride. For an intern, it was the opening of a whole new world, We had been raised to be ready for one kind of profession, and we sensed that the profession itself had changed at the moment of our entry. We knew that other molecular variations of sulfanilamide were on their way from industry, and we heard about the possibility of penicillin and other antibiotics; we became convinced, overnight, that nothing lay beyond reach for the future. Medicine was off and running.

Dr. Thomas was personally involved in this chemotherapeutic revolution. Four years later, he coauthored an article published in the *Journal of the American Medical Association* detailing the treatment of meningitis with sulfadiazine after investigating an epidemic in Halifax, Nova Scotia.

Walsh McDermott shared many of Dr. Thomas's experiences and was one of my cherished mentors. Dr. McDermott was also an intern in the 1930s, but at the Bellevue Hospital in New York. He observed personally the chemotherapeutic revolution after the introduction of the sulfonamides, and devoted his professional life to the study of microbial diseases and their profound impact on society at every level. Shortly before his death in October 1991, Dr. McDermott began work on a book of which the central theme was the influence of antimicrobial therapy on society as a new technology.

With the editorial assistance of Dr. Rogers, excerpts of this book were assembled and published after Dr. McDermott's death (41). This short article eloquently details the state of medicine before, during, and after the introduction of the sulfonamides, and it should be required reading for all students of medicine. The profound impact of sulfanilamide in the late 1930s was considered by McDermott and Rogers as follows:

> Unlike arsphenamine, the new drug was effective against several different microbial species, each the cause of a different and known serious disease. The long-wished-for drug with an action different on microbial cells and body cells was at hand. It was called 'a miracle drug,' and properly so. In the desperately ill patients, the effects produced were no different from those one might visualize were there to be a true divine intervention. So far as could be determined, nothing like them on such a scale had ever been seen before, since the beginning of time.

Dr. McDermott's discussion of the social ramifications of this chemotherapeutic revolution and ensuing changes is profound. By 1941, the sulfonamides quickly became the treatment of choice for meningococcal meningitis. The concomitant use of antimeningococcal antisera was no longer recommended. Although given by various routes, and in higher dosages, the results were similar to those reported by Schwentker and colleagues. By the early 1940s, the mortality of meningococcal meningitis was reduced to 9% to 11%. Despite the mortality rate with sulfadiazine of only 3.8% in 14,504 military personnel hospitalized in this country with meningococcal meningitis during World War II, this condition still killed more United States servicemen than any other infectious disease between 1940 and 1945. Sulfadiazine remained the agent of choice for the treatment of meningococcal meningitis for another 20 years and was a useful prophylactic agent for eradication of the carrier state, a condition relevant to the development of invasive disease, as was first described in the early 1920s (reviewed in ref. 37).

Despite these early successes, sulfadiazine and related compounds were never as effective in the treatment of pneumococcal or *Haemophilus influenzae* meningitis because of their inherent limited potency. These conditions were associated with a worse outcome than those observed in patients with meningococcal meningitis. For example, of 99 patients with pneumococcal meningitis observed at the Boston City Hospital between 1920 and 1936, not a single patient survived. Furthermore, among 78 children with *Haemophilus influenzae* meningitis described by Fothergill, a 98% mortality was observed and was reduced to only 84.6% in 221 children who were treated with antiserum (reviewed in ref. 42).

The discovery of penicillin from Fleming to Florrey and Chain and colleagues has been described in detail in multiple publications over the past 50 years. The military became the preferential benefactor of this new substance during World War II, and the new drug was used by the United States Navy for the treatment of meningococcal meningitis. One of the early reports by Rosenberg and Arling in 1944 (43) documented the extreme efficacy of this new therapy since only one of 65 patients died, despite the low doses administered intrathecally and either intravenously or intramuscularly. Prior to this intervention, extensive drainage of CSF was still considered a mainstay of therapy. For several years, a controversy arose regarding the superiority of ampicillin over sulfonamide therapy for meningitis caused by *Neisseria meningitides*. However, the use of penicillin for the treatment of meningitis was eventually driven by the spectacular results obtained in the treatment of this condition caused by other pathogenic organisms.

The discovery of penicillin and its application to medical practice has been amply demonstrated by multiple authors, in particular Harry Dowling's magnificent treatise on the introduction of antimicrobial agents in the twentieth century entitled *Fighting Infection*. An early report of the efficacy of penicillin in meningococcal meningitis was authored by Rosenberg and Arling (43); judged from today's perspective, it was an amazing affirmation of the low dosages required to eliminate penicillin-susceptible meningococci from the CSF. A total of 35 patients received a dosage of less than 100,000 units systemically while another 20 received less than 250,000 units either intramuscularly or intravenously; the remaining 16 patients received dosages of between 250,000 units and 900,000 units via the systemic route. These dosages were minuscule when compared with those recommended by contemporary authors. Furthermore, the excellent cure rate of 98.6% in this series was exemplary. Thus, for the first time, the efficacy of penicillin was demonstrated in a large series of patients with meningococcal meningitis. The excellent results helped bring penicillin into the forefront of meningitis therapy. On the other hand, as anticipated by the authors in their discussion, the mode of treatment and the route of administration proved not to be optimal, and in later years, various alternatives were sought to augment efficacy, such as continuous versus intermittent bolus administration, proper dosage and duration of administration, and adjunctive treatments to improve outcome (42).

CONCLUSIONS

Bacterial meningitis remains a relatively common disease, with substantial morbidity and mortality. Despite the introduction of new antimicrobial agents and diagnostic techniques, this disease represents a formidable therapeutic challenge. Over the millennia, multiple authors have contributed to our understanding of the etiology, epidemiology, diagnosis, and management of this condition. In recent years, extensive investigations have focused on the pathogenesis and pathophysiology of bacterial meningitis (intentionally excluded from this review, as it is beautifully detailed in the pages that follow). Nevertheless, a more thorough understanding of the pathogenesis and pathophysiology of this condition can lead to a more appropriate application of the major therapeutic principles gained during the past century and, it is hoped, an improved outcome of patients afflicted with this devastating condition.

REFERENCES

1. Tunkel AR, Scheld WM. Acute bacterial meningitis. *Lancet* 1995;346:1675–1680.
2. Quagliarello VJ, Scheld WM. Treatment of bacterial meningitis. *N Engl J Med* 1997;336:708–716.
3. Schuchat TA, Robinson K, Wenger J, et al. Bacterial meningitis in the United States in 1995. *N Engl J Med* 1997;337:970–976.

4. Adams WG, Deaver KA, Cochi SL, et al. Decline of childhood *Haemophilus influenzae* type b in the Hib vaccine era. *JAMA* 1992;269:221–226.
5. Butler JC, Shapiro ED, Carlone GM. Pneumococcal vaccines: history, current status, future directions. *Am J Med* 1999;107:69S–76S.
6. Phillips ED. *Aspects of Greek medicine.* New York: St. Martin's Press, 1973:47.
7. Phillips ED. *Aspects of Greek medicine.* New York: St. Martin's Press, 1973:105.
8. Olukoga AO, Bolode KU, Donaldson D. Cerebrospinal fluid analysis in clinical diagnosis. *J Clin Pathol* 1997;50:187–192.
9. Clarke E, O'Malley CD. The ventricular system and CSF. In: *The human brain and spinal cord.* Berkeley: University of California Press, 1968:708–755.
10. Torack RM. Historical aspects of normal and abnormal brain fluids. I. Cerebrospinal fluid. *Arch Neurol* 1982;39:197–201.
11. Viets H. Domenico Cotugno: his description of the cerebrospinal fluid. *Bull Hist Med* 1935;3:701–738.
12. Magendie F. Further notes on the cerebrospinal fluid. *J Physiol Exp Pathol* 1927;7:5–27, 66–82.
13. Roos KL, Tunkel AR, Scheld WM. Bacterial meningitis in children and adults. In: Scheld WM, Whitley RJ, Durack DT, eds. *Infections of the central nervous system,* 2nd ed. Philadelphia: Lippincott-Raven, 1997:335–401.
14. Wispelwey B, Dacey RG, Jr., Scheld WM. Brain abscess. In: Scheld WM, Whitley RJ, Durack DT, eds. *Infections of the central nervous system,* 2nd ed. Philadelphia: Lippincott-Raven, 1997:463–493.
15. Cartwright K. Introduction and historical aspects. In: Cartwright K, ed. *Meningococcal disease.* Chichester, UK: John Wiley, 1995:1–19.
16. Vieusseux G. Mémoire sur la maladie qui a régné Genève au printemps de 1805. *J Méd Chir Pharmacol* 1805;11:163–182.
17. Domingo P, Barquet M. The first epidemic of cerebrospinal meningitis. *Gesnerus* 1994;51:280–282.
18. Danielson L, Mann E. The history of a singular and very mortal disease, which lately made its appearance in Medfield. In: Adams D, ed. *The Medical and Agricultural Register for the Years 1806 and 1807.* 1806;1:65–69.
19. The first American account of cerebrospinal meningitis. *Rev Infect Dis* 1983;5:969–972.
20. North E. *A treatise on a malignant epidemic, commonly called spotted fever.* New York: T and J Swords, 1811.
21. North E. Concerning the epidemic of spotted fever in New England. *Rev Infect Dis* 1980;2:811–816.
22. Lapeyssonnie L. Milestones in meningococcal disease. In: Vedros MA, ed. *Evolution of meningococcal disease.* Boca Raton: CRC Press, 1987:1–4.
23. Verghese A, Gallemore G. Kernig's and Brudzinski's signs revisited. *Rev Infect Dis* 1987;9:1187–1192.
24. *Aphorisms of Hippocrates.* Birmingham, AL: The Classics of Medicine Library, 1982.
25. Bendiner E. Andreas Vesalius: man of mystery in life and death. *Hosp Pract* 1986;21:199–234.
26. Strong N. *An inaugural dissertation on the disease termed petechial or spotted fever.* Hartford, CT: Peter B. Gleason, 1810:4.
27. Kernig VM, Uber EN. Krankheits symptom der acuten meningitis. *St. Petersburg Med Wochenschr* 1882;7:398.
28. Brudzinski J. Un signe nouveau sur les membres inférieures dans les méningites chez les enfants sigme de la nuque. *Arch Méd Enfant* 1809;12:745–752.
29. Uchihara T, Tsukagoshi H. Jolt accentuation of headache: the most sensitive sign of CSF pleocytosis. *Headache* 1991;31:167–171.
30. Attia J, Hatala R, Cook DJ, et al. Does this adult patient have acute meningitis? *JAMA* 1999;282:175–181.
31. Williams WC. Danse pseudomacabre. In: Coles R, ed. *William Carlos Williams: the doctor stories.* New York: New Directions, 1932:88–91.
32. Weichselbaum A. Uber die aetiologie der akuten meningitis cerebrospinalis. *Fortschrift Med* 1887;5:573–583, 620–626.
33. Quinke HJ. Die lumbalpunction des hydrocephalus. *Berl Klin Wochenschr* 1891;28:929–965.
34. Mestrezat W. Le liquide céphalo-rachidien normal et pathologique, valeur clinique de l'examen chimique. *Thèse* 1911;17:35.
35. Nishimura K. The lactic acid content of blood and cerebrospinal fluid. *Proc Soc Exp Biol Med* 1924;22:322–324.
36. Nathan B, Scheld WM. The role of C-reactive protein and pro-calcitonin in the diagnosis of meningitis. In: Remington JM, Schwartz MN, eds. 2001 (*in press*).
37. Scheld WM, Mandell GL. Sulfonamides and meningitis. *JAMA* 1984;251:791–794.

38. Flexner S. The results of serum treatment in 1,300 cases of epidemic meningitis. *J Exp Med* 1913;17:553–576.
39. Schwentker FF, Gelman S, Long PH. The treatment of meningococcic meningitis with sulfanilamide: preliminary report. *JAMA* 1937;108:1407–1408.
40. Thomas L. *The youngest science: notes of a medicine watcher.* New York: Viking Press, 1983:270.
41. McDermott W, Rogers DE. Social ramifications of control of microbial disease. *Johns Hopkins Med J* 1982;151:302–312.
42. Täuber MG, Sande MA. The impact of penicillin on the treatment of meningitis. *JAMA* 1984;251: 1877–1880.
43. Rosenberg DH, Arling PA. Penicillin in the treatment of meningitis. *JAMA* 1944;125:1011–1017.

2

Epidemiology and Etiology

Bacterial meningitis is a very important and frequently devastating disease. Many bacterial pathogens have been reported to cause meningitis, although this book will deal primarily with those that produce the acute meningitis syndrome, defined by the onset of symptoms over the course of several hours up to several days. Despite the large number of bacterial pathogens that have been reported to cause acute meningitis, certain microorganisms are isolated with a higher frequency (see later). In addition, in recent years, there has been a shift in the agents that can cause bacterial meningitis. Here I will review the changes in these epidemiologic patterns, as well as the common bacteria that are etiologic agents of acute meningitis.

EPIDEMIOLOGY

Bacterial meningitis continues to be an important cause of morbidity and mortality in the United States and throughout the world, despite the availability of effective antimicrobial therapy. Therefore accurate information on the etiologic agents, populations at risk, trends in antimicrobial resistance, morbidity, and mortality is critical to develop public health measures and ensure appropriate management.

Several studies performed in the United States in the 1950s, 1960s, and 1970s characterized the epidemiology of bacterial meningitis. Annual attack rates were quite significant in these studies (Table 2.1) (1–5), although these case-finding efforts were performed in relatively small populations. In one retrospective study of 209 patients with nontuberculous bacterial meningitis at King County Hospital (serving a population of approximately one million) in Seattle, Washington, from 1955 through 1960, *Streptococcus pneumoniae, Neisseria meningitidis,* and *Haemophilus influenzae* accounted for the majority (72%) of cases (1). The high isolation frequency for these three major meningeal pathogens was verified in another review from the Massachusetts General Hospital from 1956 to 1962, in which these microorganisms were isolated in 71% of the 207 patients studied (6). Similar findings were also observed in other surveillance studies (2–5), highlighting the importance of targeting therapeutic and preventive strategies toward these microorganisms.

TABLE 2.1. *Incidence of bacterial meningitis in selected series in the United States from 1955 through 1971*

Study	Incidence (cases per 100,000)
King County Hospital, Seattle (1955–1960)	5.0
Olmstead County, Minnesota (1959–1970)	9.8
Charleston County, South Carolina (1961–1971)	10.0
Bernalillo County, New Mexico (1964–1971)	7.3
Tennessee (1963–1971)	7.0

Data from Carpenter RR, Petersdorf RG. The clinical spectrum of bacterial meningitis. *Am J Med* 1962;33:262–275; Fraser DW, Henke CE, Feldman RA. Changing patterns of bacterial meningitis in Olmsted County, Minnesota, 1935–1970. *J Infect Dis* 1973;128:300–307; Fraser DW, Darby CP, Koehler RE, et al. Risk factors in bacterial meningitis: Charleston County, South Carolina. *J Infect Dis* 1973;127:271–277; Fraser DW, Geil CC, Feldman RA. Bacterial meningitis in Bernalillo County, New Mexico: a comparison with three other American populations. *Am J Epidemiol* 1974;100:29–34; and Floyd RF, Federspiel CF, Schaffner W. Bacterial meningitis in urban and rural Tennessee. *Am J Epidemiol* 1974;99: 395–407, with permission.

In 1977, the Centers for Disease Control and Prevention (CDC), in collaboration with the Conference of State and Territorial Epidemiologists, established a nationwide surveillance system for bacterial meningitis to gather prospective epidemiologic data that would supplement retrospective hospital and community-based studies of bacterial meningitis. Three surveillance studies published by the CDC over the last 20 years have provided important information on the changing epidemiology of bacterial meningitis in the United States (Table 2.2). In the first published study, 13,974 cases of bacterial meningitis reported to the CDC from 27 states in the United States from 1978 through 1981 were analyzed (7). The overall annual attack rate for bacterial meningitis, as defined in this surveillance study, was approximately 3.0 cases

TABLE 2.2. *Etiology of bacterial meningitis in the United States*

Organism	Percentage of total cases		
	1978–1981	1986	1995
Haemophilus influenzae	48	45	7
Neisseria meningitidis	20	14	25
Streptococcus pneumoniae	13	18	47
Streptococcus agalactiae	3	6	12
Listeria monocytogenes	2	3	8
Other	8	14	—
Unknown	6	—	—

Data from Schlech WF III, Ward JI, Band JD, et al. Bacterial meningitis in the United States, 1978 through 1981. The national bacterial meningitis surveillance study. *JAMA* 1985;253:1749–1754; Wenger JD, Hightower AW, Facklam RR, et al. Bacterial meningitis in the United States, 1986: report of a multistate surveillance study. *J Infect Dis* 1990;162:1316–1323; and Schuchat A, Robinson K, Wenger JD, et al. Bacterial meningitis in the United States in 1995. *N Engl J Med* 1997;337:970–976, with permission.

per 100,000 population, although there was variability based on age, race, and sex; unfortunately, there was significant underreporting of cases in this study because no active effort was undertaken to detect cases. Attack rates were higher for males than for females (3.3 versus 2.6 cases per 100,000 population), with the highest attack rates for children under 1 year of age (76.7 cases per 100,000 population). Attack rates also varied with geographic locale, with the highest rates reported in the Pacific region (Washington and Oregon which had 4.5 cases per 100,000 population). The three common meningeal pathogens, *H. influenzae, N. meningitidis,* and *S. pneumoniae,* accounted for more than 80% of cases. In a subsequent study involving five states (Missouri, New Jersey, Oklahoma, Tennessee, and Washington) and Los Angeles County during 1986 (population of almost 34 million), an active, laboratory-based surveillance for all cases of meningitis and for invasive bacterial disease caused by the five most common etiologic agents of bacterial meningitis (*H. influenzae, S. pneumoniae, N. meningitidis,* group B streptococcus, and *Listeria monocytogenes*) was performed (8). In this study, the overall incidence of bacterial meningitis was two to three times that of the previous report, likely due to the voluntary reporting system that was used in previous study (7). *H. influenzae, N. meningitidis,* and *S. pneumoniae* continued to account for the majority of cases (77%), confirming the appropriateness of extensive vaccination campaigns against these pathogens.

With the introduction of *H. influenzae* type b conjugate vaccines in the United States and several countries throughout the world, dramatic declines in the incidence of invasive *H. influenzae* type b disease were reported. Evaluation of the epidemiology of bacterial meningitis in the United States in the era of *H. influenzae* type b vaccination was performed in a recent surveillance study conducted during 1995 in laboratories serving all the acute-care hospitals in 22 counties of four states (Georgia, Tennessee, Maryland, California) serving more than 10 million population (9). In this study, the incidence of bacterial meningitis decreased dramatically as a result of the vaccine-related decline in meningitis caused by *H. influenzae* type b, with little or no change in the incidence of meningitis caused by the other major meningeal pathogens when compared with data obtained in 1986 (Table 2.3). The median age of persons with

TABLE 2.3. *Incidence of bacterial meningitis in the United States*

Organism	Incidence (cases per 100,000 population)	
	1986	1995
Haemophilus influenzae	2.9	0.2
Streptococcus pneumoniae	1.1	1.1
Neisseria meningitidis	0.9	0.6
Group B streptococcus	0.4	0.3
Listeria monocytogenes	0.2	0.2

Data from Wenger JD, Hightower AW, Facklam RR, et al. Bacterial meningitis in the United States, 1986: report of a multistate surveillance study. *J Infect Dis* 1990;162:1316–1323; and Schuchat A, Robinson K, Wenger JD, et al. Bacterial meningitis in the United States in 1995. *N Engl J Med* 1997;337:970–976, with permission.

TABLE 2.4. *Etiology of bacterial meningitis in selected series outside of the United States*

	Percentage of total cases			
Organism	United Kingdom (1980–1984)	Cairo, Egypt (1971–1975)	Dakar, Senegal (1970–1979)	Salvador, Brazil (1973–1982)
Haemophilus influenzae	29	3	20	23
Neisseria meningitidis	25	56	11	22
Streptococcus pneumoniae	20	8	29	17
Streptococcus agalactiae	7	—	4	—
Listeria monocytogenes	2	—	<0.5	—
Other	16	1	9	20
Unknown	—	32	26	18

Data from Noah ND. Epidemiology of bacterial meningitis: UK and USA. In: Williams JD, Burnie J, eds. *Bacterial meningitis.* London: Academic Press, 1987:93–115; Greenwood BM. The epidemiology of acute bacterial meningitis in tropical Africa. In: Williams JD, Burnie J, eds. *Bacterial meningitis.* London: Academic Press, 1987:61–91; Miner WF, Edman DC. Acute bacterial meningitis in Cairo, Arab Republic of Egypt, 1 January 1971 through 31 December 1975. *Am J Trop Med Hyg* 1978;27:986–994; and Bryan JP, de Silva HR, Tavares A, et al. Etiology and mortality of bacterial meningitis in northeastern Brazil. *Rev Infect Dis* 1990;12: 128–135, with permission.

bacterial meningitis increased greatly (from 15 months in 1986 to 25 years in 1995) such that, in the United States, bacterial meningitis is now a disease predominantly of adults rather than of infants and children. These data indicate that the development of effective vaccines and other preventive strategies against other meningeal pathogens may further decrease the overall incidence of this devastating infection.

Bacterial meningitis is also a major problem in the developing world (Table 2.4) (10–13). In Dakar, Senegal, the average incidence of bacterial meningitis was 50 cases per 100,000 population; approximately one in 250 children develops bacterial meningitis during the first 5 years of life, with a mortality rate of greater than 50%. In the largest review of approximately 4,100 cases of bacterial meningitis at Hospital Couta Maia in Salvador, Brazil, from 1973 through 1982, the attack rate was 45.8 cases per 100,000 population (13). The overall case fatality rate was 33%, with 50% of deaths occurring within 48 hours of hospitalization. Children younger than 15 years of age accounted for 79% of cases; 45% of cases were in children younger than 2 years of age. *H. influenzae, N. meningitidis,* and *S. pneumoniae* accounted for 62% of the cases and 70% of the deaths. The case fatality rates for meningitis caused by the Enterobacteriaceae was 86%; more than half of these cases in children less than 24 months of age were caused by *Salmonella* species, an unusual meningeal pathogen in industrialized nations. These data underscore the need for improved therapeutic regimens and vaccine strategies to control bacterial meningitis in developing countries of the world.

The likely etiologic agents of bacterial meningitis vary, depending on the age, risk factors, and underlying disease status of the patient (Table 2.5). These parameters, and their association with specific infecting microorganisms, are discussed later.

TABLE 2.5. Common bacterial pathogens based on age and predisposing factor in patients with meningitis[a]

Predisposing factor	Common bacterial pathogens
Age	
<1 mo	Streptococcus agalactiae, Escherichia coli, Listeria monocytogenes, Klebsiella species
1–23 mo	Streptococcus pneumoniae, Neisseria meningitidis Streptococcus agalactiae, Haemophilus influenzae, Escherichia coli
2–50 yr	Neisseria meningitidis, Streptococcus pneumoniae
>50 yr	Streptococcus pneumoniae, Neisseria meningitidis, Listeria monocytogenes, aerobic gram-negative bacilli
Nosocomial acquisition	Aerobic gram-negative bacilli (including Pseudomonas aeruginosa), staphylococci (Staphylococcus aureus and coagulase-negative staphylococci)
Head trauma	
Basilar skull fracture	Streptococcus pneumoniae, Haemophilus influenzae, group A β-hemolytic streptococci
Penetrating trauma	Staphylococcus aureus, Staphylococcus epidermidis, aerobic gram-negative bacilli (including Pseudomonas aeruginosa)
Postneurosurgery	Aerobic gram-negative bacilli (including Pseudomonas aeruginosa), Staphylococcus aureus, Staphylococcus epidermidis
Cerebrospinal fluid shunt	Staphylococcus epidermidis, Staphylococcus aureus, aerobic gram-negative bacilli (including Pseudomonas aeruginosa), Propionibacterium acnes
Immunocompromised state	
Cellular immunodeficiency	Listeria monocytogenes, Nocardia species
Humoral immunodeficiency	Streptococcus pneumoniae, Haemophilus influenzae, Neisseria meningitidis, Staphylococcus aureus, other streptococci
Neutropenia	Aerobic gram-negative bacilli (including Pseudomonas aeruginosa), Staphylococcus aureus

[a] Age must always be an important parameter when considering specific etiologic agents of bacterial meningitis.

Age

In the neonate, the epidemiology of bacterial meningitis has changed considerably over the last 50 years (14). Gram-negative bacilli (primarily *Escherichia coli*) were previously the most frequently isolated microorganisms, although the group B streptococcus has recently emerged as the most common meningeal pathogen isolated during the neonatal period, accounting for 125 cases per 100,000 population in children less than 1 month of age in the United States (9). The increased frequency of isolation of this organism during the neonatal period has also been observed in other countries throughout the world (15–17), although a recent prospective study from southern Israel found that gram-negative bacilli (*E. coli* and *Klebsiella* species) were the main pathogens causing neonatal sepsis and meningitis (18). Other important bacteria isolated in neonates with bacterial meningitis include *L. monocytogenes,* staphylococci (*Staphylococcus aureus* and *Staphylococcus epidermidis*) and nonfermenting gram-negative bacilli. Many factors contribute to the development of meningitis in the neonate, although the most significant are low birth weight and premature rupture of membranes; meningitis has been more frequently observed since advances in neonatal intensive care have permitted survival of very-low-birth-weight infants. Infants may also acquire the infecting organism from the hands of hospital personnel (19).

In infants and children from 1 month to 2 years of age, the marked predominance of *H. influenzae* type b as a cause of meningitis in the preconjugate vaccine era has given way to *S. pneumoniae* and *N. meningitidis* as the more commonly isolated pathogens. In patients 2 to 29 years of age, *N. meningitidis* is the most frequently isolated bacterial cause of meningitis in the United States (9).

In patients greater than or equal to 16 years of age, most cases of community-acquired bacterial meningitis are caused by *S. pneumoniae, N. meningitidis,* and *L. monocytogenes* (Table 2.6) (20–22), although *Listeria* meningitis is uncommon in adults under 50 years of age. In this age group, case fatality rates for single episodes of community-acquired meningitis were 25% overall in a study of 253 cases of community-acquired bacterial meningitis at the Massachusetts General Hospital (20); there was no significant variability of this mortality rate over the 27-year period of the study. Risk factors for death among adult patients with community-acquired meningitis included age 60 years or older, obtunded mental status on admission, and seizures within the first 24 hours of presentation.

TABLE 2.6. *Etiology of bacterial meningitis in patients 16 yr of age and older*

	Percentage of total cases		
Organism	Massachusetts General Hospital (1962–1988)	Parkland Memorial Hospital (10-yr review)	University of Iceland (1975–1994)
Haemophilus influenzae	4	5	5
Neisseria meningitidis	14	16	56
Streptococcus pneumoniae	38	56	20
Listeria monocytogenes	11	7	6
Other[a]	20	10	—
Unknown	13	—	8

[a] Includes gram-negative bacilli, streptococci, enterococci, *Staphylococcus aureus, Neisseria gonorrhoeae,* anaerobes, and diphtheroids.

Data from Durand ML, Calderwood SB, Weber DJ, et al. Acute bacterial meningitis in adults: a review of 493 episodes. *N Engl J Med* 1993;328:21–28; Luby JP. Southwestern internal medicine conference: infections of the central nervous system. *Am J Med Sci* 1992;304:379–391; and Sigurdardottir B, Bjornsson OM, Jonsdottir KE, et al. Acute bacterial meningitis in adults: a 20-year overview. *Arch Intern Med* 1997;157:425–430, with permission.

Nosocomial Acquisition

Bacterial meningitis is a significant problem in hospitalized patients. The National Nosocomial Infection Surveillance Program documented an incidence of 5.6 non-surgical, nosocomial central nervous system infections for every 100,000 patients discharged from the hospital between 1986 and 1993; meningitis accounted for 91% of all infections (23). In a recent large series of 493 episodes of bacterial meningitis in adults 16 years of age or older at the Massachusetts General Hospital from 1962 through 1988, 40% of episodes were nosocomial in origin (20). In contrast to the likely etiologic agents in adults with community-acquired bacterial meningitis, most noso-comial cases were caused by gram-negative bacilli (38%) and staphylococci (18%). *S. pneumoniae, N. meningitidis,* and *L. monocytogenes* accounted for only 9% of cases. The overall case fatality rate for patients with single episodes of nosocomial menin-gitis was 35% and did not vary significantly over the 27-year period of the study. The most common risk factor for nosocomial meningitis is neurosurgery, with the risk of infection increasing with longer duration of operation, use of external drainage, operations through the paranasal sinuses, and need for reexploration (23). During the neonatal period, development of bacteremia, associated with use of invasive devices during hospitalization, increases the risk of secondary meningitis as a result of the neonate's immature blood-brain barrier.

Head Trauma

Bacterial meningitis is a feared complication of acute head injury and may result from various degrees of trauma, ranging from relatively minor accidents to penetrating injuries of the skull (24–26). The incidence of acute bacterial meningitis following head injury ranges from 0.2% to 17.8% in various series (mean of approximately 6% in several reports). The presence of a leak of cerebrospinal fluid (CSF), manifested clinically as rhinorrhea or otorrhea, greatly increases the risk of posttraumatic bacterial meningitis. CSF rhinorrhea and otorrhea most often occur after a basilar skull fracture and are definite signs of a dural tear. The dural tear leads to the development of a CSF fistula, and it is the fistula, not the rhinorrhea or otorrhea, that increases the risk of bacterial meningitis. Once this fistulous tract is established, any maneuver that increases intracranial pressure may force microorganisms into the intracranial space. The longer the duration of the fistula, the greater the risk for the subsequent development of bacterial meningitis. Failure to repair the dural defect may result in recurrent attacks of bacterial meningitis (8). The types of head trauma that may lead to CSF leaks and thus increase the risk of posttraumatic bacterial meningitis include accidental falls, motor vehicle accidents, blunt trauma, and gunshot wounds.

The microorganisms isolated from patients with posttraumatic bacterial meningi-tis depend upon the pathogenic mechanism responsible for the initial trauma. When meningitis occurs following basilar skull fracture and CSF rhinorrhea, the microor-ganism isolated from CSF is usually *S. pneumoniae* (55% of cases), although *H. influenzae* (16% of cases) or group A β-hemolytic streptococci (8% of cases) may occasionally be the causative agent (25,26). Staphylococci and gram-negative bacilli are exceedingly rare after basilar skull fracture unless the patient has been hospitalized for a prolonged period, or if the meningitis occurs as a complication of penetrating head trauma or open head wound.

Postneurosurgical Period

The rate of central nervous system infection following neurosurgical procedures not involving trauma is relatively low (26). The rate of bacterial meningitis in clean neurosurgical procedures using perioperative prophylactic antimicrobial therapy ranges from 0.5% to 0.7%. In clean-contaminated procedures, such as transsphenoidal approaches to the pituitary fossa, the rate of postoperative infection has been reported to range from 0.4% to 2.0%; postoperative CSF leakage has been identified as an important risk factor for meningitis after transsphenoidal surgery (27). When infection does occur, bacteria enter the meninges from contiguous sites of colonization or suppuration (e.g., wound infection at the cutaneous incision, indwelling lumbar or ventricular drains, or the sinuses). Infecting microorganisms following neurosurgical procedures include enteric gram-negative bacilli (*Klebsiella* species, *Enterobacter* species, and *Pseudomonas aeruginosa*) and staphylococci (primarily *S. epidermidis*) (26,28); respiratory tract flora should be considered as causative pathogens when operative procedures traverse the paranasal sinuses.

Cerebrospinal Fluid Shunts

The rate of CSF shunt infections has ranged from 2% to 40%, although more recent series have reported infection rates of less than 4% (26,29). CSF shunts may become infected as a result of retrograde infection from the distal end (principally involving infection of externalized devices); wound or skin breakdown overlying the shunt, allowing direct access of microorganisms; hematogenous seeding; or colonization at the time of surgery. Colonization at the time of surgery is probably the most frequent cause of CSF shunt infection, since most isolated organisms from infected shunts are commensal skin organisms. Etiologic agents of CSF shunt infections are usually staphylococcal species (65% to 85% of cases, most commonly *S. epidermidis*) and gram-negative bacilli (6% to 20% of cases); polymicrobial infection is found in 10% to 15% of cases. In recent years, the prevalence of CSF shunt infection caused by diphtheroids (especially *Propionibacterium acnes*) has increased, accounting for 50% of cases in one review (30); better culture techniques may increase the probability of isolating these organisms from infected CSF shunts.

Immunocompromised State

The risk of bacterial meningitis in the immunocompromised patient depends upon the underlying disease and its treatment, the duration of immunosuppression, and the type of immune abnormality (31–33). The four major types of host-defense abnormalities encountered in the immunosuppressed patient are defects in cell-mediated immunity, defects in humoral immunity, reduced number and/or function of neutrophils, and loss of splenic function (as a result of surgery, disease, or radiotherapy).

Patients with deficiencies in cell-mediated immunity (e.g., organ transplant recipients, patients treated with daily corticosteroids or other immunosuppressive agents, and patients with human immunodeficiency virus infection or hematologic malignancies) are more susceptible to bacterial infection with intracellular microorganisms such as *L. monocytogenes*. Patients who have defective humoral immunity (e.g., those with chronic lymphocytic leukemia, multiple myeloma, or Hodgkin's disease) or who have loss of splenic function are subject to infection with encapsulated bacteria such as *S. pneumoniae*. Neutropenic patients may be prone to central nervous system infection with enteric gram-negative bacilli such as *P. aeruginosa, Klebsiella* species, and *E. coli*.

ETIOLOGY

Streptococcus pneumoniae

Streptococcus pneumoniae is the most frequently observed etiologic agent of bacterial meningitis in the United States, now accounting for 47% of total cases (9). The mortality rate from pneumococcal meningitis ranges from 19% to 26% in the United States (7–9), with rates of about 30% to 60% in the developing world (13,34,35). Of the 84 known pneumococcal capsular serotypes, 23 account for between 85% and 94% of all invasive disease (36). In one study of 519 cases of pneumococcal meningitis in persons of all ages, 12 capsular serotypes or groups (1,3,4,6,7,8,9,12,14,18,19, and 23) were responsible for 410 (79%) cases (37). In studies examining the specific pneumococcal capsular serotypes isolated from CSF, from 74% to 90% represent the serotypes available in the 23-valent pneumococcal polysaccharide vaccine (36–38).

Patients with pneumococcal meningitis often have contiguous or distant foci of pneumococcal infection such as pneumonia (15% to 25% of cases), otitis media (30% of cases), mastoiditis, sinusitis, or endocarditis. Serious pneumococcal infection (including meningitis) may be observed during the extremes of life (persons less than 2 years and greater than 70 years of age) and in patients with various underlying conditions (e.g., splenectomy or asplenic states such as sickle cell disease, multiple myeloma, hypogammaglobulinemia, alcoholism, malnutrition, chronic liver or renal disease, malignancy, Wiskott-Aldrich syndrome, thalassemia major, and diabetes mellitus) (39–45). In one study, alcoholism was the most important risk factor in adults with invasive pneumococcal disease (40). *S. pneumoniae* is the most common etiologic agent of meningitis in patients who have suffered basilar skull fracture with CSF leak (25,26).

Neisseria meningitidis

Neisseria meningitidis most commonly causes meningitis in children and young adults, and is associated with an overall mortality rate of 3% to 13% in the United

States (7–9). Most meningococcal disease is caused by organisms in serogroups A, B, C, Y, and W135. Meningococci of serogroups B, C, and Y account for most of the endemic disease in the United States (46,47) as well as in other countries of the world (48,49). Major epidemics of invasive meningococcal disease have been reported in a number of developing countries (including Brazil, Nepal, China, and various sub-Saharan African nations) and are primarily caused by serogroup A meningococcus (50,51); attack rates during these epidemics can approach 1% of the population. A broad savannah region in Africa, extending from Gambia to Ethiopia, is known as the "meningitis belt" (Fig. 2.1). This region is uniquely susceptible to intense serogroup A meningococcal epidemics that usually occur in 8- to 14-year cycles; various host, organism, and environmental risk factors contribute to these epidemics. It has been suggested that "antigenic shifts" in serogroup A meningococcal clones may trigger

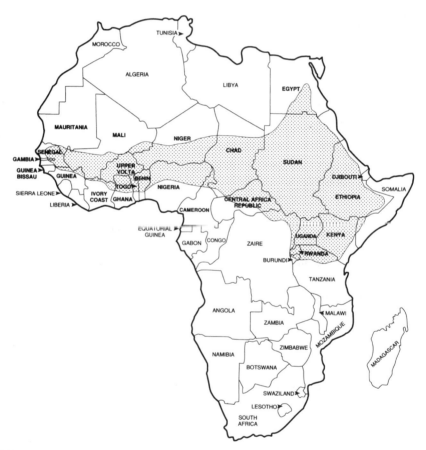

FIG. 2.1. Meningitis belt of sub-Saharan Africa. (From Moore PS. Meningococcal meningitis in sub-Saharan Africa: a model for the epidemic process. *Clin Infect Dis* 1992;14:515–525, with permission.)

an outbreak of disease by suddenly decreasing herd immunity within a population. Spread of specific clones of serogroup A meningococcus has been reported outside of the African meningitis belt (52,53).

Meningococcal disease caused by serogroup C may also occur in epidemics, although to a lesser extent than with serogroup A. However, the incidence of serogroup C disease has been increasing. Several recent outbreaks of disease caused by serogroup C meningococci have been reported in the United States, Canada, and Europe (54–56), with most caused by one strain of the electrophoretic type 37 (ET-37) termed ET-15 (54,55). Isolates of the ET-37 complex were also responsible for most cases of sporadic serogroup C meningococcal disease in another study (57). Infection caused by serogroup Y strains may be associated with pneumonia.

Nasopharyngeal carriage of *N. meningitidis* is an important factor that leads to the development of invasive disease (46,58). By a conservative estimate, 500 million out of the 6 billion people in the world carry *N. meningitidis* in the nasopharynx, with the rate of carriage lowest in children and highest in adolescents and young adults. Up to 10% of patients with meningococcal meningitis have had contact with another known case. The estimated prevalence of meningococcal carriage in the United States is 5% to 10% under nonepidemic conditions. In closed populations, such as military recruits, carriage rates can reach levels as high as 40% to 90%. Household contacts exposed to a patient with meningococcal disease have a 500 to 4,000-fold increased risk of developing invasive disease; 70% to 80% of secondary cases occur within 14 days of the primary case, often developing within 5 days of the index case. Coincident upper respiratory tract infection may increase the risk of developing invasive meningococcal disease (59,60). Transmission of *N. meningitidis* has also been documented in campus bars, sports clubs, and dance clubs (61–63).

Patients with deficiencies in the terminal complement components (C5, C6, C7, C8, and perhaps C9), the so-called membrane attack complex, have an increased incidence of neisserial infections (64–70), including that caused by *N. meningitidis*. In one review (64), patients with late complement component deficiencies had a markedly increased frequency of meningococcal disease (42% versus 0.0072% in the general population), although mortality rates caused by meningococcal disease were lower than those in patients with an intact complement system (3% versus 19% in the general population), perhaps because endotoxin release induced by serum from these deficient patients is decreased, thereby avoiding development of extensive tissue damage (71). An increased risk of invasive meningococcal disease has also been described in a Dutch family with dysfunctional properdin (72) and in patients with familial properdin deficiency (73), suggesting a potential role for the alternative pathway in complement-mediated resistance against meningococci. The patients with familial properdin deficiency had a high mortality rate (75%) compared with those with late complement component deficiencies (3%), possibly because complement-enhanced phagocytosis remains intact in patients with late complement component deficiencies. In properdin-deficient serum, there is not only an impairment in the elimination of microorganisms by means of serum bactericidal activity, but also a defect in complement-dependent phagocytosis.

Streptococcus agalactiae

The group B streptococcus (*S. agalactiae*) is a common cause of meningitis in neonates, with 52% of all cases in the United States reported during the first month of life (9). The incidence of neonatal sepsis and meningitis caused by group B streptococcus is 0.5 to 3.0 cases per 1,000 live births (74,75), although there are substantial geographic and racial differences; disease occurs substantially more often in African American infants than in other racial groups. In the United States, the overall mortality rate of group B streptococcal meningitis ranges from 7% to 27% (7–9).

Group B streptococcal infections in infants are restricted to very early infancy (74,75). Early-onset disease is most often manifest in the first days of life, in which newborns acquire the organism from their mothers, who are colonized in their genital tracts. The group B streptococcus has been isolated from vaginal or rectal cultures of 15% to 35% of asymptomatic pregnant women (74–76); colonization rates do not vary during pregnancy and may be chronic (40% of women), transient, or intermittent. The risk of perinatal transmission from the mother to her infant is increased when the inoculum of organisms and number of sites of maternal colonization are increased; the route of delivery does not influence transmission. Infection occurs following ascending spread of the organism into the amniotic fluid, where aspiration of contaminated amniotic fluid may lead to invasive disease. Perinatal transmission can also occur across intact membranes. Late-onset infections occur in infants between 1 week and 2 to 3 months of age (75). The pathogenesis of late-onset infection is less well understood, although some cases probably reflect acquisition of the organism during passage of the infant through the birth canal. Horizontal transmission has also been documented from the hands of nursery personnel to the infant. Most cases of neonatal group B streptococcal meningitis are caused by subtype III organisms and occur after the first week of life.

The group B streptococcus can also cause meningitis in adults (77–82). Disease in adults tends to occur in association with severe underlying conditions and has been associated with a high mortality rate (27% to 34%) (78,80). Risk factors for infection in adults include age more than 60 years, diabetes mellitus, pregnancy or the postpartum state, cardiac disease, collagen-vascular diseases, malignancy, alcoholism, hepatic failure, renal failure, previous stroke, neurogenic bladder, decubitus ulcers, and corticosteroid therapy. In one review of group B streptococcal meningitis in adults, no underlying illnesses were found in 43% of patients (78).

Listeria monocytogenes

Listeria monocytogenes causes 8% of cases of bacterial meningitis in the United States and carries a mortality rate of 15% to 29% (7–9). In a recently published review of adult patients with community-acquired bacterial meningitis, *L. monocytogenes* was responsible for 11% of cases (20). *Listeria* has been isolated from dust, soil, water, sewage, decaying vegetable matter (including animal feed and silage), and fecal flora of many mammals (83). Outbreaks of *Listeria* infection have been associated with consumption of contaminated cole slaw, raw vegetables, milk, and cheese, with sporadic cases traced to contaminated cheese, turkey franks, rillettes, and alfalfa tablets (83–90); these outbreaks point to the intestinal tract as the usual portal of entry of this organism. The importance of food as a source of sporadic outbreaks is supported by the CDC finding that 11% of all refrigerator food samples were contaminated with *L. monocytogenes,* 64% of patients' refrigerators contained at least one contaminated food item, and *Listeria* isolates from the food and the infected patients had the same multilocus-enzyme-electrophoresis type in 33% of instances (83). Serotypes 1/2b and 4b have been implicated in up to 80% of meningitis cases caused by this organism.

Patients at the extremes of age are especially prone to listerial infection, with most cases of meningitis seen in infants less than 1 month of age and adults greater than 50 years of age (Fig. 2.2) (83,90). Although colonization rates are low, pregnant women (who account for 25% of all cases of listeriosis) may harbor the organism asymptomatically in their genital tract and rectum and transmit the infection to their infants. Other predisposing conditions include alcoholism, malignancy, use of corticosteroid therapy, immunosuppression (e.g., following renal transplantation), diabetes mellitus, liver disease, chronic renal disease, collagen-vascular diseases, and conditions associated with iron overload (83,84,90–95). A similar spectrum of predisposing factors

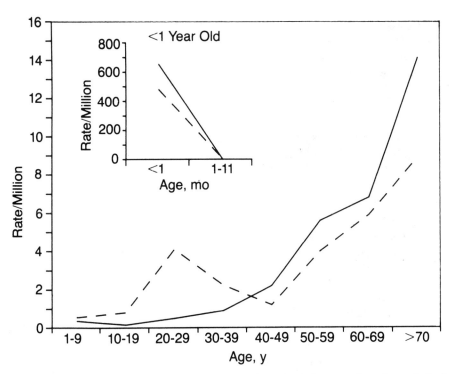

FIG. 2.2. Age-specific incidence of listeriosis, by sex. Solid line indicates male patients; dashed line, female patients. (From Ciesielski CA, Hightower AW, Parsons SK, et al. Listeriosis in the United States: 1980–1982. *Arch Intern Med* 1988;148:1416–1419, with permission.)

TABLE 2.7. *Predisposing factors and comorbid conditions among 458 patients with meningitis or meningoencephalitis caused by* Listeria monocytogenes

Predisposing factor/comorbid condition	Number of patients (% of total)
Malignancy[a]	111 (24)
Transplantation[b]	94 (17)
Alcoholism and/or liver disease	58 (13)
Immunosuppression/steroid treatment	49 (11)
HIV/AIDS	34 (7)
Diabetes mellitus	35 (8)
Autoimmune disorders	18 (4)
Iron overload	5 (1)
Other	9 (2)
No predisposing factor	166 (36)

[a] Hematologic malignancy in 64/111 patients; solid tumors in 31/111 patients.
[b] Renal transplantation in 80/94 patients.
Data from Mylonakis E, Hohmann EL, Calderwood SB. Central nervous system infection with *Listeria monocytogenes*: 33 years' experience at a general hospital and review of 776 episodes from the literature. *Medicine* 1998;77:313–336, with permission.

and comorbid conditions was found in a review of 458 patients with meningitis or meningoencephalitis caused by *L. monocytogenes* (Table 2.7) (96). However, *Listeria* meningitis can occur throughout life and in patients without predisposing conditions (36% of cases). *Listeria* meningitis is found infrequently in patients with human immunodeficiency virus (HIV) infection (96–99), despite the increased incidence of listeriosis in patients with deficiencies in cell-mediated immunity.

Haemophilus influenzae

Haemophilus influenzae was previously isolated in 15% to 18% of all cases of bacterial meningitis in the United States (7,8); this organism is now isolated in only 7% of cases (9). The overall mortality rate is 3% to 6% (7–9). Most episodes of meningitis previously occurred in infants and children under the age of 6 years (peak incidence of 6 to 12 months), with 90% of cases caused by capsular type b strains. In recent years, there has been a profound reduction in the incidence of invasive infections (including bacterial meningitis) caused by *H. influenzae* type b in the United States and Western Europe (Fig. 2.3) (9,100–108). This reduction is primarily attributed to the recent widespread use of conjugate vaccines against *H. influenzae* type b that have been licensed for routine use in all children beginning at 2 months of age. The number of cases of *H. influenzae* type b meningitis since introduction of vaccination has decreased more than 85%, with reductions of more than 95% noted in several studies (107,108). Similar reductions in the rate of infection have also been witnessed in countries where vaccine uptake has been only moderate (50% to 75%), suggesting that herd immunity is enhanced by vaccination. This result may lie in the ability of conjugate vaccines to reduce nasopharyngeal carriage of *H. influenzae* type b and subsequently reduce transmission (109). In developing countries, use of *H. influenzae*

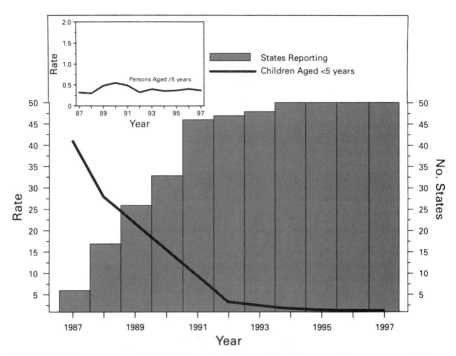

FIG. 2.3. Incidence rate per 100,000 of invasive *Haemophilus influenzae* disease among children less than 5 years of age and persons ≥5 years of age in the United States, 1987–1997. (From Centers for Disease Control and Prevention. Progress toward elimination of *Haemophilus influenzae* type b disease among infants and children—United States, 1987–1997. *MMWR* 1998;47:993–998, with permission.)

type b conjugate vaccines has not been extensively studied. However, one recently published trial in Gambian infants demonstrated that *H. influenzae* type b conjugate vaccine prevented most cases of meningitis caused by this organism, with an overall efficacy of more than 90% (110,111).

Isolation of *H. influenzae* as a cause of meningitis in older children and adults may be associated with the presence of certain preexisting conditions, including sinusitis, otitis media, epiglottitis, and pneumonia, suggesting that contiguous spread from local infection is a frequent pathogenic route to the central nervous system. Predisposing conditions in patients with *H. influenzae* meningitis include diabetes mellitus, alcoholism, splenectomy or asplenic states, head trauma with CSF leak, multiple myeloma, and immune deficiency (e.g., hypogammaglobulinemia) (112–116).

Aerobic Gram-Negative Bacilli

The aerobic gram-negative bacilli (e.g., *Klebsiella* species, *E. coli, Enterobacter* species, *Acinetobacter* species, *Serratia marcescens, P. aeruginosa, Salmonella* species) have become increasingly important as etiologic agents in patients with

TABLE 2.8. *Specific etiologic agents in patients with gram-negative bacillary meningitis*

	Percentage of total cases	
Organism	Dallas, Texas (1969–1989); N = 98 cases in neonates and infants	Massachusetts General Hospital (1962–1988); N = 57 cases in adults
Escherichia coli	53	30
Klebsiella–Enterobacter	16	N/A
Klebsiella species	N/A	23
Enterobacter species	N/A	9
Citrobacter diversus	9	4
Salmonella species	9	0
Proteus mirabilis	4	4
Serratia marcescens	3	9
Pseudomonas species	0	10
Acinetobacter species	0	10
Other[a]	5	1

[a] Includes *Bacteroides fragilis* and *Aeromonas* species from neonates and infants, and "coliform" bacteria and nonenteric gram-negative bacilli from adults.

Data from Durand ML, Calderwood SB, Weber DJ, et al. Acute bacterial meningitis in adults: a review of 493 episodes. *N Engl J Med* 1993;328:21–28; and Unhanand M, Mustafa MM, McCracken GH Jr., et al. Gram-negative enteric bacillary meningitis: a twenty-one-year experience. *J Pediatr* 1993;122:15–21, with permission.

bacterial meningitis (Table 2.8) (20,117–124); mortality rates range from about 30% to 80%. In a review of 98 cases of gram-negative enteric bacillary meningitis in neonates and infants at Parkland Memorial Hospital and Children's Medical Center in Dallas, Texas, from 1969 through 1989 (117), the most commonly isolated organism was *E. coli* (53% of cases). Most cases (75%) of *E. coli* meningitis are caused by strains possessing the K1 antigen. Neural tube defects and urinary tract abnormalities were identified as the most common predisposing factors to development of gram-negative meningitis in this study. *Citrobacter diversus* was isolated from 9% of patients; isolation of this organism has important implications because of the propensity for infants with *C. diversus* meningitis to also have one or more brain abscesses (76% of cases in one large review) (125,126).

In a review of 493 episodes of bacterial meningitis in adults at the Massachusetts General Hospital from 1962 through 1988, gram-negative bacilli were significantly more common in nosocomial than in community-acquired cases (38% versus 9%, respectively) (20). In addition, there was an increase in the relative frequency of isolation of gram-negative bacilli as a cause of meningitis throughout the period of the study (from 11% in the 1960s to 24% in the 1980s; $P < 0.01$), which may be related to the increase in the relative frequency of nosocomial meningitis principally as a result of numbers of patients undergoing neurosurgical procedures.

Aerobic gram-negative bacilli may also be isolated from the CSF of patients following head trauma and from patients who are elderly, are immunosuppressed, have gram-negative septicemia, or have received endoscopic injection sclerotherapy for esophageal varices (20,117–124,127). Some cases have been associated with disseminated strongyloidiasis in the hyperinfection syndrome, in which meningitis caused by enteric gram-negative bacilli occurs secondary to seeding of the meninges during persistent or recurrent bacteremias associated with the migration of infective larvae (128). Alternatively, the larvae may carry enteric organisms on their surfaces or within their own gastrointestinal tracts as they exit the intestine and subsequently invade the meninges.

Staphylococci

Meningitis caused by *Staphylococcus aureus* accounts for 1% to 9% of cases of bacterial meningitis in previously published reports, with mortality rates ranging from 14% to 77% (129–132). Meningitis usually occurs in patients following neurosurgical procedures or after head trauma, and in those with CSF shunts (12% to 29% of cases). Underlying conditions in patients with no prior central nervous system disease include diabetes mellitus, alcoholism, chronic renal failure requiring hemodialysis, injection drug use, and malignancies. In one epidemiologic study (130), 55% of cases were observed in patients with various central nervous system disorders (prior neurosurgery, CSF shunt, stroke, trauma, hemorrhage, seizure disorder, neoplasm, hydrocephalus, and arteriovenous malformation). Other underlying conditions in patients with community-acquired *S. aureus* meningitis include sinusitis, endocarditis, abscess, cellulitis, osteomyelitis, and pneumonia. Mortality rates in patients with *S. aureus* meningitis have been reported to be higher when the pathogenesis of meningitis is hematogenous rather than postoperative (56% versus 18%) (131).

Staphylococcus epidermidis is the most common cause of meningitis in patients with CSF shunts (29,133), accounting for 47% to 64% of cases. The propensity of this organism to cause infection in CSF shunts is likely a result of specific virulence factors that allow it to adhere directly to prosthetic devices and to produce substances that are protective against phagocytosis (134,135).

Anaerobes

Anaerobic meningitis is a rare entity, accounting for less than 1% of cases of bacterial meningitis (136–139). The mortality rates in small series have ranged from 25% to 30%. Anaerobic meningitis may occur as a complication of brain abscess that ruptures into a ventricle or surface of the brain, although it more commonly results from a contiguous focus of infection (i.e., in patients with otitis media, mastoiditis, sinusitis, pharyngeal suppuration, infections of the teeth or oral cavity, head and neck malignancy, recent head and neck surgery or wound infection, head trauma, and recent laminectomy or neurosurgery). A variety of anaerobic bacteria have been reported to cause meningitis, most commonly *Bacteroides* species (especially *B. fragilis*), *Peptostreptococcus* species, *Fusobacterium,* and *Clostridium* species (136–146). In many cases more than one organism may be recovered. Anaerobes should be looked for, and the CSF cultured appropriately, in patients with meningitis and a focus of potential anaerobic infection.

Other Bacterial Causes of Meningitis

Despite the frequency with which the viridans streptococci cause bacteremia, they are uncommon causes of meningitis, accounting for 0.3% to 5% of culture-proven cases (147,148); *S. salivarius* may be the viridans streptococcus most commonly associated with meningitis. The source of these organisms is usually the patient's endogenous flora, although the portal of entry cannot always be identified. Predisposing conditions for viridans streptococcal meningitis include ear, nose, or throat pathology; endocarditis; primary extracranial infection; head trauma; neurosurgery; lumbar puncture; spinal-epidural analgesia; gastrointestinal pathology; gastrointestinal manipulation; and severe immunocompromise following chemotherapy (147–151).

Group A streptococcal meningitis is uncommon and usually occurs in association with other illnesses, most often pharyngitis and otitis media (152,153). Meningitis has been reported to be caused by other β-hemolytic streptococci, including those from groups C, F, and G (148,154); cases are usually associated with infective endocarditis. *Streptococcus bovis* has also been described as a cause of meningitis, usually in association with gastrointestinal disease, endocarditis, or oral lesions (155).

Enterococci are unusual etiologic agents of bacterial meningitis, accounting for only 0.3% to 0.8% of cases (20,156). In one review, the majority of adult patients with enterococcal meningitis had underlying illnesses; disease was associated with immunosuppressive therapy (63% of cases), CNS trauma or surgery, and/or an enterococcal infection outside the central nervous system (31% of cases) (157). Most (69%) of the pediatric patients with enterococcal meningitis had underlying central nervous system pathology, which appears to be a major associated condition in this age group; 25% of patients had primary enterococcal meningitis without an associated condition. The overall mortality rate was 13% in this series.

Diphtheroids, particularly *Propionibacterium acnes,* have become important etiologic agents of meningitis in patients with CSF shunt infections (29), accounting for up to 50% of cases in one series (30). Positive culture results with these organisms in patients with CSF shunts or external drainage devices cannot be ignored or considered to be contaminants even if the patient is without symptoms. *Corynebacterium jeikeium* has also been reported to be a rare cause of infection of ventricular CSF shunts (158).

A recent review of 28 cases of nocardial meningitis revealed the presence of predisposing conditions, usually reflecting depression of cell-mediated immunity, in approximately 75% of patients (159). These included immunosuppressive drug therapy, malignancy, head trauma, central nervous system procedures, chronic granulomatous disease, and sarcoidosis. The overall mortality was 57% in this review, with survivors tending to be younger, to be less likely to have associated brain abscess, and to have lower CSF glucose concentrations at initial presentation.

Many other bacterial pathogens have been reported to cause meningitis, as described in small case series or single case reports. These unusual bacterial causes of acute meningitis have included *Brucella* species (160), *Bordetella bronchiseptica* (161), *Flavobacterium meningosepticum* (162), *Stomatococcus mucilaginosus* (163,164), *Leuconostoc* species (165), other *Neisseria* species (166,167), *Pasteurella* species (168–171), *Campylobacter fetus* (172), and *Abiotrophia defectiva* (173). With continued increases in numbers of immunocompromised patients and/or use of invasive diagnostic or therapeutic devices involving the central nervous system, other bacterial pathogens may also be reported as etiologic agents of acute meningitis.

REFERENCES

1. Carpenter RR, Petersdorf RG. The clinical spectrum of bacterial meningitis. *Am J Med* 1962;33: 262–275.
2. Fraser DW, Henke CE, Feldman RA. Changing patterns of bacterial meningitis in Olmsted County, Minnesota, 1935–1970. *J Infect Dis* 1973;128:300–307.
3. Fraser DW, Darby CP, Koehler RE, et al. Risk factors in bacterial meningitis: Charleston County, South Carolina. *J Infect Dis* 1973;127:271–277.
4. Fraser DW, Geil CC, Feldman RA. Bacterial meningitis in Bernalillo County, New Mexico: a comparison with three other American populations. *Am J Epidemiol* 1974;100:29–34.
5. Floyd RF, Federspiel CF, Schaffner W. Bacterial meningitis in urban and rural Tennessee. *Am J Epidemiol* 1974;99:395–407.
6. Swartz MN, Dodge PR. Bacterial meningitis—a review of selected aspects. I. General clinical features, special problems and unusual meningeal reactions mimicking bacterial meningitis. *N Engl J Med* 1965;272:725–730, 842–848.
7. Schlech WF III, Ward JI, Band JD, et al. Bacterial meningitis in the United States, 1978 through 1981. The national bacterial meningitis surveillance study. *JAMA* 1985;253:1749–1754.
8. Wenger JD, Hightower AW, Facklam RR, et al. Bacterial meningitis in the United States, 1986: report of a multistate surveillance study. *J Infect Dis* 1990;162:1316–1323.
9. Schuchat A, Robinson K, Wenger JD, et al. Bacterial meningitis in the United States in 1995. *N Engl J Med* 1997;337:970–976.
10. Noah ND. Epidemiology of bacterial meningitis: UK and USA. In: Williams JD, Burnie J, eds. *Bacterial meningitis*. London: Academic Press, 1987:93–115.
11. Greenwood BM. The epidemiology of acute bacterial meningitis in tropical Africa. In: Williams JD, Burnie J, eds. *Bacterial meningitis*. London: Academic Press, 1987:61–91.
12. Miner WF, Edman DC. Acute bacterial meningitis in Cairo, Arab Republic of Egypt, 1 January 1971 through 31 December 1975. *Am J Trop Med Hyg* 1978;27:986–994.
13. Bryan JP, de Silva HR, Tavares A, et al. Etiology and mortality of bacterial meningitis in northeastern Brazil. *Rev Infect Dis* 1990;12:128–135.
14. De Louvois J. Acute bacterial meningitis in the newborn. *J Antimicrob Chemother* 1994;34:61–73.
15. Francis BM, Gilbert GL. Survey of neonatal meningitis in Australia: 1987–1989. *Med J Aust* 1992; 156:240–243.
16. Hervas JA, Alomar A, Salva F, et al. Neonatal sepsis and meningitis in Mallorca, Spain, 1977–1991. *Clin Infect Dis* 1993;16:719–724.
17. Ishikawa T, Asano Y, Morishima T, et al. Epidemiology of bacterial meningitis in children: Airchi Prefecture, Japan, 1984–1993. *Pediatr Neurol* 1996;14:244–250.
18. Greenberg D, Shinwell ES, Yagupsky P, et al. A prospective study of neonatal sepsis and meningitis in southern Israel. *Pediatr Infect Dis J* 1997;16:768–773.
19. Smith AL. Neonatal bacterial meningitis. In: Scheld WM, Whitley RJ, Durack DT, eds. *Infections of the central nervous system,* 2nd ed. Philadelphia: Lippincott-Raven Publishers, 1997:313–334.
20. Durand ML, Calderwood SB, Weber DJ, et al. Acute bacterial meningitis in adults: a review of 493 episodes. *N Engl J Med* 1993;328:21–28.
21. Luby JP. Southwestern internal medicine conference: infections of the central nervous system. *Am J Med Sci* 1992;304:379–391.
22. Sigurdardottir B, Bjornsson OM, Jonsdottir KE, et al. Acute bacterial meningitis in adults. A 20-year overview. *Arch Intern Med* 1997;157:425–430.
23. Farr BM, Scheld WM. Nosocomial meningitis. *Ochner Clin Rep* 1998;10:1–7.
24. Tenney JH. Bacterial infections of the central nervous system in neurosurgery. *Neurol Clin* 1986;4: 91–114.
25. Tunkel AR, Scheld WM. Acute infectious complications of head trauma. In: Braakman R, ed. *Handbook of clinical neurology, head injury.* Amsterdam: Elsevier Science Publishing, 1990:317–326.
26. Kaufman BA, Tunkel AR, Pryor JC, et al. Meningitis in the neurosurgical patient. *Infect Dis Clin North Am* 1990;4:677–701.

27. Van Aken MO, de Marie S, vander Lely AJ, et al. Risk factors for meningitis after transsphenoidal surgery. *Clin Infect Dis* 1997;25:852–856.
28. Mangi RJ, Quintiliani R, Andriole VT. Gram-negative bacillary meningitis. *Am J Med* 1975;59: 829–836.
29. Kaufman BA. Infections of cerebrospinal fluid shunts. In: Scheld WM, Whitley RJ, Durack DT, eds. *Infections of the central nervous system,* 2nd ed. Philadelphia: Lippincott-Raven, 1997: 555–577.
30. Rekate HL, Ruch T, Nulsen FE. Diphtheroid infections of cerebrospinal fluid shunts. *J Neurosurg* 1980;52:553–556.
31. Armstrong D, Wong B. Central nervous system infections in immunocompromised hosts. *Annu Rev Med* 1982;33:291–308.
32. Rubin RH, Hooper DC. Central nervous system infections in the compromised host. *Med Clin North Am* 1985;69:281–293.
33. Tunkel AR, Scheld WM. Central nervous system infection in the compromised host. In: Rubin RH, Young LS, eds. *Clinical approach to infection in the compromised host,* 3rd ed. New York: Plenum, 1994:163–210.
34. Greenwood BM. Selective primary health care: strategies for control of disease in the developing world. XIII: Acute bacterial meningitis. *Rev Infect Dis* 1984;6:374–389.
35. O'Dempsey TJD, McArdle TF, Lloyd-Evans N, et al. Pneumococcal disease among children in a rural area of West Africa. *Pediatr Infect Dis J* 1996;15:431–437.
36. Urwin G, Yuan MF, Hall LMC, et al. Pneumococcal meningitis in the North East Thames region UK: epidemiology and molecular analysis of isolates. *Epidemiol Infect* 1996;117:95–102.
37. Austrian R. Some observations on the pneumococcus and on the current status of pneumococcal disease and its prevention. *Rev Infect Dis* 1981;3:S1–S17.
38. Nielsen SV, Henrichsen J. Capsular types of *Streptococcus pneumoniae* isolated from blood and CSF during 1982–1987. *Clin Infect Dis* 1992;15:794–798.
39. Geiseler PJ, Nelson KE, Levin S, et al. Community-acquired purulent meningitis: a review of 1,316 cases during the antibiotic era, 1954–1976. *Rev Infect Dis* 1980;2:725–745.
40. Burman LA, Norrby R, Trollfors B. Invasive pneumococcal infections: incidence, predisposing factors, and prognosis. *Rev Infect Dis* 1985;7:133–142.
41. Henneberger PK, Galaid EI, Marr JS. The descriptive epidemiology of pneumococcal meningitis in New York City. *Am J Epidemiol* 1983;117:484–491.
42. Olopoenia L, Frederick W, Greaves W, et al. Pneumococcal sepsis and meningitis in adults with sickle cell disease. *South Med J* 1990;83:1002–1004.
43. Godeau B, Bachir D, Schaeffer A, et al. Severe pneumococcal sepsis and meningitis in human immunodeficiency virus-infected adults with sickle cell disease. *Clin Infect Dis* 1992;15:327–329.
44. Musher DM. Infections caused by *Streptococcus pneumoniae*. clinical spectrum, pathogenesis, immunity, and treatment. *Clin Infect Dis* 1992;14:801–809.
45. Kragsbjerg P, Kallman J, Olcen P. Pneumococcal meningitis in adults. *Scand J Infect Dis* 1994;26: 659–666.
46. Riedo FX, Plikaytis BD, Broome CV. Epidemiology and prevention of meningococcal disease. *Pediatr Infect Dis J* 1995;14:643–657.
47. Pinner RW, Onyango F, Perkins BA, et al. Epidemic meningococcal disease in Nairobi, Kenya, 1989. *J Infect Dis* 1992;166:359–364.
48. Block C, Roitman M, Bogokowsky B, et al. Forty years of meningococcal disease in Israel: 1951–1990. *Clin Infect Dis* 1993;17:126–132.
49. Scholten RJPM, Bijlmer HA, Poolman JT, et al. Meningococcal disease in the Netherlands, 1958–1990: a steady increase in the incidence since 1982 partially caused by new serotypes and subtypes of *Neisseria meningitidis*. *Clin Infect Dis* 1993;16:237–246.
50. Moore PS. Meningococcal meningitis in sub-Saharan Africa: a model for the epidemic process. *Clin Infect Dis* 1992;14:515–525.
51. Pinner RW, Gellin BG, Bibb WF, et al. Meningococcal disease in the United States—1986. *J Infect Dis* 1991;164:368–374.
52. Luo N, Perera C, Holton J, et al. Spread of *Neisseria meningitidis* group A clone III-I meningitis epidemic into Zambia. *J Infect* 1998;36:141–143.
53. McGee L, Koornhof HJ, Caugant DA. Epidemic spread of subgroup III of *Neisseria meningitidis* serogroup A to South Africa in 1996. *Clin Infect Dis* 1998;27:1214–1220.
54. Jackson LA, Schuchat A, Reeves MW, et al. Serogroup C meningococcal outbreaks in the United States: an emerging threat. *JAMA* 1995;273:383–389.

55. Whalen CM, Hockin JC, Ryan A, et al. The changing epidemiology of invasive meningococcal disease in Canada, 1985 through 1992: emergence of a virulent clone of *Neisseria meningitidis*. *JAMA* 1995;273:390–394.
56. Berron S, La Fuente LD, Martin E, et al. Increasing incidence of meningococcal disease in Spain associated with a new variant of serogroup C. *Eur J Clin Microbiol Infect Dis* 1998;17:85–89.
57. Raymond NJ, Reeves M, Ajello G, et al. Molecular epidemiology of sporadic (endemic) serogroup C meningococcal disease. *J Infect Dis* 1997;176:1277–1284.
58. Stephens DS. Uncloaking the meningococcus: dynamics of carriage and disease. *Lancet* 1999; 353:941–942.
59. Moore PS, Hierholzer J, DeWitt W, et al. Respiratory viruses and *Mycoplasma* as cofactors for epidemic group A meningococcal meningitis. *JAMA* 1990;264:1271–1275.
60. Harrison LH, Armstrong CW, Jenkins SR, et al. A cluster of meningococcal disease on a school bus following epidemic influenza. *Arch Intern Med* 1991;151:1005–1009.
61. Imrey PB, Jackson LA, Ludwinski PH, et al. Meningococcal carriage, alcohol consumption, and campus bar patronage in a serogroup C meningococcal disease outbreak. *Antimicrob Agents Chemother* 1995;33:3133–3137.
62. Cookson ST, Corrales JL, Lotero JO, et al. Disco fever: epidemic meningococcal disease in northeastern Argentina associated with disco patronage. *J Infect Dis* 1998;178:266–269.
63. Koh YM, Barnes GH, Kaczmarski E, et al. Outbreak of meningococcal disease linked to a sports club. *Lancet* 1998;352:706–707.
64. Ross SC, Densen P. Complement deficiency states and infection: epidemiology, pathogenesis and consequences of neisserial and other infections in an immune deficiency. *Medicine* 1984;64:243–273.
65. Ellison RT III, Kohler PF, Curd JG, et al. Prevalence of congenital or acquired complement deficiency in patients with sporadic meningococcal disease. *N Engl J Med* 1983;308:913–916.
66. Rosen MS, Lorber B, Myers AR. Chronic meningococcal meningitis: an association with C5 deficiency. *Arch Intern Med.* 1988;148:1441–1442.
67. Fijen CAP, Kuijper EJ, Hannema AJ, et al. Complement deficiencies in patients over ten years old with meningococcal disease due to uncommon serogroups. *Lancet* 1989;2:585–588.
68. Zoppi M, Weiss M, Nydegger UE, et al. Recurrent meningitis in a patient with congenital deficiency of the C9 component of complement: first case of C9 deficiency in Europe. *Arch Intern Med* 1990;150:2395–2399.
69. Fijen CAP, Kuijper EJ, Tjia HG, et al. Complement deficiency predisposes for meningitis due to nongroupable meningococci and *Neisseria*-related bacteria. *Clin Infect Dis* 1994;18:780–784.
70. Fijen CAP, Kuijper EJ, te Bulte MT, et al. Assessment of complement deficiency in patients with meningococcal disease in the Netherlands. *Clin Infect Dis* 1999;28:98–105.
71. Lehner PJ, Davies KA, Walport MJ, et al. Meningococcal septicaemia in a C6-deficient patient and effects of plasma transfusion on lipopolysaccharide release. *Lancet* 1992;340:1379–1381.
72. Sjäholm AG, Kuijper EJ, Tijssen CC, et al. Dysfunctional properdin in a Dutch family with meningococcal disease. *N Engl J Med* 1988;319:33–37.
73. Densen P, Weiler JM, Griffiss JM, et al. Familial properdin deficiency and fatal meningococcemia: correction of the bactericidal defect by vaccination. *N Engl J Med* 1987;316:922–926.
74. Schuchat A. Group B streptococcus. *Lancet* 1999;353:51–56.
75. Schuchat A. Epidemiology of group B streptococcal disease in the United States: shifting paradigms. *Clin Microbiol Rev* 1998;11:497–513.
76. Regan JA, Klebanoff MA, Nugent RP, et al. The epidemiology of group B streptococcal colonization in pregnancy. *Obstet Gynecol* 1991;77:604–610.
77. Farley MM, Harvey RC, Stull T, et al. A population-based assessment of invasive disease due to group B streptococci in nonpregnant adults. *N Engl J Med* 1993;328:1807–1811.
78. Dunne DW, Quagliarello V. Group B streptococcal meningitis in adults. *Medicine* 1993;72:1–10.
79. Jackson LA, Hilsdon R, Farley MM, et al. Risk factors for group B streptococcal disease in adults. *Ann Intern Med* 1995;123:415–420.
80. Domingo P, Barquet N, Alvarez M, et al. Group B streptococcal meningitis in adults: report of twelve cases and review. *Clin Infect Dis* 1997;25:1180–1187.
81. Robibaro B, Vorbach H, Weigel G, et al. Group B streptococcal meningoencephalitis after colonization in a nonpregnant woman. *Clin Infect Dis* 1998;26:1243–44.
82. Barile AJ, Kallen AJ, Wallace MR. Fatal group B streptococcal meningitis in a previously healthy adult. *Clin Infect Dis* 1999;28:151.
83. Lorber B. Listeriosis. *Clin Infect Dis* 1997;24:1–11.
84. Gellin BG, Broome CV. Listeriosis. *JAMA* 1989;261:1313–1320.

85. Cherubin CE, Appleman MD, Heseltine PNR, et al. Epidemiological spectrum and current treatment of listeriosis. *Rev Infect Dis* 1991;13:1108–1114.
86. Schuchat A, Deaver KA, Wenger JD, et al. Role of foods in sporadic listeriosis. I. Case-control study of dietary risk factors. *JAMA* 1992;267:2041–2045.
87. Pinner RW, Schuchat A, Swaminathan B, et al. Role of foods in sporadic listeriosis. II. Microbiologic and epidemiologic investigation. *JAMA* 1992;267:2046–2050.
88. Bula CJ, Bille J, Glauser MP. An epidemic of food-borne listeriosis in western Switzerland: description of 57 cases involving adults. *Clin Infect Dis* 1995;20:66–72.
89. Goulet V, Rocourt J, Rebiere I, et al. Listeriosis outbreak associated with the consumption of rillettes in France in 1993. *J Infect Dis* 1998;177:155–160.
90. Ciesielski CA, Hightower AW, Parsons SK, et al. Listeriosis in the United States: 1980–1982. *Arch Intern Med* 1988;148:1416–1419.
91. Anaissie E, Kontoyiannis DP, Kantarjian H, et al. Listeriosis in patients with chronic lymphocytic leukemia who were treated with fludarabine and prednisone. *Ann Intern Med* 1992;117:466–469.
92. Skogberg K, Syrjänen J, Jahkola M, et al. Clinical presentation and outcome of listeriosis in patients with and without immunosuppressive therapy. *Clin Infect Dis* 1992;14:815–821.
93. Kessler SL, Dajani AS. Listeria meningitis in infants and children. *Pediatr Infect Dis J* 1990;9:61–63.
94. Salata RA, King RE, Gose F, et al. *Listeria* monocytogenes cerebritis, bacteremia, and cutaneous lesions complicating hairy cell leukemia. *Am J Med* 1986;81:1068–1072.
95. Calder JAM. *Listeria* meningitis in adults. *Lancet* 1997;350:307–308.
96. Mylonakis E, Hohmann EL, Calderwood SB. Central nervous system infection with *Listeria monocytogenes*: 33 years' experience at a general hospital and review of 776 episodes from the literature. *Medicine* 1998;77:313–336.
97. Mascola L, Lieb L, Chiu J, et al. Listeriosis: an uncommon opportunistic infection in patients with acquired immunodeficiency syndrome: a report of five cases and a review of the literature. *Am J Med* 1988;84:162–164.
98. Decker CF, Simon GL, DiGioia RA, et al. *Listeria monocytogenes* infections in patients with AIDS: report of five cases and review. *Rev Infect Dis* 1991;13:413–417.
99. Berenguer J, Solera J, Diaz MD, et al. Listeriosis in patients infected with human immunodeficiency virus. *Rev Infect Dis* 1991;13:115–119.
100. Adams WG, Deaver KA, Cochi SL, et al. Decline of childhood *Haemophilus influenzae* type b (Hib) disease in the Hib vaccine era. *JAMA* 1993;269:221–226.
101. Shapiro ED. Infections caused by *Haemophilus influenzae* type b. The beginning of the end? *JAMA* 1993;269:264–266.
102. Centers for Disease Control and Prevention. Progress toward elimination of *Haemophilus influenzae* type b disease among infants and children—United States, 1987–1997. *MMWR* 1998;47:993–998.
103. Robbins JB, Schneerson R, Anderson P, et al. Prevention of systemic infections, especially meningitis, caused by *Haemophilus influenzae* type b. *JAMA* 1996;276:1181–1185.
104. Urwin G, Yuan MF, Feldman RA. Prospective study of bacterial meningitis in North East Thames region, 1991–3, during introduction of *Haemophilus influenzae* vaccine. *Br Med J* 1994;309:1412–1414.
105. Peltola H, Kilpi T, Anttila M. Rapid disappearance of *Haemophilus influenzae* type b meningitis after routine childhood immunisation with conjugate vaccines. *Lancet* 1992;340:592–594.
106. Garpenholt O, Silfverdal SA, Hugosson S, et al. The impact of *Haemophilus influenzae* type b vaccination in Sweden. *Scand J Infect Dis* 1996;28:165–169.
107. Van Alphen L, Spanjaard L, van der Ende A, et al. Effect of nationwide vaccination of 3-month-old infants in The Netherlands with conjugate *Haemophilus influenzae* type b vaccine: high efficacy and lack of herd immunity. *J Pediatr* 1997;131:869–873.
108. Booy R, Heath PT, Slack MPE, et al. Vaccine failures after primary immunisation with *Haemophilus influenzae* type-b conjugate vaccine without booster. *Lancet* 1997;349:1197–1202.
109. Booy R, Kroll JS. Is *Haemophilus influenzae* finished? *J Antimicrob Chemother* 1997;40:149–153.
110. Mulholland K, Hilton S, Adegbola R, et al. Randomised trial of *Haemophilus influenzae* type-b tetanus protein conjugate for prevention of pneumonia and meningitis in Gambian infants. *Lancet* 1997;349:1191–1197.
111. Steinhoff MC. *Haemophilus influenzae* type b infections are preventable everywhere. *Lancet* 1997;349:1186–1187.
112. Spagnuolo PJ, Ellner JJ, Lerner PI, et al. *Haemophilus influenzae* meningitis: the spectrum of disease in adults. *Medicine* 1982;61:74–85.

113. Crowe HM, Levitz RE. Invasive *Haemophilus influenzae* disease in adults. *Arch Intern Med* 1987;147:241–244.
114. Takala AK, Eskola J, van Alphen L. Spectrum of invasive *Haemophilus influenzae* type b disease in adults. *Arch Intern Med* 1990;150:2573–2576.
115. Farley MM, Stephens DS, Brachman PS, et al. Invasive *Haemophilus influenzae* disease in adults: a prospective, population-based surveillance. *Ann Intern Med*. 1992;116:806–812.
116. Morris JT, Longfield RN. Meningitis and bacteremia due to nontypeable *Haemophilus influenzae* in adults. *Clin Infect Dis* 1992;14:782–783.
117. Unhanand M, Mustafa MM, McCracken GH Jr, et al. Gram-negative enteric bacillary meningitis: a twenty-one-year experience. *J Pediatr* 1993;122:15–21.
118. Cherubin CE, Marr JS, Sierra MF, et al. *Listeria* and gram-negative bacillary meningitis in New York City, 1972–1979. *Am J Med* 1981;71:199–209.
119. Gower DJ, Barrows AA III, Kelly DL, et al. Gram-negative bacillary meningitis in the adult: review of 39 cases. *South Med J* 1986;79:1499–1502.
120. Campbell JR, Diacovo T, Baker CJ. *Serratia marcescens* meningitis in neonates. *Pediatr Infect Dis J* 1992;11:881–886.
121. Ventura G, Tumbarello M, Tacconelli E, et al. Gram-negative bacillary meningitis in adults. *J Chemother* 1995;7[Suppl 4]:177–179.
122. Tang LM, Chen ST. *Klebsiella oxytoca* meningitis: frequent association with neurosurgical procedures. *Infection* 1995;23:163–167.
123. Papadakis KA, Vartivarian SE, Vassilaki ME, et al. *Stenotrophomonas maltophilia* meningitis: report of two cases and review of the literature. *J Neurosurg* 1997;87:106–108.
124. Lu CH, Chang WN, Chuang YC, et al. The prognostic factors of adult gram-negative bacillary meningitis. *J Hosp Infect* 1998;40:27–34.
125. Forman SD, Smith EE, Ryan NJ, et al. Neonatal *Citrobacter* meningitis: pathogenesis of cerebral abscess formation. *Ann Neurol* 1984;16:655–659.
126. Kline MW. *Citrobacter* meningitis and brain abscess in infancy: epidemiology, pathogenesis, and treatment. *J Pediatr* 1988;113:430–434.
127. Wang WM, Chen CY, Jan CM, et al. Central nervous system infection after endoscopic injection sclerotherapy. *Am J Gastroenterol* 1990;85:865–867.
128. Cameron ML, Durack DT. Helminthic infections of the central nervous system. In: Scheld WM, Whitley RJ, Durack DT, eds. *Infections of the central nervous system*, 2nd ed. Philadelphia: Lippincott-Raven Publishers, 1997:845–878.
129. Gordon JJ, Harter DH, Phair JP. Meningitis due to *Staphylococcus aureus*. *Am J Med* 1985;78:965–970.
130. Schlesinger LS, Ross SC, Schaberg DR. *Staphylococcus aureus* meningitis: a broad-based epidemiologic study. *Medicine* 1987;66:148–156.
131. Jensen AG, Espersen F, Skinhoj P, et al. *Staphylococcus aureus* meningitis: a review of 104 nationwide, consecutive cases. *Arch Intern Med* 1993;153:1902–1908.
132. Lerche A, Rasmussen N, Wandall JH, et al. *Staphylococcus aureus* meningitis: a review of 28 consecutive community-acquired cases. *Scand J Infect Dis* 1995;27:560–573.
133. Bayston R. Hydrocephalus shunt infections. *J Antimicrob Chemother* 1994;34:75–84.
134. Quie PG, Belani KK. Coagulase-negative staphylococcal adherence and persistence. *J Infect Dis* 1987;156:543–547.
135. Dougherty SH. Pathobiology of infection in prosthetic devices. *Rev Infect Dis* 1988;10:1102–1117.
136. Heerema MS, Ein ME, Musher DM, et al. Anaerobic bacterial meningitis. *Am J Med* 1979;67:219–227.
137. Tarnvik A. Anaerobic meningitis in children. *Eur J Clin Microbiol* 1986;5:271–274.
138. Law DA, Aronoff SC. Anaerobic meningitis in children: case report and review of the literature. *Pediatr Infect Dis J* 1992;11:968–971.
139. Stephenson JR, Hopper P, Tabaqchali S. Anaerobic bacterial meningitis. *J Infect* 1986;13:37–39.
140. Feder HM Jr. *Bacteroides fragilis* meningitis. *Rev Infect Dis* 1987;9:783–786.
141. Odugbemi T, Jatto SA, Afolabi K. *Bacteroides fragilis* meningitis. *J Clin Microbiol* 1985;21:282–283.
142. Long JG, Preblud SR, Keyserling HL. *Clostridium perfringens* meningitis in an infant: case report and literature review. *Pediatr Infect Dis J* 1987;6:752–754.
143. Heidemann SM, Meert KL, Perrin E, et al. Primary clostridial meningitis in infancy. *Pediatr Infect Dis J* 1989;8:126–128.
144. Korman TM, Athan E, Spelman DW. Anaerobic meningitis due to *Peptostreptococcus* species: case report and review. *Clin Infect Dis* 1997;25:1462–1464.

145. Hawkey PM, Jewes LA. How common is meningitis caused by anaerobic bacteria? *J Clin Microbiol* 1985;22:325.
146. Frank GR, Rubin LG. Mixed meningitis with *Bacteroides ovatus* caused by an occult congenital dermal sinus. *Pediatr Infect Dis J* 1989;8:401–403.
147. Hoyne AL, Herzon H. *Streptococcic viridans* meningitis: a review of the literature and report of nine recoveries. *Ann Intern Med* 1950;33:879–902.
148. Johnson CC, Tunkel AR. Viridans streptococci and groups C and G streptococci. In: Mandell GL, Bennett JE, Dolin R, eds. *Principles and practice of infectious diseases,* 5th ed. Philadelphia: Churchill-Livingstone, 2000:2167–2183.
149. Schneeberger PM, Janssen M, Voss A. Alpha-hemolytic streptococci: a major pathogen of iatrogenic meningitis following lumbar puncture: case reports and review of the literature. *Infection* 1996;24:29–33.
150. Carley NH. *Streptococcus salivarius* bacteremia and meningitis following upper gastrointestinal endoscopy and cauterization for gastric bleeding. *Clin Infect Dis* 1992;14:947–948.
151. Bouhemad B, Dounas M, Mercier FJ, et al. Bacterial meningitis following combined spinal-epidural analgesia for labor. *Anaesthesia* 1998;53:290–295.
152. Chow JW, Muder RR. Group A streptococcal meningitis. *Clin Infect Dis* 1992;14:418–421.
153. Asnis DS, Knez T. Group A streptococcal meningitis. *Arch Intern Med* 1998;158:810–814.
154. Sepkowitz KA, Kasemsri T, Brown AE, et al. Meningitis due to β-hemolytic non-A, non-D streptococci among adults at a cancer hospital: report of four cases and review. *Clin Infect Dis* 1992;14:92–97.
155. Cohen LF, Dunbar SA, Sirbasku DM, et al. *Streptococcus bovis* infection of the central nervous system: report of two cases and review. *Clin Infect Dis* 1997;25:819–823.
156. Quaade F, Kristensen KP. Purulent meningitis: a review of 658 cases. *Acta Med Scand* 1962;171:543–550.
157. Stevenson KB, Murray EW, Sarubbi FA. Enterococcal meningitis: report of four cases and review. *Clin Infect Dis* 1994;18:233–239.
158. Greene KA, Clark RJ, Zabramski JM. Ventricular CSF shunt infections associated with *Corynebacterium jeikeium*: report of three cases and review. *Clin Infect Dis* 1993;16:139–141.
159. Bross JE, Gordon G. Nocardial meningitis: case reports and review. *Rev Infect Dis* 1991;13:160–165.
160. McLean DR, Russell N, Khan MY. Neurobrucellosis: clinical and therapeutic features. *Clin Infect Dis* 1992;15:582–590.
161. Chang KC, Zakheim RM, Cho CT, et al. Posttraumatic purulent meningitis due to *Bordetella bronchiseptica*. *J Pediatr* 1975;86:639–640.
162. Uchihara T, Yokota T, Watabiki S, et al. *Flavobacterium meningosepticum* meningitis in an adult. *Am J Med* 1988;85:738–739.
163. Langbaum M. *Stomatococcus mucilaginosus* septicemia and meningitis in a premature infant. *Pediatr Infect Dis J* 1992;11:334–335.
164. Souillet G, Chomarat M, Barbe G, et al. *Stomatococcus mucilaginosus* meningitis in a child with leukemia. *Clin Infect Dis* 1992;15:1045.
165. Friedland IR, Snipelisky M, Khoosal M. Meningitis in a neonate caused by *Leuconostoc* sp. *J Clin Microbiol* 1990;28:2125–2126.
166. Stotka JL, Rupp ME, Meier FA, et al. Meningitis due to *Neisseria mucosa*: case report and review. *Rev Infect Dis* 1991;13:837–841.
167. Denning DW, Gill SS. *Neisseria lactamica* meningitis following skull trauma. *Rev Infect Dis* 1991;13:216–218.
168. Armengol S, Mesalles E, Domingo C, et al. A new case of meningitis due to *Pasteurella multocida*. *Rev Infect Dis* 1991;13:1254.
169. Roberts SR, Esther JW, Brewer JH. Posttraumatic *Pasteurella multocida* meningitis. *South Med J* 1988;81:675–676.
170. Belardi FG, Pascoe JM, Beegle ED. *Pasteurella multocida* meningitis in an infant following occipital dog bite. *J Fam Pract* 1982;14:778–782.
171. Minton EJ. *Pasteurella pneumotropica:* meningitis following a dog bite. *Postgrad Med J* 1990;66:125–126.
172. Dronda F, Garcia-Arata I, Navas E, et al. Meningitis in adults due to *Campylobacter fetus* subspecies *fetus*. *Clin Infect Dis* 1998;27:906–907.
173. Schlegel L, Merlet C, Larouche JM, et al. Iatrogenic meningitis due to *Abiotrophia defectiva* after myelography. *Clin Infect Dis* 1999;28:155–156.

3

Pathogenesis and
Pathophysiology

Knowledge of the pathogenesis and pathophysiology of bacterial meningitis has increased dramatically over the last 30 years (Fig. 3.1) (1–5). We now have a better understanding of the mechanisms by which meningeal pathogens initially colonize the host and lead to invasive disease, the importance of virulence factors of the pathogen that allow it to evade host defense mechanisms and enter the central nervous system (CNS), and the bacterial and host determinants that cause breakdown of the blood-brain barrier (BBB), induce subarachnoid space inflammation, produce cerebral edema, increase intracranial pressure, and lead to altered cerebral blood flow and neuronal injury in patients with bacterial meningitis. The following sections review the models used to study the pathogenesis and pathophysiology of bacterial meningitis, and detail the relationships between specific bacterial virulence factors and host defense mechanisms that are responsible for the acquisition and clinical expression of disease.

EXPERIMENTAL ANIMAL MODELS

Experimental animal models have been extremely important to learn about the pathogenic and pathophysiologic mechanisms operable in bacterial meningitis (3,6). Although these models differ from natural infection by the route of bacterial inoculation employed, the bacterial pathogen administered, and the animal host selected, they have allowed investigators to elucidate the various bacterial virulence factors important for bacterial colonization and local invasion, intravascular survival, and CNS invasion, and helped to understand the host defense mechanisms that attempt to control and/or eradicate these infections.

The infant rat model has been the one most often studied to elucidate the early pathogenic events of bacterial meningitis. In this model, infant rats (albino Sprague-Dawley suckling rats) have been shown to develop meningitis following atraumatic intranasal inoculation with *Haemophilus influenzae* type b (7). Following inoculation

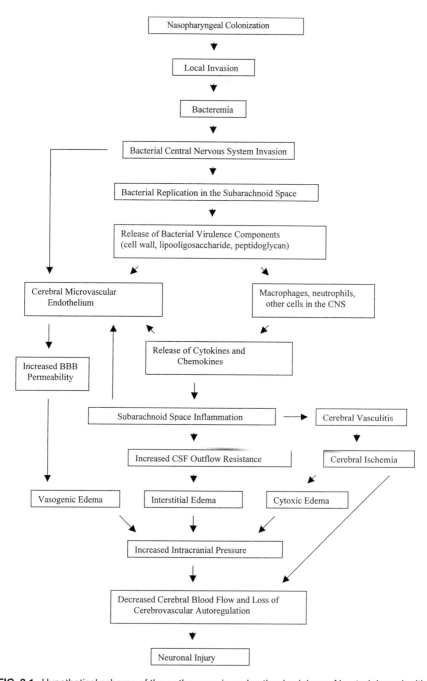

FIG. 3.1. Hypothetical scheme of the pathogenesis and pathophysiology of bacterial meningitis.

of 5-day-old rats with 10^7 colony-forming units (CFU) of *H. influenzae* type b, 73% of rats were bacteremic after 2 days and 81% were bacteremic after 7 days. Similar results were obtained with rats that were 10 or 20 days old. The incidence of meningitis, irrespective of rat host age, was directly related to the intensity of the bacteremia, and the incidence of bacteremia fell when the inoculum size was decreased (8). This model has several similarities with human disease, since there is an initial nasopharyngeal focus of infection, and bacteremia is required for the development of meningitis. Infant rats have also been shown to develop meningitis following challenge with *Escherichia coli* via the orogastric, subcutaneous, or intraperitoneal routes (6). This model has similarities to newborn infection with *E. coli,* including host age and the importance of bacteremia for the development of meningitis. Disadvantages of the infant rat model, however, are the animal's small size, which permits only small samples (7 to 25 μL) of cerebrospinal fluid (CSF) and blood to be obtained from rats 5 to 10 days old, the variable time course in the development of meningitis, and the low case fatality rate. Therefore these models have been used primarily to study the early pathogenic sequences of bacterial meningitis (i.e., the determinants of colonization and translocation into the bloodstream, intravascular survival and bacteremia, and mechanisms of meningeal invasion). Infant primates have also been used to study bacterial meningitis following atraumatic intranasal inoculation with *H. influenzae* type b, with bacteremia and meningitis developing in 89% and 94% of animals, respectively (9). However, this animal model is employed infrequently because of expense.

Adult animals are most often utilized to study the pathophysiologic consequences of meningitis once bacteria have reached the subarachnoid space. In these models, meningitis is usually induced following the intracisternal inoculation of bacteria or their products to establish infection and/or inflammation. Three animal species have been employed to study these mechanisms. In the adult rabbit model, New Zealand white rabbits are anesthetized and a helmet is formed with dental acrylic that is attached to the skull by screws (6,10); the helmet allows the animal to be placed in a stereotactic frame that holds a geared electrode introducer with a spinal needle to facilitate cisternal punctures. Lethal infections are reliably established in this model with a predictable time course after intracisternal challenge with an appropriate inoculum of live bacteria; animals can also be challenged with purified bacterial products or various host factors. The animal's large size permits easy handling, the ability to sample CSF at multiple time points, the possibility of using different inocula (i.e., live pathogen, bacterial products, inflammatory mediators), and the ability to measure multiple pathophysiologic parameters (e.g., white blood cell counts, protein, inflammatory cytokines, and intracranial pressure). However, the pathogenesis of meningitis is artificial in this model, since the normal bacteremia-to-meningitis sequence is bypassed.

An adult rat model of meningitis has been developed utilizing adult Wistar rats, in which CSF can be removed and various inoculations performed using a micromanipulator fitted to a 25-gauge needle (11). This model has been modified by other investigators, permitting it to be used to measure a variety of pathophysiologic parameters (e.g., cerebral blood flow and intracranial pressure) and maintain standardized controlled conditions, with continuous monitoring of mean arterial blood pressure, body temperature, and end-tidal carbon dioxide tension (12). A disadvantage of this model (compared with the rabbit model) is that the number of CSF determinations is limited because of smaller CSF volume in the rat. An adult mouse model has been developed, primarily for the study of *Listeria monocytogenes* meningoencephalitis, in which the organism is inoculated intracerebrally through the right orbital surface of the zygomatic bone (13). This model has also been utilized to study the effects of inflammatory cytokines in the CNS after administration via lumbar puncture (14).

The following sections will discuss information obtained from the animal models described earlier, which has led to a greater understanding of the pathogenesis and pathophysiology of bacterial meningitis. Modification of these models and development of *in vitro* models utilizing cell culture systems have also been developed to improve our understanding of this devastating disease.

COLONIZATION AND INVASION

The early pathogenic events that result in bacterial meningitis depend on an interplay between specific virulence factors and host defense mechanisms (Table 3.1). The initiation of infection with meningeal pathogens usually begins with host acquisition of

TABLE 3.1. *Potential factors contributing to the pathogenesis of bacterial meningitis*

Pathogenic event	Factors that enhance bacterial virulence	Host defense mechanisms
Mucosal colonization	Fimbriae, polysaccharide capsule, IgA protease production, bacteriocins, viral upper respiratory tract infection, lack of specific antibody to meningeal pathogens	Integrity of mucosal epithelium, secretory IgA, ciliary activity, anticapsular polysaccharide antibodies
Intravascular survival	Polysaccharide capsule, absence of a spleen	Complement activation, organism-specific antibodies
Central nervous system invasion	High-density bacteremia, fimbriae, polysaccharide capsule, association with monocytes, changes in cytoskeleton of cells of the blood-brain barrier, *ibe10* gene, platelet-activating factor receptor, pneumococcal choline-binding protein A	Blood-brain barrier
Survival within the subarachnoid space	Polysaccharide capsule, low concentrations of complement and immunoglobulins, degradation of complement components	Complement, immunoglobulins

a new organism by nasopharyngeal colonization (3). These events have been studied in an *in vitro* model of human nasopharyngeal cells in culture infected with *Neisseria meningitidis* or *H. influenzae* type b, in which the following events were observed (15): (a) association of the microorganism with mucus; (b) cytotoxicity characterized by breakdown of epithelial cell tight junctions, sloughing of ciliated cells, and ciliostasis; (c) selective attachment of microorganisms to nonciliated epithelial cells; (d) multiplication and formation of microcolonies on the epithelial surface; (e) invasion of the epithelium by the intracellular (for *N. meningitidis*) or intercellular (for *H. influenzae*) routes; and (f) passage of microorganisms to the submucosa. These events require viable microorganisms and are not completed by commensal species. The bacterial virulence factors and host defense mechanisms important for these events are discussed in detail later.

Bacterial Virulence Factors

Adherence represents a relatively stable attachment of bacteria to a surface. This may occur through adhesive surface structures called adhesins, which are ligand molecules that bind specifically to complementary receptors on host mucosal cells. Many bacteria, however, possess specific organelles called "fimbriae" or "pili" that mediate adherence to mucosal surfaces (16). Typically, a bacterium has 50 to 400 of these filaments projecting from its surface; each filament has a hydrophobic tip that makes contact with other cells. The phenotypic expression of fimbriae also manifests phase variation *in vitro* and *in vivo,* such that under certain cultural conditions proportions of bacterial populations are either fimbriated or nonfimbriated, allowing the fimbriated forms to survive at phagocyte-poor sites such as mucosal surfaces while permitting the nonfimbriated forms to reach phagocyte-rich sites in deep tissues (17).

Fimbriae are important to many of the major meningeal pathogens to enhance adherence of these microorganisms to mucosal surfaces. The fimbriae of *N. meningitidis* are important to mediate adherence of this organism to nasopharyngeal epithelial cells; these fimbriated strains accounted for 80% of primary meningococcal isolates from nasopharyngeal carriers and from the CSF of patients with meningococcal meningitis (3), although all fimbriae were lost on serial subculture in the laboratory. The fimbriae appear morphologically as aggregated bundles or single filaments (18); aggregated bundles are found primarily among disease isolates exhibiting a low degree of adherence to human buccal epithelial cells, whereas the single filaments have medium to high adherence characteristics, being found predominantly among colonizing isolates. Once meningococci attach to nonciliated nasopharyngeal epithelial cells via a specific cell surface receptor, they are transported across these cells within a phagocytic vacuole (15), a process that appears to be essential for subsequent hematogenous dissemination.

Fimbriae have also been implicated in the attachment of *H. influenzae* to upper tract respiratory epithelial cells (19,20). Lack of fimbrial expression impairs the ability of *H. influenzae* type b to colonize the nasopharynx (21), although fimbriae have not been found on isolates from the CSF or blood of patients with invasive disease, suggesting that their presence is not necessary for development of invasive disease, including meningitis (22). This contrasts with the finding that meningococci isolated from blood and CSF are heavily fimbriated, suggesting an additional role for fimbriae in meningococcal pathogenesis (15). Furthermore, the type of fimbriae expressed by *H. influenzae* type b strains may facilitate adherence to selected nasopharyngeal sites: α-fimbriae enhance adherence in the anterior nasopharynx, whereas β-fimbriae facilitate the process more posteriorly (4). Following nasopharyngeal colonization, invasion into the bloodstream by *H. influenzae* appears to occur via breakdown in tight junctions between epithelial cells (in contrast to *N. meningitidis,* which invades via parasite-directed endocytosis), leading to invasion by an intercellular mechanism (15).

In addition, acquisition and colonization by *H. influenzae* type b or *N. meningitidis* may be promoted following respiratory tract infection by viral agents such as influenza A Victoria and respiratory syncytial virus (23), which causes loss of host defenses by a decrease in ciliated cells. Epidemics of meningitis caused by *N. meningitidis* in sub-Saharan Africa coincide with the dry periods of the year, when the protective barrier of the mucous membrane is compromised (5). However, the precise role of a preceding upper respiratory viral infection in the enhancement of nasopharyngeal colonization by these microorganisms is controversial.

Surface encapsulation may be another important virulence factor for nasopharyngeal colonization and systemic invasion of meningeal pathogens. There are six encapsulated types of *H. influenzae* (a through f), although type b strains cause more than 95% of systemic and meningeal infections (24). In an experimental infant rat model utilizing laboratory transformants, it has been demonstrated that, although all encapsulated strains of *H. influenzae* had the potential for systemic invasion after intraperitoneal inoculation, type b strains were the most virulent and were the only capsular types capable of systemic invasion following intranasal inoculation (24,25). Indeed, the presence of antibodies to type b capsule, which are almost uniformly detected in humans by the age of 4 years even in the absence of known exposure to *H. influenzae* type b, usually confers protection against invasive disease (26); lack of sufficient antibody concentrations correlates with an increased risk for invasive disease. The presence of these antibodies may also relate to the ability of some unencapsulated strains to produce some type b capsular material, perhaps from new DNA acquired from microorganisms colonizing the gastrointestinal tract. For example, *E. coli* K100 possesses a capsule that is immunologically nearly identical to the type b capsule of *H. influenzae* and may stimulate the production of cross-reacting anticapsular antibodies (27,28). Polysaccharide capsule may also be an important virulence factor for development of invasive disease by *Streptococcus pneumoniae.* Eighteen pneumococcal serotypes are responsible for 82% of cases of bacteremic pneumococcal pneumonia, with a close correlation between bacteremic subtypes and those implicated in meningitis (29,30). The factors that mediate dissemination from a recently colonized site are largely unknown, but lack of specific antibody appears critical for the development of invasive pneumococcal disease. In addition, *in vivo* capsular transformation events may equip pneumococcal strains with highly virulent blood invasive phenotypes, increasing the seriousness of pneumococcal infection, especially that caused by multidrug-resistant strains (31). However, adherence may be less important in the pathogenicity of pneumococcal infections, because low degrees of adherence have been observed among strains isolated from patients with serious infections such as septicemia and meningitis (32). A study of *S. pneumoniae* nasopharyngeal adherence in children showed that these microorganisms were more often found on desquamated cells than on cells taken from intact epithelium (33). Nasopharyngeal mucus may provide a protected nidus from which pneumococci can spread (17), although the various factors responsible for enhanced invasiveness among certain pneumococcal serotypes remain undefined.

Other bacterial surface components have been examined to determine their roles in the early stages of the pathogenesis of bacterial meningitis (3). The lipooligosaccharide (LOS) and outer membrane proteins (OMPs) of *H. influenzae* have been particularly studied in this regard; antibodies directed against these components confer protection after repeated challenge with this organism. Hemocin, the bacteriocin produced by *H. influenzae,* may also play a role in host nasopharyngeal colonization and/or systemic invasion by this organism. Following intranasal inoculation of infant rats with an equal mixture of a non–hemocin-producing strain and its hemocin-producing counterpart, hemocin-producing organisms predominated in isolates from both nasopharyngeal and blood cultures (34). However, the precise role of these and other surface components of meningeal pathogens in development of mucosal colonization and systemic invasion remains undefined.

Host Defense Mechanisms

The adherence of microorganisms to mucosal surfaces may be inhibited by natural antibodies, such as IgA, found in mucosal secretions. However, it appears that the presence of high concentrations of circulating IgA antibodies to *N. meningitidis* may permit the development or progression of invasive disease by preferentially binding to the organism and blocking the beneficial effects of IgG and IgM antibodies (17). In addition, species of many pathogenic bacteria (e.g., *Neisseria, Haemophilus, Streptococcus*) produce IgA1 proteases (35) that cleave IgA in the hinge region and facilitate adherence of bacterial strains to mucosal surfaces through local destruction of IgA (36). Support for the importance of this enzyme in the pathogenesis of meningitis came from a study in which antibody production against the IgA1 protease of *N. meningitidis* was stimulated by disease or acquisition of carriage, with antibody concentrations remaining constant upon continued carriage (37). However, the exact role of IgA1 protease production in this pathogenic sequence remains unclear.

The presence of anticapsular polysaccharide antibodies may also be effective in decreasing nasopharyngeal carriage of meningeal pathogens. In an intralitter transmission model in which infant rats were intranasally inoculated with *S. pneumoniae* and placed in a cage with other infant rats, pretreatment of uninoculated rats with systemic IgG antibodies to pneumococcal polysaccharide reduced intralitter transmission of *S. pneumoniae* (38), suggesting that IgG antibodies to pneumococcal polysaccharide may be sufficient to reduce pneumococcal nasopharyngeal carriage in humans.

INTRAVASCULAR SURVIVAL

Bacterial Virulence Factors

Once bacteria cross the mucosal barrier and gain access to the bloodstream, they must overcome additional host defense mechanisms to survive. The presence of bacterial capsule, by effectively inhibiting neutrophil phagocytosis and resisting classic complement-mediated bactericidal activity, may enhance bloodstream survival of the organism, thereby facilitating intravascular replication (3). The most common meningeal pathogens (*H. influenzae, N. meningitidis, S. pneumoniae, E. coli, S. agalactiae*) are all encapsulated. In addition, certain capsular types are disproportionately associated with development of meningitis. For example, about 84% of cases of neonatal *E. coli* meningitis are caused by strains bearing the K1 antigen (39,40); in the absence of specific host antibody to the K1 capsule, these organisms are profoundly resistant to phagocytosis. The presence of the K1 capsule and the high degree of bacteremia are key determinants in the development of *E. coli* meningitis (41), suggesting that there may be specific sites in the brain that have an affinity for K1 capsule and are responsible for entry of this microorganism into the meninges. The K1 antigen of *E. coli* shares antigenic characteristics with capsular material from other organisms (e.g., serogroup B meningococci and type III group B streptococci); human monoclonal antibodies with reactivity against specific epitopes on the K1 capsule of *E. coli* or on the group B polysaccharide of *N. meningitidis* may prove to be effective in the therapy and/or prevention of bacteremia caused by these organisms (42).

The specific chemical constituents of the capsular polysaccharide may play an important role in promoting infection. Sialic acid is a prominent component of the capsular polysaccharides of type III group B streptococci, *E. coli* K1, and serogroups B and C meningococci (43); these microorganisms are prominent causes of neonatal and infant sepsis and meningitis. Since sialic acid is also a component of host cells, these organisms do not activate the alternative complement pathway and are a poor stimulus of host antibody production (see later).

Host Defense Mechanisms

The host possesses several defense mechanisms to counteract the antiphagocytic effects of bacterial capsule (3). Through the humoral immune response, antibodies bind to specific microbial antigens, and this antigen-antibody complex can then enlist the aid of effector cells or activate the complement cascade (44). Complement activation can occur via the classical or alternative complement pathways. The classical pathway is triggered by antigen-antibody complexes and proceeds through activation of the three early recognition components C1, C4, and C2, with the formation of C3 convertase. However, the alternative pathway may be activated on the surface of many bacteria in the absence of specific antibody. Both pathways converge at C3, with the sequential activation of C5, C6, C7, C8, and C9 to form the membrane attack complex. To limit tissue damage, these factors must be directed against the bacterial pathogen when it is in an extracellular location; this can be accomplished by opsonization, by which organisms are coated with antibody and/or specific complement fragments, thereby facilitating the phagocytic process (45). Although both antipneumococcal cell-wall antibody and antipneumococcal capsular antibody promote the efficient deposition of C3b on the pneumococcal surface, the C3b deposited on the surface of the pneumococcal capsule is a more efficient opsonin *in vitro* and *in vivo* than is C3 deposited by anti-cell-wall antibody (46,47). However, the pneumococcal cell wall, rather than the polysaccharide capsule, appears to play a major role in the activation of the alternative pathway; the alternative pathway is not activated by the capsule because of inefficient binding of factor B to C3b deposited on the capsule (48). Impairment of the alternative complement pathway (e.g., in patients with sickle cell anemia and those who have undergone splenectomy) predisposes to the development of pneumococcal meningitis.

Haemophilus influenzae type b also activates the complement cascade (49). Experimental studies in an experimental rat model have shown that following intravenous or intraperitoneal challenge with *H. influenzae* of varying serotypes (a, b, c, or d), rats depleted of C3 developed a greater incidence and magnitude of bacteremia. Although the incidence of bacteremia caused by type b organisms increased from 63% to 95% in complement-depleted rats, complement depletion did not affect the incidence and severity of meningitis (50–52).

Complement system activation is also an essential host defense mechanism against invasive disease caused by *N. meningitidis*. Patients with deficiencies in the components of the membrane attack complex (C5, C6, C7, C8, and C9) are particularly prone to neisserial infections, with an 8,000-fold greater risk of invasive meningococcal disease than persons with an intact complement system, although usually with a more favorable outcome when appropriate therapy is instituted (1.6% to 2.7% versus 19%) (53). The reasons for the worse outcome in patients with an intact complement system are unclear, although it has been suggested that the presence of complement-activating products, in concert with other mediators, may contribute to the development of multisystem organ failure and death. A qualitative relationship exists between the concentration of circulating meningococcal LOS, a fatal outcome, and the degree of complement activation (54). Therefore the ability to assemble the membrane attack complex may contribute to mortality in patients with invasive meningococcal infections.

CENTRAL NERVOUS SYSTEM INVASION
AND REPLICATION

Bacterial Virulence Factors

The mechanism(s) by which meningeal pathogens gain access to the CNS remain unknown. One factor may be the concentration of microorganisms in the blood. In an infant rat model, the intranasal inoculation of *H. influenzae* type b initially led to a low-grade bacteremia of approximately 10^2 CFU/mL (7); at this concentration, no organisms were present in CSF. Bacterial replication occurred at a rapid rate, and meningitis developed in 100% of animals at bacterial densities of 10^5 CFU/mL. In a monkey model, high-density bacteremia ($\geq 10^4$ CFU/mL) led to the appearance of meningitis within 48 hours, whereas a lower-density bacteremia ($< 10^4$ CFU/mL) took an average of 7 days before meningitis occurred (55). In another study, culture-positive meningitis was produced in an experimental infant rat model only after an intense bacteremia ($> 10^3$ CFU/mL) had been present for at least 6 hours (56). However, sustained bacteremia cannot be the sole factor responsible for meningeal invasion because many other organisms (e.g., viridans streptococci) that produce high-grade bacteremia during infective endocarditis rarely produce meningitis. The presence of the K1 capsule and a high degree of bacteremia were found to be key determinants in the development of *E. coli* meningitis in an experimental animal model, suggesting that there may be specific binding sites in the brain that have an affinity for the K1 capsule to permit the organism to cross the meninges (41).

The site of CNS invasion by meningeal pathogens is unclear. Early studies in the infant rat model of *H. influenzae* type b meningitis using fluorescein-conjugated rabbit antiserum suggested that invasion from the bloodstream was via the dural venous sinus system. However, other experiments suggested that the site of invasion was above the cribriform plate or via the choroid plexi (due to their exceptionally high rate of blood flow of approximately 200 mL/g/min) (55), implying that more microorganisms would be delivered to this site per unit time than to most other anatomic locations in the body. In addition, when CSF compartments were sampled early in the course of bacterial meningitis, higher bacterial densities were found in the lateral ventricles than in the cisterna magna, lumbar subarachnoid space, or supracortical subarachnoid space, although there was equilibration in these other locations with time.

Recent experimental studies, however, have demonstrated that receptors for some meningeal pathogens are present on cells of the choroid plexi and cerebral capillaries that may facilitate movement of pathogens into the subarachnoid space. In cryostat sections of infant rat brain cortical slices, *E. coli* strains possessing S fimbriae have been shown to bind specifically to the luminal surfaces of the vascular endothelium and the epithelium lining the choroid plexi and brain ventricles (57). Binding was abolished by pretreatment of the brain sections with neuraminidase or the trisaccharide receptor analog of S fimbriae. In a subsequent series of experiments, 1 hour after intraperitoneal challenge with an S-fimbriated population of *E. coli,* about 50% of organisms in the CSF were S-fimbriated and 50% were nonfimbriated (58), indicating that phase variation to the nonfimbriated form was necessary for these bacteria to invade the CNS. *Neisseria meningitidis* was also shown to adhere *in vivo* to the endothelium of both the choroid plexus and meninges in a fatal case of meningococcemia (59); isolates obtained from the CSF expressed significantly more PilC protein than the blood isolates, suggesting that PilC plays an important role for this organism to cross the BBB. Despite these studies, the importance of adherence of meningeal pathogens to sites within the CNS requires further study.

To understand the cellular mechanisms important for CNS invasion, the invasion of *E. coli* into endothelial and epithelial cell cultures was studied. It appeared that microtubule-dependent and/or microfilament-dependent pathways, which rearrange the cell cytoskeleton, may be important for bacterial uptake and crossing of the BBB (60). This has also been examined for *Listeria monocytogenes,* in which invasion of human brain microvascular endothelial cells in culture required a rearrangement of actin filaments (61). The ability of strains of *E. coli* to invade endothelial cells was investigated at the molecular level. Recently, a gene (termed *ibe10*) has been cloned and found to encode an 8.2-kDa protein, which permits *E. coli* to invade brain microvascular endothelial cells both *in vitro* and *in vivo* (62). The prevalence of *ibe10* was also increased in *E. coli* isolates from CSF, compared with those in feces or blood (63). In addition, the *aslA* gene product of *E. coli* K12 has been shown to have homology to the DNA adjacent to the *TnphoA* insertion site, which potentially contributes to the invasion process of meningitic *E. coli* across the BBB (64). However, none of the determinants described thus far is sufficient by itself to account for all the virulence properties of *E. coli* strains causing neonatal meningitis. In one study examining the phylogenetic relationships of 69 strains of *E. coli* causing neonatal meningitis, coexistence of the *pap* and *sfa/foc* adhesin-encoding operons, the *aer* operon, the *ibe10* gene, the K1 antigen, and the presence of the 14.9-kb *Hin* dIII fragment was significantly higher in meningitic strains of *E. coli* (65), suggesting that these factors are essential in the pathogenesis of neonatal *E. coli* meningitis. However, because some cases of meningitis in normal-risk neonates were caused by isolates that lacked these determinants, further studies are needed to assess the role of these virulence determinants in meningeal invasion.

Other microbial virulence factors may be important for bacterial invasion of the CNS. The liberation of LOS of *N. meningitidis* may contribute to its pathogenicity in invasive infections (66). The importance of OMPs, however, is less clear. A recent report suggested that *H. influenzae* strains with OMP subtype 1c caused more episodes of meningitis and fewer episodes of epiglottitis than strains of subtype 1, perhaps as a result of the ability of each subtype to release LOS under appropriate circumstances (67). Additional studies are needed to examine these concepts in further detail.

Another pathogenic mechanism postulated to promote CNS invasion by meningeal pathogens is association of the organism with circulating monocytes. Utilizing histologic and scanning microscopic techniques to examine the neuraxes of pigs inoculated with a strain of *Streptococcus suis* type 2, the only pathologic lesions detected were associated with the choroid plexus, manifested as brush border disruption, decrease in the number of Kolmer cells, and exudation of fibrin and inflammatory cells into the ventricles (68). Intracellular bacteria were demonstrated in the parenchyma of the choroid plexus, in the ventricular monocytes, and within circulating peripheral blood monocytes, suggesting that bacteria may gain access to the CSF in association with monocytes migrating along normal pathways.

Recently, transcytosis through microvascular endothelial cells has been investigated as another possible mechanism of meningeal invasion during bacterial meningitis. In an *in vitro* model utilizing rat and human brain microvascular endothelial cells (69), the transparent phase variants of pneumococci that gained access to an intracellular vesicle from the apical side of the microvascular endothelial cell monolayer were able to transcytose to the basal surface of these cells in a manner dependent on the platelet-activating factor (PAF) receptor and the presence of pneumococcal choline-binding protein A; remaining transparent bacteria entering the cell underwent a previously unrecognized recycling to the apical surface. These data suggest that interaction of pneumococci with the PAF receptor results in sorting so as to transcytose bacteria across the cell (rather than passing between cells), whereas non-PAF receptor entry shunts bacteria for exit and reentry on the apical surface. This bidirectional trafficking of pneumococci represents an important potential bioprobe to investigate transport across mammalian cells.

Host Defense Mechanisms

Once meningeal pathogens enter the subarachnoid space, host defense mechanisms are generally inadequate to control the infection, allowing bacteria to replicate to huge densities (3). CSF concentrations of complement components are absent or present in minimal concentrations (70–72). Meningeal inflammation leads to increased, although low, CSF complement concentrations, and observations in experimental animal models and in patients with meningitis have revealed absent or barely detectable opsonic and bactericidal activities. For example, in an experimental rabbit model, opsonization of a serum-sensitive *E. coli* strain was absent *in vitro* during incubation with CSF from animals challenged with *E. coli* K1, although CSF from animals with *Staphylococcus aureus* meningitis was opsonically active *in vitro* against *E. coli* (73).

This relative complement deficiency may be of critical importance, since specific antibody and/or complement is essential for opsonization of encapsulated meningeal pathogens and efficient phagocytosis. Possible explanations for these low concentrations of complement components during bacterial meningitis are unclear but include insufficient traversal across the BBB, variable subarachnoid space inflammation, and low production rates in the CNS. It has also been suggested that complement components crossing the BBB may be degraded by leukocyte proteases, resulting in inefficient opsonic activity at the site of infection. Leukocyte proteases have been shown to degrade functional complement components (e.g., C3b) in CSF samples from patients with meningococcal meningitis, with the formation of nonopsonic products (e.g., C3d) (74). In addition, in an experimental rabbit model of pneumococcal meningitis, the intracisternal inoculation of a nonspecific protease inhibitor (phenylmethylsulfonyl fluoride) led to a decline in pneumococcal concentrations in CSF compared with saline-inoculated controls (75), perhaps by influencing leukocyte-protease-mediated complement destruction in the CSF. Despite the fact that there is low functional and bactericidal activity in purulent CSF, the presence of some measurable opsonic activity may correlate with a favorable outcome, as demonstrated in concentrated CSF samples from 15 of 27 patients with bacterial meningitis (76), suggesting that some complement-mediated opsonic activity appears in CSF during bacterial meningitis, particularly in patients who completely recover.

Immunoglobulin concentrations are also low in normal CSF (average blood:CSF ratio of IgG normally about 800:1), and, although concentrations increase during bacterial meningitis, they remain low compared with simultaneous serum concentrations (74,77). There is evidence of local CSF antibody synthesis in some forms of infectious meningitis, which may be critical in local host defense. In an experimental rabbit model, the intravenous administration of a bactericidal monoclonal antibody against the polyribosyl-ribitol phosphate of *H. influenzae* type b produced high serum antibody concentrations (approximately 1,000 to 6,000 ng/mL), but BBB permeability was poor ($\leq 5.5\%$) even in the presence of meningeal inflammation (78), suggesting that systemic administration of type-specific antibodies alone is likely to be suboptimal in the therapy of bacterial meningitis. In the preantibiotic era, outcome of bacterial meningitis was improved by CSF instillation of immune serum supplemented with complement (79), although it remains to be determined whether intrathecal administration of type-specific monoclonal antibodies is currently useful in patients with bacterial meningitis.

As bacteria continue to multiply in the subarachnoid space during bacterial meningitis, a number of pathophysiologic consequences ensue, which depend upon the interplay between specific bacterial virulence characteristics and host factors (Table 3.2). These are discussed in detail in the following sections.

ALTERATIONS OF THE BLOOD-BRAIN BARRIER

Bacterial meningitis, like many other disease states of the CNS, increases permeability of the BBB. The barrier separates the brain from the intravascular compartment and maintains homeostasis within the CNS (80,81). The major sites of the BBB are the arachnoid membrane, choroid plexus epithelium, and cerebral microvascular endothelium. Previous morphologic studies have demonstrated an intact arachnoid membrane in animals with bacterial meningitis (82), such that the increased BBB permeability seen in bacterial meningitis must occur at the level of the choroid plexus epithelium, cerebral microvascular endothelium, or both. The endothelial cells of the cerebral microvasculature have been the site of intensive study in bacterial meningitis. The distinguishing features of cerebral capillaries, as opposed to other systemic capillaries, are that adjacent endothelial cells are fused together by pentalaminar tight junctions that prevent intercellular transport, pinocytotic vesicles are rare or absent, and mitochondria are abundant. Therefore the increased BBB permeability seen in bacterial meningitis might result from separation of intercellular tight junctions, from increased pinocytosis, or from both alterations; the bacterial virulence factors and host response are discussed in detail later.

Bacterial Virulence Factors

Utilizing an adult experimental rat model, the propensity for meningeal pathogens to induce functional and morphologic alterations of the BBB was examined (11). Morphologic alterations of BBB integrity were assessed by methods for harvesting cerebral microvessels and examination by transmission electron microscopy, and functional alterations were assessed by measuring the blood-to-CSF transfer of circulating

TABLE 3.2. *Potential factors contributing to the pathophysiology of bacterial meningitis*

Pathophysiologic parameters	Bacterial virulence factors	Host factors
Increased blood-brain barrier permeability	Cell wall, lipooligosaccharide, outer membrane vesicles, peptidoglycan	Interleukin-1β, tumor necrosis factor-α, matrix metalloproteinases, reactive nitrogen intermediates, peroxynitrite
Subarachnoid space inflammation	Cell wall, lipooligosaccharide, outer membrane vesicles, peptidoglycan	Complement components (e.g., C5a), prostaglandins (PGE$_2$, prostacyclin), interleukins (IL-1β, IL-6, IL-8, IL-12), interferon-γ, growth-related protein-α, tumor necrosis factor-α, platelet activating factor, macrophage inflammatory proteins 1 and 2, monocyte chemotactic protein-1, reactive nitrogen intermediates, peroxynitrite
Leukocyte traversal across the blood-brain barrier	Lipooligosaccharide, cell wall	Immunoglobulin superfamily (intercellular adhesion molecule-1), leukocyte integrins (CD18), leukocyte selectins (endothelial leukocyte adhesion molecule 1, CD62, leukocyte-adhesion molecule 1), endothelin
Increased intracranial pressure	Cell wall, lipooligosaccharide, outer membrane vesicles, peptidoglycan, pneumococcal strain variability	PGE$_2$, IL-1β, TNF-α, endothelin, reactive oxygen species, reactive nitrogen intermediates, bradykinin, peroxynitrite
Altered cerebral blood flow	Cell wall, lipooligosaccharide	Cerebrospinal fluid leukocytes, endothelin, reactive oxygen species, reactive nitrogen intermediates, bradykinin
Neuronal injury	Cell wall, lipooligosaccharide	Reactive oxygen species, reactive nitrogen intermediates, peroxynitrite, excitatory amino acids

Although various bacterial virulence factors and host factors are listed separately under individual pathophysiologic parameters, there is likely overlap in the factors responsible for these pathophysiologic manifestations.

radioactive albumin, a molecule normally excluded by an intact BBB. Following the intracisternal inoculation of either *E. coli, S. pneumoniae,* or *H. influenzae* type b, alterations of the BBB were found with all three pathogens, manifested morphologically by an early and sustained increase in pinocytotic vesicle formation and a progressive separation of intercellular tight junctions; these morphologic changes correlated with the functional penetration of albumin into CSF. Following intracisternal inoculation of an unencapsulated strain of *H. influenzae,* there was an increase in pinocytotic vesicle formation without separation of intercellular tight junctions, suggesting that encapsulation of *H. influenzae* was not essential for BBB injury but facilitated its progression by avoidance of host defense mechanisms (i.e., deficient opsonic mechanisms in CSF permitted sustained concentrations of encapsulated strains). The increased BBB permeability was observed both in normal animals and in animals rendered leukopenic by the intraperitoneal injection of cyclophosphamide (83), although permeability was augmented by the presence of leukocytes at least late (18 hours after inoculation) in the disease course.

Since surface encapsulation was not an essential virulence factor for production of BBB injury, BBB permeability was examined following the intracisternal inoculation of purified *H. influenzae* type b LOS (84). Purified LOS was shown to increase BBB permeability in an experimental rat model in both a dose- and time-dependent manner (maximum change at a dose of 20 ng at 4 hours after intracisternal inoculation), with a close correlation between permeability and CSF pleocytosis 4 hours after intracisternal inoculation. There was significant inhibition of the LOS effect on BBB permeability by preincubation of the LOS with polymyxin B (a cationic antibiotic that binds to the lipid A region of the LOS molecule) or neutrophil acyloxyacyl hydrolase (which removes nonhydroxylated fatty acids from the lipid A region of LOS), but not by monoclonal antibodies directed against the oligosaccharide portion of the molecule, indicating the importance of the lipid A region of the LOS in increasing BBB permeability. Increased BBB permeability was also observed following the intracisternal inoculation of *H. influenzae* type b outer membrane vesicles (85), an effect that was blocked by preincubation with polymyxin B but not by a monoclonal antibody directed against the oligosaccharide side chain of the LOS; no change in permeability was observed in leukopenic animals. *H. influenzae* type b peptidoglycan has also been shown to induce meningeal inflammation and BBB permeability in an infant rat model (86).

The effects of LOS on BBB permeability have also been examined in an *in vitro* model by growing purified preparations of cerebral microvascular endothelium on a semipermeable support (87–89). Several investigators have demonstrated increased permeability across this monolayer after exposure of the monolayers to *H. influenzae* type b or purified LOS. The mechanism for this increased permeability is unclear. It may be related to a direct cytotoxic effect of LOS (89), or by the LOS-induced formation of various second messengers (e.g., cyclic AMP or cyclic GMP) by the cerebral microvascular endothelial cells (3).

The site of BBB injury was subsequently examined by *in situ* tracer perfusion and immunolabeling procedures to identify the topography and microvascular exit pathways of bovine serum albumin (BSA) (90). After intracisternal challenge of rats with *E. coli* (O111:B4) LOS, an inducible increase in immunodetectable monomeric BSA binding to the luminal membranes of all microvascular segments in the pia-arachnoid and superficial brain cortex was demonstrated by transmission electron microscopy. Exit of both perfused colloidal gold-BSA and immunodetectable BSA was through open intercellular junctions of venules in the pia-arachnoid, specifically and topographically localizing the BBB injury in bacterial meningitis to the meningeal venules.

Host Factors

Further experiments utilizing the experimental rat model demonstrated that LOS did not directly mediate the increased BBB permeability in bacterial meningitis, but did so by inducing the production of various inflammatory cytokines within the CNS; intracisternal inoculation of purified LOS led to increased CSF concentrations of both interleukin-1 (IL-1) and tumor necrosis factor (TNF) within 30 to 120 minutes (3). Furthermore, the intracisternal inoculation of human recombinant IL-1β into rats led to a peak increase in BBB permeability about 3 hours after inoculation (91), earlier than the peak response obtained following inoculation with LOS (4 hours); increased BBB permeability was significantly attenuated by preincubation of the cytokine with a monoclonal antibody to IL-1 and totally abolished in leukopenic animals. No permeability changes were induced following the intracisternal inoculation of human recombinant TNF-α, although all available evidence suggests that these cytokines act synergistically, since inoculation with submaximal doses of IL-1β plus TNF-α, at concentrations that produced no changes individually, enhanced BBB permeability. In contrast, in a study of patients with bacterial meningitis (92), CSF concentrations of TNF-α, but not IL-1β, correlated with BBB disruption (assessed by CSF protein concentrations); synergy between IL-1β and TNF-α was also noted in this study.

Matrix metalloproteinases (MMPs), a family of zinc-dependent endopeptidases that degrade components of the extracellular matrix, may also be involved in the increased BBB permeability during bacterial meningitis. In a rat model of meningococcal meningitis, an increase in CSF concentrations of MMP-9 was seen 6 hours after meningococcal challenge (93). An MMP inhibitor, batimastat, significantly reduced BBB disruption and intracranial pressure but failed to significantly reduce CSF white blood cell counts. Matrix metalloproteinases may alter BBB permeability by degrading components of the extracellular matrix that contribute to the integrity of the BBB. In a subsequent study utilizing the same experimental rat model of meningococcal meningitis, the mRNA expression pattern of various MMPs was investigated (94). The results demonstrated increased mRNA expression of gelatinase B (MMP-9), as well as collagenase-3 and stromelysin-1, indicating that MMPs may play a critical role in disruption of the BBB in experimental meningitis. Further studies are needed to determine whether these compounds are important targets for adjunctive therapy in bacterial meningitis.

SUBARACHNOID SPACE INFLAMMATION

Bacterial meningitis is characterized by the development of a neutrophilic pleocytosis within the CSF. Various chemoattractants have been investigated for their role in subarachnoid space inflammation. The complement component C5a has been suggested as one chemotactic component, with chemotactic activity appearing 2 to 4 hours before neutrophil influx into CSF (95). In an experimental rabbit model, the intracisternal inoculation of C5a led to an influx of leukocytes into CSF, peaking 1 hour after inoculation (96), a response that was attenuated by coadministration of prostaglandin E$_2$

(PGE$_2$) in a dose- and time-dependent manner, suggesting a direct antiinflammatory action of PGE$_2$ on C5a-induced CSF pleocytosis during bacterial meningitis. Elevated CSF concentrations of two alternative pathway complement activation proteins, C3 and factor B, have also been found in mice and in patients with bacterial meningitis (97,98). In the mouse model of *Listeria* meningitis (97), intrathecal synthesis of C3 and factor B occurred during the course of the disease. Recent studies have examined various chemokines (chemotactic cytokines) and their role in mediating CSF chemotactic activity. In an experimental mouse model of *Listeria* meningoencephalitis, macrophage inflammatory proteins MIP-1α and MIP-2 were important in the recruitment of leukocytes into the CSF (99). Elevated CSF concentrations of MIP-1α and MIP-1β, as well as other chemokines (interleukin-8, growth-related protein-α, and monocyte chemotactic protein-1), have also been found to be increased in patients with bacterial meningitis (100,101). However, no significant correlation was found between CSF leukocyte counts and chemokine concentrations or chemotactic activity mediated by CSF, suggesting that other factors influence the extent of CSF pleocytosis *in vivo*. In another study, elevated CSF concentrations of IL-8 and growth related protein-α significantly correlated with the number of immigrated granulocytes into the CSF of patients with bacterial meningitis (102), suggesting the importance of these chemokines in recruitment of leukocytes into the subarachnoid space.

The induction of a marked subarachnoid space inflammatory response by meningeal pathogens contributes to many of the pathophysiologic consequences of bacterial meningitis (Table 3.3) and, therefore, significant morbidity and mortality from this disorder. For example, development of a subarachnoid space inflammatory response may be crucial in the pathogenesis of sensorineural deafness in patients with bacterial meningitis. In an infant rat model of pneumococcal meningitis, multiple intraperitoneal inocula of *S. pneumoniae* into 5-day-old rats led to bacteremia and meningitis in 50% and 40% of animals, respectively (103). Hematoxylin and eosin-stained sections of brain tissue in rats with positive CSF cultures revealed inflammation in the

TABLE 3.3. *Consequences of subarachnoid space inflammation*

Increased blood-brain barrier permeability
Vasogenic cerebral edema
Cytotoxic cerebral edema
Interstitial cerebral edema
Cerebral vasculitis
Increased cerebrospinal fluid outflow resistance
Increased intracranial pressure
Altered cerebral blood flow
Loss of cerebrovascular autoregulation
Cerebral cortical ischemia
Cerebrospinal fluid acidosis
Increased cerebrospinal fluid lactate
Decreased cerebrospinal fluid glucose
Neuronal injury
Cranial and spinal nerve dysfunction
Encephalopathy

meninges and scala tympani, but not in the scala media; perilymphatic inflammation also occurred more significantly than endolymphatic inflammation. These data suggest that bacteria reach the cochlea via the cochlear duct, which provides a connection between perilymphatic fluid and CSF.

Recent experimental studies have focused on the virulence factors of meningeal pathogens, and the specific host factors they induce, to learn more about the mechanisms responsible for subarachnoid space inflammation and leukocyte traversal across the BBB (Table 3.2).

Bacterial Virulence Factors

Despite the importance of the polysaccharide capsule of bacteria in the intravascular and subarachnoid space survival of meningeal pathogens, capsular polysaccharides are remarkably noninflammatory, even when inoculated in purified form into the CSF of animals. In contrast, the cell walls of *S. pneumoniae* are potent inducers of CSF inflammation (104). In addition, the independent intracisternal inoculation of the major components of the pneumococcal cell wall, teichoic acid and peptidoglycan, induces CSF inflammation (105); teichoic acid had the highest specific activity of the cell wall fractions tested, with peak subarachnoid space inflammation occurring 5 hours after CSF instillation. These findings lend support to the concept that release of pneumococcal cell wall lytic products during antibiotic-induced autolysis during treatment of bacterial meningitis contributes to an accentuated host inflammatory response in the subarachnoid space. This CSF inflammatory response was reduced by inhibition of the cyclooxygenase pathway of arachidonic acid metabolism (106). Simultaneous treatment with methylprednisolone and oxindanac were particularly effective in decreasing inflammation induced by pneumococcal cell walls, whereas another inhibitor, diclofenac sodium, was effective at 5 and 7 hours after CSF inoculation but was not inhibitory 24 hours after cell wall challenge. Nordihydroguaiaretic acid, an inhibitor of the lipoxygenase pathway, was ineffective in preventing cell wall–induced inflammation. When tested against natural infection after challenge with live pneumococci, cyclooxygenase inhibitors, in conjunction with ampicillin, also reduced inflammation associated with release of inflammatory bacterial products during ampicillin-induced bacterial lysis. There was a correlation between CSF concentrations of the arachidonic acid metabolite PGE_2 and leukocytes after inoculation of live pneumococci or pneumococcal cell walls, and inhibition of the cyclooxygenase pathway reduced both the CSF concentrations of PGE_2 and CSF inflammation. Therefore it was suggested that use of these antiinflammatory agents, in conjunction with antimicrobial therapy, might improve outcome in bacterial meningitis by reduction of the CSF inflammatory response. Pneumolysin, an intracellular polypeptide toxin of *S. pneumoniae* released after bacterial cell lysis, does not appear to play a role in meningeal inflammation following administration of antimicrobial therapy (107).

Subarachnoid space inflammation is also induced by the intracisternal inoculation of purified *H. influenzae* type b LOS. In an experimental rabbit model, the intracisternal inoculation of purified LOS produced a dose-dependent increase in CSF white blood cell concentrations and protein (108), whereas no inflammation was induced with purified *H. influenzae* type b capsular polysaccharide. This response was blocked by pretreatment of the LOS with polymyxin B or neutrophil acyloxyacyl hydrolase, but not by a monoclonal antibody to epitopes on the oligosaccharide portion of the LOS molecule, supporting the importance of the lipid A region of the LOS molecule in the induction of inflammation. Similar results were obtained in an experimental rat model (84), with a maximal degree of CSF inflammation observed 8 hours after challenge with a 20-ng LOS dose. However, *H. influenzae* type b LOS does not exist in a free state in nature, but rather in the form of outer membrane vesicles that may represent a relevant nonreplicating vehicle for delivery of the toxic moieties of LOS to host cells. In experimental models utilizing rabbits and rats, the intracisternal inoculation of *H. influenzae* type b outer membrane vesicles also induced meningeal inflammation in a dose- and time-dependent manner (85,109). This response was blocked by polymyxin B but not by two monoclonal antibodies directed against the surface epitopes of LOS within outer membrane vesicles, supporting the concept that LOS carried via outer membrane vesicles leads to the induction of CSF inflammation.

Host Factors

Recently, however, experimental evidence has supported the concept that pneumo-coccal cell wall or LOS does not directly induce subarachnoid space inflammation, but does so through the local CNS release of inflammatory mediators such as IL-1, TNF, and/or prostaglandins. In an experimental rat model, the intracisternal inoculation of purified *H. influenzae* type b LOS led to elevated CSF concentrations of IL-1 and TNF within 30 to 120 minutes (3). Elevated CSF concentrations of TNF have also been found in an experimental rabbit model (110), with peak activity at 2 hours and persistence for about 5 hours; simultaneous analysis of serum revealed no TNF activity, indicating that the TNF was produced principally within the CNS. The administration of intravenous dexamethasone or intracisternal anti-TNF antibodies, concomitant with the inoculation of *H. influenzae* type b LOS, resulted in a significantly decreased CSF inflammatory response. These experiments were then extended in the experimental rabbit model following the intracisternal inoculation of live *H. influenzae* type b (111). The administration of ceftriaxone 6 hours after initiation of experimental infection provoked rapid bacterial lysis, followed by greatly increased CSF concentrations of LOS and TNF (peak TNF activity at 2 hours). The simultaneous administration of dexamethasone with ceftriaxone did not affect LOS release, but there was a substantial attenuation of CSF TNF activity and the CSF inflammatory response. Tumor necrosis factor was produced principally within the CNS (i.e., no TNF activity was detected in serum samples) in this experimental animal model, a finding that has also been observed in patients with bacterial meningitis (112). In addition, the presence of TNF-α in CSF appears to be indicative of a bacterial etiology (113–116), although the absence of TNF-α does not exclude the diagnosis of bacterial meningitis. Furthermore, elevated CSF concentrations of PGE$_2$, prostacyclin, IL-1β, and TNF have been found in the majority of infants and children with bacterial meningitis (117).

The direct intracisternal inoculation of these inflammatory mediators can also induce CSF inflammation. In an experimental rabbit model, injection of purified rabbit TNF-α or human recombinant IL-1β produced significant CSF inflammation (118). This effect was synergistic when lower doses of each cytokine were administered simultaneously, with more rapid and significantly increased leukocyte influx than when each cytokine was administered alone. In contrast, in an experimental rabbit model of pneumococcal meningitis, the parameters of CSF leukocytosis, BBB permeability, and brain edema were induced by intracisternal inoculation of human recombinant TNF-α, macrophage inflammatory proteins 1 and 2, and IL-1α, but not by IL-1β (119); leukocytosis and brain edema were inhibited by antibodies homologous to each mediator as well as in rabbits treated with a monoclonal antibody to CD18 to render neutrophil-endothelial cell interactions dysfunctional. Platelet-activating factor (PAF) is also inflammatory in the CNS, causing significant BBB permeability and cerebral edema (119); at higher doses, these effects are accompanied by CSF leukocytosis, which can be inhibited by administration of antibody to the CD18 family of leukocyte adhesion molecules. In an experimental rabbit model, treatment with a PAF receptor antagonist decreased CSF cytochemical values induced by intracisternal challenge with pneumococci but not *H. influenzae* (120), suggesting a specific role for PAF in pneumococcal disease. In addition, another study utilizing an experimental rat model found that PAF augmented the meningeal inflammation and BBB permeability elicited by *H. influenzae* type b LOS (121).

These findings have implications with regard to prognosis in patients with bacterial meningitis. Outcome from gram-negative bacillary meningitis has been correlated with persistence of organisms and higher concentrations of endotoxin (as measured by the *Limulus* lysate assay) in CSF (122). In children with *H. influenzae* type b meningitis treated with ceftriaxone, CSF concentrations of free LOS correlated positively with the number of bacteria killed in CSF, the Herson-Todd severity score, and number of febrile hospital days (123), suggesting that release of free LOS with antimicrobial therapy enhanced the host inflammatory response in the subarachnoid space. In an experimental rabbit model of *E. coli* meningitis, a single intravenous dose of an antimicrobial agent (cefotaxime, cefpirome, meropenem, chloramphenicol, or gentamicin) caused a 2- to 10-fold increase in free CSF LOS concentrations within 2 hours, although free LOS concentrations increased almost 100-fold in untreated animals 4 hours later as bacteria continued to multiply (124). However, antimicrobial therapy enhanced the CSF inflammatory response significantly in comparison with the untreated animals. The degree of elevated CSF concentrations of IL-1β also correlated with outcome from neonatal gram-negative bacillary meningitis (125). In infants and children with predominantly *H. influenzae* type b meningitis, patients with CSF concentrations of IL-1β of 500 pg/mL or more were more likely to develop neurologic sequelae, whereas elevated CSF concentrations of TNF were not associated with outcome (126). CSF IL-1β concentrations were reduced when the patients were treated with dexamethasone, suggesting that dexamethasone exerted its antiinflammatory effects in the subarachnoid space by inhibiting IL-1β gene expression. Elevated CSF concentrations of PAF have also been demonstrated in children with *H.*

influenzae meningitis (127), correlating with bacterial density and with CSF concentrations of LOS and TNF-α; these increased concentrations of TNF-α and PAF were associated with severity of disease. This was confirmed in more recent studies that demonstrated that elevated CSF concentrations of TNF-α and soluble TNF receptor (sTNFR), the natural homeostatic regulator of the actions of TNF-α, were important for predicting neurologic sequelae in bacterial meningitis (128,129).

Other agents that reduce subarachnoid space inflammation have also been examined in experimental animal models as possible adjuncts in the therapy of bacterial meningitis (Table 3.4). Pentoxifylline, a phosphodiesterase inhibitor, decreases endotoxin-induced TNF-α production, attenuates the inflammatory action of IL-1 and TNF on leukocyte function, and blocks the LOS-induced release of TNF and IL-1 from microglial cell cultures. In an experimental rabbit model of *H. influenzae* type b meningitis, administration of pentoxifylline 20 minutes before intracisternal challenge with *H. influenzae* type b LOS significantly reduced CSF concentrations of leukocytes, protein, and lactate (130). However, dexamethasone was superior to pentoxifylline in modulation of these CSF inflammatory changes, and no appreciable synergism was observed when both agents were simultaneously administered. Thalidomide, which also inhibits TNF-α production, was recently studied in an experimental rabbit model of meningitis. Thalidomide reduced TNF-α production following intracisternal challenge with either *H. influenzae* type b or *S. pneumoniae*, although it had a relatively greater effect on the inflammatory response to *S. pneumoniae* (131). Bactericidal/permeability-increasing protein (BPI), which is present in the azurophilic granules of neutrophils and binds to and neutralizes the biologic activity of the lipid A portion of LOS, has also been studied for its effects on CSF inflammation in bacterial meningitis. In an experimental rabbit model, the intracisternal inoculation of recombinant BPI significantly reduced CSF inflammation in response to meningococcal endotoxin (132); this effect was not seen following systemic administration, likely because of failure of BPI to cross the BBB. IL-1 receptor antagonist (IL-1RA) and sTNFR have also been studied in an experimental rabbit model, in which the intracisternal inoculation of rabbit recombinant IL-1β and TNF-α combined with IL-1RA and sTNFR produced less inflammation in rabbits than after inoculation of either of these cytokines alone (133). However, IL-1RA and sTNFR did not reduce the meningeal inflammatory response associated with intracisternal inoculation of *H. influenzae* type b LOS, indicating that these cytokine inhibitors may not be effective in modulating inflammation induced by a broad inflammatory stimulus such as gram-negative bacteria or their products.

More recently, other cytokines have been studied for their role in the subarachnoid space inflammatory response in bacterial meningitis. Elevated CSF concentrations of IL-6, which is induced by IL-1, have been observed in the CSF of patients with bacterial meningitis (134–137). These increased concentrations occurred after release of TNF-α and before neutrophilic infiltration into CSF (138), but the presence of IL-6 did not correlate with any of the indices of meningeal inflammation or severity of disease. IL-8, a cytokine with potent chemoattractant and activating effects on neutrophils, has been detected in CSF of patients with bacterial meningitis (139–141);

TABLE 3.4. *Agents that attenuate the subarachnoid space inflammatory response and other pathophysiologic parameters in experimental animal models of bacterial meningitis*

Nonsteroidal antiinflammatory agents
  Oxindanac
  Diclofenac sodium
  Indomethacin
Corticosteroids
  Methylprednisolone
  Dexamethasone
Antiendotoxin agents
  Polymyxin B
  Neutrophil acyloxyacyl hydrolase
  Bactericidal/permeability-increasing protein
Anti-cytokine agents
  Anti-TNF monoclonal antibody
  Anti-IL-1β monoclonal antibody
  Platelet-activating factor receptor antagonist
  Interleukin 1 receptor antagonist
  Soluble tumor necrosis factor receptor
  Pentoxifylline
  Thalidomide
  Interleukin-10
Monoclonal antibodies against leukocyte adhesion molecules
  Anti-ICAM-1 (CD54)
  Anti-CD18 (IB4)
  Anti-CD11 (1B6)
Inhibitors of leukocyte rolling
  Fucoidin
  Heparin
Endothelin antagonists
  BQ-788
  BQ-123
Matrix metalloproteinase inhibitors
  Batimastat
  GM6001
Inhibitors of biologic activity of reactive oxygen species
  Superoxide dismutase
  Catalase
  Deferoxamine
  N-acetyl-L-cysteine
  α-phenyl-tert-butyl nitrone
  C60 (carboxyfullerence)
  Trylizad-mesylate
  Rifampin
Inhibitors of nitric oxide synthase
  N-nitro-L-arginine
  7-nitroindazole
  Aminoguanidine
  Bradykinin B$_2$ receptor antagonist
  Interleukin-10
  S-methyl-isothiourea
Inhibitors of peroxynitrite
  Uric acid
Inhibitors of excitatory amino acids
  Kynurenic acid

IL-8 may also have a role as a neutrophil chemotactic factor in nonbacterial meningitis. IL-10, an antiinflammatory protein formed by T lymphocytes and monocytes, inhibits the production of pro-inflammatory cytokines such as TNF-α and has been detected in the CSF of animals and humans with bacterial meningitis (142–145). In an experimental rabbit model, IL-10 modulated the CSF TNF-α concentrations in experimental meningitis caused by *H. influenzae* type b LOS, *H. influenzae* type b, or *L. monocytogenes*, an effect that was maximal when IL-10 was combined with dexamethasone (146). Finally, the production of interferon-gamma (IFN-γ) was induced by IL-12 (which is produced by phagocytic cells in response to infection and stimulates adaptive immunity) with TNF-α as a costimulator and inhibited by IL-10 (147); IFN-γ production may contribute to the natural immunity against microorganisms in CSF during the acute phase of bacterial meningitis.

Therefore it appears that release of inflammatory mediators in the CNS is responsible for induction of a marked subarachnoid space inflammatory response (Figs. 3.2 and 3.3) and may correlate with morbidity and mortality in patients with bacterial meningitis.

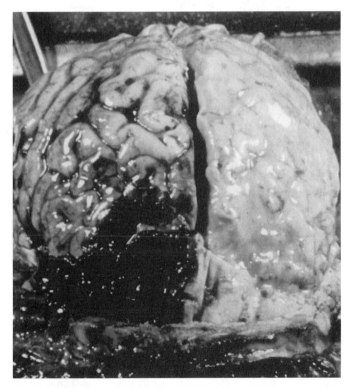

FIG. 3.2. Brain removed at autopsy in a patient with bacterial meningitis. There is the presence of purulent exudate over the right cerebral hemisphere, as well as evidence of a left occipital contusion. (Courtesy of Sidney E. Croul, M.D.)

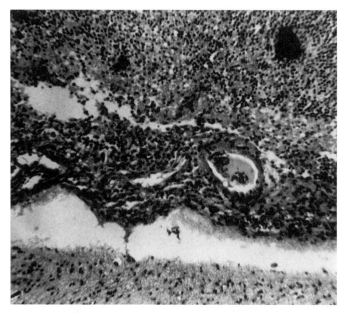

FIG. 3.3. Histopathology of the brain of a patient with bacterial meningitis. There is purulent exudate composed of neutrophils above a layer of cerebral cortex. (Courtesy of Sidney E. Croul, M.D.)

Leukocyte Traversal

The precise pathway of leukocyte traversal into the CSF is unknown, although adherence to cerebral vascular endothelial cells is a likely prerequisite. Pretreatment of noncerebral endothelial cells in culture (primarily derived from the umbilical vein) with LOS or cytokines (IL-1 or TNF) induces adherence and transendothelial passage of neutrophils (148–152). This adherence may be mediated by three families of adhesion molecules: the immunoglobulin superfamily, the integrin family, and the selectin family. The immunoglobulin superfamily includes the antigen-specific receptors of B and T lymphocytes and two intercellular adhesion molecules (ICAM-1 and ICAM-2); ICAM-1 is induced on endothelium within 10 to 24 hours of exposure to inflammatory cytokines (153). Adhesion molecules of the integrin family are composed of α and β subunits and can be classified on the basis of their subunits into β_1, β_2, and β_3 integrins; members of the β_2 (CD18) subfamily (also known as leukocyte integrins) are expressed only on leukocytes, with the degree of expression increased within minutes by chemoattractants (153). The selectin family includes endothelial leukocyte adhesion molecule 1 (ELAM-1), which is transiently inducible on endothelial cells after stimulation with IL-1 and TNF (154); neutrophil adhesion occurs independently of ICAMs and integrins. Other selectins include GMP-140 (or CD62), which is stored in endothelial cells and quickly mobilized (within 10 minutes) to the cell surface after stimulation with thrombin or histamine to facilitate adhesion of neutrophils and monocytes to endothelial cells, and the leukocyte-adhesion molecule 1 (LAM-1), which mediates adhesion of unstimulated lymphocytes and neutrophils even under shear stress in conditions of flow (153). The binding affinity of LAM-1 for its receptor on endothelial cells is increased within minutes by neutrophil activation, or by exposure to TNF or granulocyte-macrophage colony-stimulating factor (GM-CSF), but LAM-1 is subsequently shed from the cell surface.

These adhesion molecules may be involved in the process of neutrophil entry into CSF via mechanisms involving neutrophils and cerebrovascular endothelium. In an infant mouse model of hematogenous bacterial meningitis, mice genetically deficient in the gene coding for ICAM-1 production had a significantly higher incidence of *H. influenzae* type b bacteremia than wild-type mice ($P = 0.007$), and more ICAM-1-deficient mice had positive CSF cultures (155). In contrast, the incidence of *S. pneumoniae* bacteremia was equivalent in both groups of mice, and all were CSF culture positive, although mortality was significantly higher for ICAM-1-deficient mice at 24 hours ($P = 0.0003$). These results suggested that ICAM-1 deficiency may be protective early in *H. influenzae* type b infection but detrimental in *S. pneumoniae* infection. In an experimental rat model, a monoclonal antibody (CD54) directed against ICAM-1 significantly reduced the accumulation of leukocytes in CSF during the early phase of bacterial meningitis (156), making this adhesion molecule a promising target in the development of adjunctive strategies in the therapy of bacterial meningitis.

Other families of leukocyte receptors have also been studied to determine their role in leukocyte-mediated damage in bacterial meningitis. In an experimental rabbit model, the intravenous inoculation of a monoclonal antibody (IB4) directed against the CD18 family of receptors on leukocytes (leukocyte integrins) blocked the accumulation of leukocytes in CSF despite the intracisternal inoculation of *H. influenzae* type b, *N. meningitidis,* pneumococcal cell wall, or LOS (157). In addition, this monoclonal antibody blocked the parameters of BBB permeability (i.e., influx of serum proteins into CSF), and the development of cerebral edema and death in animals challenged with lethal doses of *S. pneumoniae*. Cerebrospinal fluid penetration of antibiotics, CSF bactericidal concentrations, and bactericidal response to ampicillin therapy were not affected by administration of the monoclonal antibody, although the onset of bacteremia was delayed and there was an attenuated CSF inflammatory response after ampicillin-induced bacterial killing. In a second study utilizing an experimental rabbit model of *H. influenzae* type b meningitis, the concomitant administration of dexamethasone and IB4 led to a marked attenuation of all indices of meningeal inflammation and a reduction in brain water content compared with the results obtained in untreated animals or when each agent was used alone (158). Clinical trials with this agent, perhaps in conjunction with dexamethasone, will be needed to determine whether outcome (i.e., morbidity or mortality) can be improved by administration of IB4 in patients with bacterial meningitis.

Selectins also play an important role in promoting the margination and reversible rolling of leukocytes at sites of tissue inflammation. Following intravenous administration of prokaryotic peptides that mimic selectins (the S2 and S3 subunits of pertussis toxin) and competitively inhibit adherence of neutrophils to endothelial cells *in vitro,* recruitment of leukocytes into CSF of rabbits with pneumococcal meningitis was disrupted, suggesting that these peptides have therapeutic antiinflammatory potential (159). An anti-CD11b monoclonal antibody (1B6) was studied in an infant rat model of *H. influenzae* sepsis and meningitis; 1B6 played a role in inhibiting neutrophil emigration to sites of inflammation within the CNS but was not beneficial in decreasing mortality in this model (160). Furthermore, in an experimental cytokine-induced model of meningitis, mice deficient in P- and E-selectins displayed a near complete inhibition in CSF leukocyte accumulation and BBB permeability, versus only partial inhibition in P-selectin-deficient mice (161). In an *in vitro* model examining *L. monocytogenes* invasion of human brain microvascular endothelial cells, infection of these monolayers stimulated monocyte and neutrophil adhesion, and an anti-CD18 monoclonal antibody completely blocked neutrophil adhesion to brain microvascular endothelial cells (161), indicating that CD18-mediated binding is the predominant mechanism for neutrophil adhesion to infected human brain microvascular endothelial cells under static conditions. In additional studies, after intravenous treatment with the polysaccharide fucoidin, a homopolymer of sulfated L-fucose known to block the function of the leukocyte "rolling receptor" L-selectin (162), leukocyte rolling was rapidly and profoundly reduced (confirmed by intravital microscopy in muscle), and the accumulation of both leukocytes and plasma proteins into CSF of rabbits challenged intrathecally with pneumococcal antigen was profoundly reduced. These findings suggest that inhibition of selectin-mediated leukocyte rolling may also be an effective therapeutic approach to attenuation of leukocyte-mediated damage during bacterial meningitis (163).

The dynamic aspects of these leukocyte–endothelial cell interactions were also examined in a meningitis model by means of confocal laser scanning microscopy, a new microscopic technique with much-improved depth discrimination properties. In an experimental model of pneumococcal meningitis, the behavior of rhodamine 6G-labeled leukocytes in pial vessels was determined (164). Compared with controls, the number of adherent leukocytes significantly ($P < 0.05$) increased within 1 hour following intracisternal challenge with *S. pneumoniae,* with further increases noted up to 6 hours after infection; adherence occurred in pial venules but not in arterioles. Pretreatment with dexamethasone significantly attenuated adherence and transendothelial passage of leukocytes. In another study utilizing this technique, heparin was found to significantly attenuate leukocyte rolling after the induction of pneumococcal meningitis (165). Therefore this technique has potential usefulness in the investigation of the efficacy of antiinflammatory agents that may interfere with leukocyte adherence to cerebral microvascular endothelium.

INCREASED INTRACRANIAL PRESSURE

Cerebral edema is the major element contributing to the increased intracranial pressure during bacterial meningitis. The cerebral edema may be vasogenic, cytotoxic, and/or interstitial in origin. However, all three elements probably contribute to cerebral edema during bacterial meningitis and may result in life-threatening cerebral herniation and other serious complications (Fig. 3.4) (3). Vasogenic cerebral edema is primarily a consequence of increased BBB permeability (see earlier). Cytotoxic cerebral edema

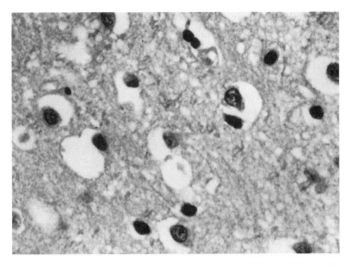

FIG. 3.4. Histopathology of the cerebral cortex from a patient with bacterial meningitis demonstrating edematous changes. There are large empty spaces around cells, representing neuropil retracting from cells. (Courtesy of Sidney E. Croul, M.D.)

results from swelling of the cellular elements of the brain most likely due to release of toxic factors from neutrophils or bacteria or both, with a subsequent increase in intracellular water content from alteration in the membranes of brain cells, resulting in potassium leakage, glucose utilization via anaerobic glycolysis, and lactate production (166). Interstitial cerebral edema reflects obstruction of the flow of normal CSF as in hydrocephalus. This last factor has been examined in an experimental rabbit model of pneumococcal or *E. coli* meningitis in which the CSF outflow resistance (defined as factors that inhibit the flow of CSF from the subarachnoid space to the major dural sinuses) was markedly elevated and remained elevated for as long as 2 weeks despite rapid CSF sterilization with penicillin therapy (167). The early administration of methylprednisolone (30 mg/kg intramuscularly) at 16 and 20 hours after intracisternal inoculation of microorganisms rapidly lowered CSF outflow resistance toward control values, suggesting that attenuation of the normal CSF absorptive mechanisms during bacterial meningitis might decrease the ability of the brain to compensate in situations of increased intracranial pressure.

These concepts have been examined in greater detail in an experimental animal model of pneumococcal meningitis by measuring the brain water content (indicative of cerebral edema if elevated), CSF lactate concentrations, and CSF pressure (168). All three parameters were elevated in infected animals. Although treatment with ampicillin rapidly sterilized the CSF and normalized brain water content and CSF pressure within 24 hours, the CSF lactate concentration remained elevated. Both methylprednisolone and dexamethasone completely reversed the development of brain edema, but only dexamethasone led to a reduction in CSF pressure and lactate, suggesting that increased CSF outflow resistance is not the only determinant of increased intracranial pressure in bacterial meningitis. However, neither agent was superior to therapy with ampicillin alone in reducing cerebral edema or intracranial pressure, and no comparison was made between ampicillin alone and the combination of ampicillin plus corticosteroids, a comparison that would have been relevant to the potential clinical usefulness of adjunctive corticosteroid therapy in patients with bacterial meningitis. A subsequent study did examine treatment with ceftriaxone versus ceftriaxone plus dexamethasone in an experimental rabbit model of *H. influenzae* meningitis (169). Although combination therapy consistently reduced the brain water content, CSF pressure, and CSF lactate to a greater degree than ceftriaxone alone, the differences were not statistically significant, and by 29 hours the values were comparable whether the animals received antibiotic alone, dexamethasone alone, or the combination. The authors suggested, however, that adjunctive dexamethasone might be more beneficial if administered early, or even before antibiotic-induced bacterial lysis and release of microbial products. In a subsequent analysis using the experimental rabbit model of *H. influenzae* type b meningitis (112), ceftriaxone administration led to a significant increase in CSF endotoxin concentrations 2 hours after administration, which was followed by a rise in CSF TNF concentrations. Simultaneous administration of dexamethasone and ceftriaxone did not affect release of endotoxin into CSF, but markedly attenuated CSF concentrations of TNF measured 8 hours later. Adjunctive dexamethasone therapy also resulted in a significant decrease in CSF leukocytosis and a trend toward earlier improvement in CSF concentrations of glucose, lactate, and protein. These parameters improved without any apparent decrease in the rate of bacterial killing within the CSF *in vivo*. Other antiinflammatory agents have also been studied for their role in affecting these parameters. Administration of indomethacin decreased both the brain water content and CSF concentrations of PGE_2 during experimental pneumococcal meningitis, although intracranial pressure was not reduced (170). In addition, the administration of either dexamethasone or oxindanac lessened the massive influx of serum albumin and other proteins of high and low molecular weight into the CSF during the early stages of experimental pneumococcal meningitis (171).

The factors responsible for production of brain edema were subsequently examined in an experimental animal model of *E. coli* meningitis in which infected animals were treated with either cefotaxime or chloramphenicol (172). Both antibiotics were effective in reducing CSF bacterial concentrations, although therapy with cefotaxime, but not chloramphenicol, induced a marked rise in CSF endotoxin concentrations that were associated with increased brain water content. The increases were neutralized by polymyxin B and by a monoclonal antibody to lipid A, suggesting that antimicrobial therapy with bacteriolytic antibiotics may be important in the pathogenesis of cerebral edema in bacterial meningitis. The peptidoglycan of the *H. influenzae* cell wall also induced cerebral edema without perturbing the other parameters of inflammation (i.e., increased BBB permeability) (173), suggesting that peptidoglycan induces cytotoxic rather than vasogenic cerebral edema. However, other investigators have found that peptidoglycan does induce BBB permeability (86). The role of the neutrophil in this process is unclear. Neutrophils appeared to contribute to development of cerebral edema if adequately stimulated in a model of sterile meningitis induced by N-formyl-methionyl-leucyl-phenylalanine (174), although the parameters of increased intracranial pressure and increased CSF concentrations of lactate and protein were unrelated to the presence of neutrophils; no increase in brain water content was observed in neutropenic animals. However, this area remains controversial because neutrophils are required for the increased BBB permeability seen in response to the intracisternal inoculation of bacterial virulence factors and inflammatory mediators (84,91).

Variability among bacterial strains may also be an important determinant in the production of the subarachnoid space inflammatory response and brain edema in bacterial meningitis. Intracisternal inoculation of three different pneumococcal isolates resulted in pronounced differences in the pathophysiologic profiles 24 hours after challenge (175). When pneumococcal cell wall fragments were inoculated intracisternally, the chemical composition of the fragments (specifically, the degree of teichoication) influenced the induction of brain edema. In a subsequent study in an experimental rabbit model (176), serotype-specific characteristics of pneumococci were found to play a major role in the subarachnoid space inflammatory process, although significant differences in brain water content were only observed with one of the serotypes tested. It is unclear, however, whether these differences affect the clinical expression of disease in patients with bacterial meningitis.

The infusion of hypertonic mannitol to treat increased intracranial pressure has been evaluated in a rabbit model of *H. influenzae* type b meningitis (177). In all animals, mannitol consistently reduced intracisternal pressure, although the magnitude of reduction was greater in infected animals and brain water content was no different in mannitol-treated animals. In contrast, in an experimental rat model of pneumococcal meningitis, mannitol modulated changes in cerebral blood flow, intracranial pressure, and brain water content (178), perhaps by a mechanism of scavenging hydroxyl radicals, which have been shown to be involved in the pathogenesis and pathophysiology of cerebral ischemia and neuronal injury in bacterial meningitis (see later).

ALTERATIONS IN CEREBRAL BLOOD FLOW AND NEURONAL INJURY

Bacterial meningitis exerts profound effects on blood vessels coursing through the subarachnoid space (3), and the resulting vasculitis leads to narrowing and/or thrombosis of cerebral blood vessels and the propensity for ischemia and/or infarction of underlying brain (Fig. 3.5). When arteriography was performed in children with bacterial meningitis, leakage of contrast material resulting from vascular involvement was observed, but these changes reverted to normal following successful antimicrobial therapy (179). With involvement of large arteries at the base of the brain, severe neurologic complications (e.g., hemiparesis, quadriparesis) with permanent neurologic sequelae may ensue (180). There may also be release of humoral factors elaborated within the CSF or blood vessel wall, with subsequent vasospasm progressing to vasodilatation and thrombotic stenosis later in the disease course (181). Phlebitis of major cortical draining vessels and/or dural sinuses may result in thrombosis with secondary brain infarction, focal neurologic deficits, and seizure activity in patients with bacterial meningitis. In combination with increased intracranial pressure, these changes may result in altered cerebral blood flow in patients with bacterial meningitis. It has been

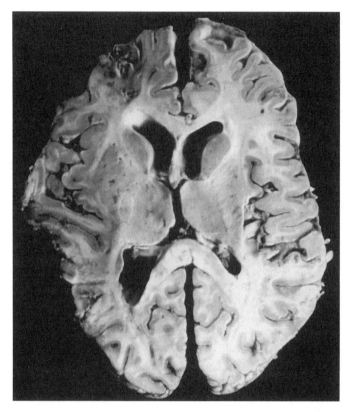

FIG. 3.5. Brain from a patient with bacterial meningitis, demonstrating a secondary left middle cerebral artery infarct with cerebral edema. (Courtesy of Sidney E. Croul, M.D.)

demonstrated in an infant rhesus monkey model of *H. influenzae* meningitis that there is cerebral cortical hypoperfusion (measured by an autoradiographic technique utilizing ^{14}C-antipyrine) during meningitis with resultant relative cerebral anoxia (55); certain areas of the cortex (postcentral, temporal, and occipital) were hypoperfused relative to the hypothalamus and midbrain while the brain stem was hyperperfused, suggesting that one of the initial physiologic changes in *H. influenzae* meningitis is cerebral cortical hypoperfusion with resultant relative cerebral anoxia.

Cerebrovascular Autoregulation

Cerebrovascular autoregulation is also lost during experimental bacterial meningitis, in which cerebral blood flow was increased when systemic pressure was increased and decreased when blood pressure was lowered (182), indicating that flow was pressure-passive. Furthermore, studies in an experimental rabbit model of pneumococcal meningitis have demonstrated that animals given a lower intravenous fluid regimen (50 mL/kg per 24 hours) of normal saline had a lower mean arterial pressure, lower cerebral blood flow, and higher concentration of CSF lactate compared with animals that received a higher fluid regimen (150 mL/kg per 24 hours) (183). In the first 4 to 6 hours of antibiotic administration, rabbits receiving lower fluid regimens had a significant decrease in mean arterial pressure and cerebral blood flow and a significant increase in CSF lactate concentrations than rabbits receiving higher fluid regimens. These results, in combination with other experimental studies that have noted an increase in cerebral blood flow within the first few hours of intracisternal inoculation of either live pneumococci or pneumococcal cell wall fragments (184), have suggested that maintenance of adequate intravascular volume and minimization of stimuli that increase systemic blood pressure may be important in the treatment of bacterial meningitis. These findings may also be of potential clinical relevance, since inadvertent increases in mean arterial pressure directly increase cerebral blood flow and intracranial pressure; depletion of intravascular volume with decreases in mean arterial pressure can cause parallel decreases in cerebral blood flow and reduction of substrate delivery to the brain. Therefore the brain is at risk from either hypoperfusion or hyperperfusion. Using near-infrared spectroscopy in conjunction with measurement of cerebral blood flow, in an experimental rabbit model of pneumococcal meningitis, infected animals had a relative increase in the deoxygenated hemoglobin fraction and a decrease in the oxygenated hemoglobin fraction (185), supporting the possibility of cerebral venous engorgement in bacterial meningitis, which may contribute to intracranial hypertension in this disorder.

Additional studies have examined the importance of the subarachnoid space inflammatory response in alterations of cerebral blood flow during bacterial meningitis. In an experimental rabbit model of *H. influenzae* type b meningitis, CSF leukocytes were found not to be responsible for the hyperemic response (186), suggesting that cerebral hyperemia in bacterial meningitis is induced directly by bacterial components or indirectly by components of the inflammatory cascade. More recently, endothelin (which has been found to regulate vascular tone and integrity and act as a mediator of inflammation) has been investigated as a possible mediator of the cerebrovascular complications in bacterial meningitis. In an experimental rat model of pneumococcal meningitis, endothelin contributed to the increased cerebral blood flow (as measured by laser Doppler flowmetry), intracranial pressure, brain water content, and CSF pleocytosis (187). Elevated CSF concentrations of endothelin have also been found in patients during the acute stage of bacterial meningitis (188), suggesting a potential role for endothelin in mediation of meningitis-induced cerebral hypoperfusion and brain infarction.

Cerebral blood flow has been measured in patients with bacterial meningitis. In an early study, measurement of cerebral blood flow (by the xenon-133 intraarterial injection method) revealed a 30% to 40% reduction in average total blood flow in five patients with pneumococcal meningitis (mean age of 54 years) but not in five patients with meningococcal meningitis (mean age of 20 years) (189). An inverse relationship between cerebral blood flow velocity (measured by Doppler techniques through the anterior fontanelle) and intracranial pressure was observed in infants with bacterial meningitis (190). Among eight patients, alterations were noted only in the four older infants (age range of 3 to 10 months) and not in the four neonates (age range of 5 to 30 days), in whom no changes in cerebral blood flow velocity were detected. In another study of 17 children (ages 8 days to 6 years) with bacterial meningitis, transcranial Doppler ultrasound monitoring demonstrated an improvement in cerebral blood flow velocity with resolution of meningitis (190). This suggests that in the early phase of bacterial meningitis, increased cerebrovascular resistance may contribute to a relative impairment of cerebral perfusion; transcranial Doppler ultrasound may be a useful technique for early detection of deterioration in cerebral hemodynamics.

Other studies have also supported the importance of cerebral blood flow abnormalities in patients with bacterial meningitis. In a study in 20 children seriously ill with bacterial meningitis (191), total and regional cerebral blood flow measured by stable xenon computed tomography revealed a global decrease in flow and even more regional variability. Although autoregulation of cerebral blood flow was preserved in the patients studied, hyperventilation reduced flow below the ischemic threshold, raising important concerns about the routine use of hyperventilation in the management of increased intracranial pressure in patients with bacterial meningitis (192). In another study of 86 adult patients with bacterial meningitis (193), cerebral angiography was performed in 27 patients who had focal deficits (either clinically, on cranial computed tomography, or both) and who had persistent coma without explained cause despite 3 days of antimicrobial therapy; 13 of the patients who underwent angiography had alterations of the blood vessel system associated with a poor prognosis. However, the definitive changes in cerebral blood flow during bacterial meningitis are controversial and may vary with stage of disease. These blood flow alterations may lead to regional hypoxia (Fig. 3.6), increased lactate concentrations in the brain secondary to utilization of glucose by anaerobic glycolysis, and CSF acidosis, which may be a precursor to encephalopathy (194). In a recent study of *E. coli* meningitis in newborn piglets, it was suggested that increased anaerobic glycolysis in the subarachnoid space (induced by TNF-α and leukocytes) leads to hypoglycorrhachia and elevated CSF lactate concentrations; induced hyperglycemia attenuated the CSF inflammatory response (195), suggesting that induced hyperglycemia might be beneficial by increasing glucose delivery to meet increasing demands. This issue requires further study, however.

Reactive Oxygen Species

Recent data have accumulated suggesting that reactive oxygen species may contribute to the increased brain water content, intracranial pressure, and changes in regional blood flow (see later) in bacterial meningitis (4,5). Reactive oxygen species are a family of molecules derived from the partial reduction of molecular oxygen. Because of their free radical nature (i.e., the presence of an unpaired electron) and loss of spin restriction, reactive oxygen species are chemically more reactive with organic molecules than oxygen and are cytotoxic. Under normal conditions, host cells are

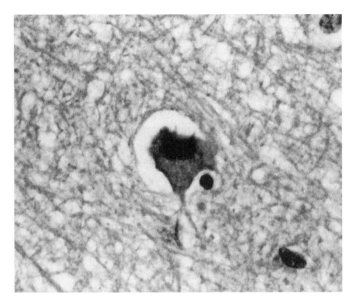

FIG. 3.6. Histopathology of the cerebral cortex in a patient with bacterial meningitis, revealing a hypoxic ischemic neuron. There is a condensed nucleus undergoing cell death; the nucleus is pyknotic and the cytoplasm is shrunken and hypereosinophilic. (Courtesy of Sidney E. Croul, M.D.)

protected from the toxic effects of reactive oxygen species by enzymatic and nonenzymatic antioxidants, which include superoxide dismutase, catalase, and glutathione peroxidase. The importance of reactive oxygen species has been examined in experimental models of bacterial meningitis. In an experimental rat model of pneumococcal meningitis following intracisternal inoculation of live pneumococci or pneumococcal cell wall components (196), the increases in brain water content and intracranial pressure were prevented; the increase in regional blood flow was significantly attenuated by conjugated superoxide dismutase and deferoxamine. Catalase, which eliminates hydrogen peroxide, also significantly attenuated the increase in regional blood flow and brain water content, although there was only a trend in reduction of intracranial pressure (197). Furthermore, in a neonatal rat model of group B streptococcal meningitis, generation of reactive oxygen intermediates (localized to cells constituting the subarachnoid and ventricular inflammation and to the cerebral vasculature) was a major contributor to cerebral ischemia and necrotic and apoptotic neuronal injury (198). The free radical scavenger α-phenyl-tert-butyl nitrone inhibited the biologic effect of the reactive oxygen intermediates, thereby improving cerebral cortical perfusion and reducing the extent of both necrotic and apoptotic neuronal injury. It also appeared that TNF-α plays a critical role in neuronal apoptosis in the hippocampus in rats with group B streptococcal meningitis (199), although it was not essential for the development of inflammation and cortical injury. Recently, the effect of a water-soluble malonic acid derivative of carboxyfullerence (C60), which has avid reactivity with free radicals and is a potent free-radical scavenger, against *E. coli*-induced meningitis was evaluated (200). C60 was found to protect mice from *E. coli*-induced death in a dose-dependent manner, and treated mice had less TNF-α and IL-1β production as assessed by staining of brain tissue. C60 also inhibited *E. coli*-induced increases in BBB permeability and CSF neutrophil infiltration, suggesting the potential of this compound as a therapeutic agent for bacterial meningitis.

Other agents that interfere with reactive oxygen intermediates have also been examined for their efficacy in experimental animal models of bacterial meningitis. Rifampin, an antimicrobial agent that releases smaller quantities of pro-inflammatory compounds from *S. pneumoniae* than β-lactam agents, was shown to reduce the release of reactive oxygen intermediates and decrease secondary brain injury in an experimental rabbit model of pneumococcal meningitis (201). In another study that evaluated three clinically used antioxidants (N-acetylcysteine, deferoxamine, and trylizad-mesylate), all reduced cortical injury (but not hippocampal injury) in an experimental pneumococcal meningitis model (202). Despite this beneficial effect, treatment did not reduce the inflammatory response, as measured by CSF concentrations of TNF-α congruent with the lack of neuroprotection in the hippocampus. The authors concluded that antioxidant strategies were clearly promising for the adjunctive therapy of bacterial meningitis, although an ideal agent should act at both the cortex and hippocampus. Further studies with other antioxidants may establish their role in the adjunctive therapy of patients with bacterial meningitis.

Nitric Oxide

Evidence has also accumulated that reactive nitrogen intermediates may play a role in the inflammatory process and other pathophysiologic events during bacterial meningitis (203,204). Nitric oxide is derived from conversion of L-arginine to L-citrulline by nitric oxide synthase (NOS). The presence of inducible nitric oxide synthase (iNOS) has been demonstrated after induction by cytokines and bacterial products; once expressed, iNOS continuously produces high concentrations of nitric oxide that can act as a microbicidal agent or cause cytotoxicity. In an experimental rat model of pneumococcal meningitis utilizing treatment with the NOS inhibitor N-nitro-L-arginine, it was determined that nitric oxide accounted for regional cerebral blood flow changes and pial arteriolar vasodilation in the early phase of meningitis and was involved as a mediator of brain edema and meningeal inflammation (205). Stimulation of cerebral endothelial cells with pneumococci released nitric oxide, presumably via iNOS. In addition, inhibition of the neuronal NOS pathway with 7-nitroindazole prevented pneumococci-induced pial arteriolar vasodilation (206). Similarly, in another rat model of meningitis, CSF concentrations of nitrite (a major metabolic product of nitric oxide *in vivo*) rose after challenge with live *H. influenzae* type b or *H. influenzae* type b LOS, in direct correlation with increased BBB permeability (207). This was confirmed in another study in an experimental rat model, in which excessive nitric oxide production contributed to BBB disruption (208). Administration of aminoguanidine, an inhibitor of iNOS, during meningeal inflammation significantly diminished meningeal nitric oxide production, attenuated white blood cell migration into the CSF, and maintained normal BBB permeability. A subsequent study also demonstrated that inhibition of nitric oxide production with aminoguanidine increased cortical hypoperfusion and ischemic neuronal injury (209), suggesting that nitric oxide attenuates the development of cortical ischemia and neuronal injury in bacterial meningitis. Taken together, these studies suggest an important but dynamic role of nitric oxide at the level of the cerebral vasculature during bacterial meningitis (5). Early on, this potent vasodilator is responsible for the hyperemia induced by subarachnoid space inflammation. Later, as cerebral blood flow tends to progressively decline under the influence of vasoconstrictive events, nitric oxide produced in the vasculature has some protective effect against ischemia. Nitric oxide inhibition further pushes the balance between vasoconstrictive and vasodilatative elements toward the vasoconstrictive side, with a subsequent increase in cerebral ischemia and neuronal injury. Therefore any attempts to downmodulate nitric oxide production during bacterial meningitis are potentially dangerous.

Locally produced inflammatory mediators may have effects on these processes in bacterial meningitis. Bradykinin has been shown to be involved as a mediator in the early phase of pneumococcal meningitis in the rat and contributes to the increase in regional blood flow, intracranial pressure, and brain water content (210). Administration of a bradykinin B_2 receptor antagonist may prevent nitric oxide release. In addition, systemic administration of IL-10 may interfere with the production of reactive nitrogen intermediates, thereby attenuating the pathophysiologic changes (increased regional cerebral blood flow, brain water content, intracranial pressure, and CSF white blood cell counts) during the early phase of experimental pneumococcal meningitis (211).

The role of nitric oxide has also been examined in patients with bacterial meningitis. It has been suggested that nitric oxide may contribute to anaerobic glycolysis and neurologic damage in children with bacterial meningitis (212). The induction of nitric oxide synthase, and consequently the production of nitric oxide, may be induced by TNF in CSF (213), which in turn mediates the increased BBB permeability in bacterial meningitis.

Current interest is focusing on the role of peroxynitrite in the development of neuronal injury in bacterial meningitis (5). Peroxynitrite is a powerful oxidative agent formed by the reaction of superoxide and nitric oxide, and exerts its cytotoxic effects by various mechanisms (including DNA damage, tyrosine nitration, and lipid peroxidation). Peroxynitrite is produced by the brain parenchyma during bacterial meningitis; inhibition of its effect on mitochondria appears to be neuroprotective. In an adult rat model of pneumococcal meningitis, treatment of infected rats with uric acid (a scavenger of peroxynitrite) significantly attenuated intracranial pressure, CSF white blood cell count, and BBB leakage (214). These data suggest that peroxynitrite is a central mediator in the pathophysiology of bacterial meningitis and that blockade of its toxicity may have a beneficial effect on these pathophysiologic alterations.

Excitatory Amino Acids

Finally, the potential role of excitatory amino acids (which mediate neuronal injury in a variety of brain disorders) in the pathogenesis of brain injury in bacterial meningitis has been proposed. In an experimental rabbit model, intracisternal inoculation of *S. pneumoniae* led to significant increases in CSF concentrations of glutamate, aspartate, glycine, taurine, and alanine (215). Elevated glutamate concentrations were also found in the brain extracellular space, suggesting that excitotoxic neuronal injury may play a role in bacterial meningitis. In an experimental rat model of group B streptococcal meningitis, administration of kynurenic acid (a nonselective inhibitor of the neurotoxic effects of excitatory amino acids) attenuated the toxic effects of glutamate by inhibition of neuronal excitatory amino acid receptors. Treated animals showed significantly less neuronal injury in the cortex and hippocampus than untreated controls (216), demonstrating the important contribution of glutamate to neurotoxicity in bacterial meningitis. Excess CSF concentrations of glutamate have also been detected in patients with bacterial meningitis (217,218). A prolonged increase in CSF glutamate concentrations may predict a poor outcome in patients with bacterial meningitis, possibly because of the sustained neurotoxic effects of this excitatory neurotransmitter.

Further studies are needed to clearly identify the mediators of neuronal injury in bacterial meningitis. It is hoped that this will lead to potent new adjunctive treatment strategies for this disorder.

REFERENCES

1. Tunkel AR, Wispelwey B, Scheld WM. Bacterial meningitis: recent advances in pathophysiology and treatment. *Ann Intern Med* 1990;112:610–623.
2. Quagliarello V, Scheld WM. Bacterial meningitis: pathogenesis, pathophysiology, and progress. *N Engl J Med* 1992;327:864–872.
3. Tunkel AR, Scheld WM. Pathogenesis and pathophysiology of bacterial meningitis. *Clin Microbiol Rev* 1993;6:118 136.
4. Pfister HW, Fontana A, Täuber MG, et al. Mechanisms of brain injury in bacterial meningitis: workshop summary. *Clin Infect Dis* 1994;19:463–479.
5. Lieb SL, T"uber MG. Pathogeneis of bacterial meningitis. *Infect Dis Clin North Am* 1999;13:527–548.
6. Koedel U, Pfister HW. Models of experimental bacterial meningitis: role and limitations. *Infect Dis Clin North Am* 1999;13:549–577.
7. Moxon ER, Smith AL, Averill DR, et al. *Haemophilus influenzae* meningitis in infant rats after intranasal inoculation. *J Infect Dis* 1974;129:154–162.
8. Moxon ER, Ostrow PT. *Haemophilus influenzae* bacteremia in infant rats: role of bacteremia in pathogenesis of age dependent inflammatory response in cerebrospinal fluid. *J Infect Dis* 1977;135:303–307.
9. Scheifele DW, Daum RS, Syriopoulou VP, et al. *Haemophilus influenzae* bacteremia and meningitis in infant primates. *J Lab Clin Med* 1980;95:450–462.
10. Dacey RG, Sande MA. Effect of probenecid on cerebrospinal fluid concentrations of penicillin and cephalosporin derivatives. *Antimicrob Agents Chemother* 1974;6:437–441.
11. Quagliarello VJ, Long WJ Jr, Scheld WM. Morphologic alterations in the blood-brain barrier with experimental meningitis in the rat: temporal sequence and role of encapsulation. *J Clin Invest* 1986;77:1084–1095.
12. Pfister HW, Koedel U, Haberl RL, et al. Microvascular changes during the early phase of experimental bacterial meningitis. *J Cereb Blood Flow Metab* 1990;10:914–922.
13. Tsai YH, Hirth RS, Leitner F. A murine model for listerial meningitis and meningoencephalomyelitis: therapeutic evaluation of drugs in mice. *Chemotherapy* 1980;26:196–206.

14. Tang T, Frenette PS, Hynes RO, et al. Cytokine-induced meningitis is dramatically attenuated in mice deficient in endothelial selectins. *J Clin Invest* 1996;97:2485–2490.
15. Stephens DS, Farley MM. Pathogenic events during infection of the human nasopharynx with *Neisseria meningitidis* and *Haemophilus influenzae*. *Rev Infect Dis* 1991;13:22–33.
16. Beachey EH. Bacterial adherence: adhesin-receptor interactions mediating the attachment of bacteria to mucosal surfaces. *J Infect Dis* 1981;143:325–345.
17. Tunkel AR, Scheld WM. Pathogenesis and pathophysiology of bacterial infections. In: Scheld WM, Whitley RJ, Durack DT, eds. *Infections of the central nervous system,* 2nd ed. Philadelphia: Lippincott-Raven, 1997:297–312.
18. Greenblatt JJ, Floyd K, Philipps MW, et al. Morphologic differences in *Neisseria meningitidis* pili. *Infect Immun* 1988;56:2356–2362.
19. Mason EO, Kaplan SL, Wiedermann BL, et al. Frequency and properties of naturally occurring adherent piliated strains of *Haemophilus influenzae* type b. *Infect Immun* 1985;49:98–103.
20. Stull TL, Mendelman PM, Haas JL, et al. Characterization of *Haemophilus influenzae* type b fimbriae. *Infect Immun* 1984;46:787–796.
21. Weber A, Harris K, Lohrke S, et al. Inability to express fimbriae results in impaired ability of *Haemophilus influenzae* type b to colonize the nasopharynx. *Infect Immun* 1991;59:4724–4728.
22. Pichichero ME, Loeb M, Anderson P, et al. Do pili play a role in pathogenicity of *Haemophilus influenzae* type b? *Lancet* 1982;2:960–962.
23. Smith AL. Pathogenesis of *Haemophilus influenzae* meningitis. *Pediatr Infect Dis J* 1987;6:783–786.
24. Moxon ER, Vaughn KA. The type b capsular polysaccharide as a virulence determinant of *Haemophilus influenzae*: studies using clinical isolates and laboratory transformants. *J Infect Dis* 1981;143:517–524.
25. Roberts M, Stull TL, Smith AL. Comparative virulence of *Haemophilus influenzae* with a type b or type d capsule. *Infect Immun* 1981;32:518–524.
26. Anderson P, Johnston RB, Smith DH. Human serum activities against *Haemophilus influenzae* type b. *J Clin Invest* 1972;51:31–38.
27. Moxon ER, Anderson P. Meningitis caused by *Haemophilus influenzae* in infant rats: protective immunity and antibody priming by gastrointestinal colonization with *Escherichia coli*. *J Infect Dis* 1979;140:471–478.
28. Schneerson R, Robbins JB. Induction of serum *Haemophilus influenzae* type b capsular antibodies in adult volunteers fed cross-reacting *Escherichia coli* O75:K100:H5. *N Engl J Med* 1975;292: 1093–1096.
29. Broome CV, Facklam RR, Allen JR, et al. Epidemiology of pneumococcal serotypes in the United States. *J Infect Dis* 1980;141:119–123.
30. Gray BM, Converse GM III, Dillon HC Jr. Serotypes of *Streptococcus pneumoniae* causing disease. *J Infect Dis* 1979;140:979–983.
31. Nesin M, Ramirez M, Tomasz A. Capsular transformation of a multidrug-resistant *Streptococcus pneumoniae in vitro*. *J Infect Dis* 1998;177:707–713.
32. Andersson B, Eriksson B, Falsen E, et al. Adhesion of *Streptococcus pneumoniae* to human pharyngeal epithelial cells *in vitro*: differences in adhesive capacity among strains isolated from subjects with otitis media, septicemia, or meningitis or from healthy carriers. *Infect Immun* 1981;32:311–317.
33. Lundberg C, Lonnroth J, Nord CE. Adherence in the colonization of *Streptococcus pneumoniae* in the nasopharynx of children. *Infection* 1982;10:63–69.
34. LiPuma JJ, Richman H, Stull TL. Haemocin, the bacteriocin produced by *Haemophilus influenzae*: species distribution and role in colonization. *Infect Immun* 1990;58:1600–1605.
35. Plaut AG. The IgA1 proteases of pathogenic bacteria. *Annu Rev Microbiol* 1983;37:603–622.
36. Mulks MH, Kornfeld SJ, Frangione B, et al. Relationship between the specificity of IgA proteases and serotypes in *Haemophilus influenzae*. *J Infect Dis* 1982;146:266–274.
37. Brooks GF, Lammel CJ, Blake MS, et al. Antibodies against IgA1 protease are stimulated both by clinical disease and asymptomatic carriage of serogroup A *Neisseria meningitidis*. *J Infect Dis* 1992;166:1316–1321.
38. Malley R, Stack AM, Ferretti ML, et al. Anticapsular polysaccharide antibodies and nasopharyngeal colonization with *Streptococcus pneumoniae* in infant rats. *J Infect Dis* 1998;178:878–882.
39. Robbins JB, McCracken GH Jr, Gotschlich EL, et al. *Escherichia coli* K1 capsular polysaccharide associated with neonatal meningitis. *N Engl J Med* 1974;290:1216–1220.
40. Cross AS, Gemski P, Sadoff JC, et al. The importance of the K1 capsule in invasive infections caused by *Escherichia coli*. *J Infect Dis* 1984;149:184–193.

41. Kim KS, Itabashi H, Gemski P, et al. The K1 capsule is the critical determinant in the development of *Escherichia coli* meningitis in the rat. *J Clin Invest* 1992;90:897–905.

42. Raff HV, Devereux D, Shuford W, et al. Human monoclonal antibody with protective activity for *Escherichia coli* K1 and *Neisseria meningitidis* group B infections. *J Infect Dis* 1988;157:118–126.

43. Fearon DT, Austen KF. The alternative pathway of complement: a system for host resistance to microbial infection. *N Engl J Med* 1980;303:259–263.

44. Frank MM, Joiner K, Hammer C. The function of antibody and complement in the lysis of bacteria. *Rev Infect Dis* 1987;9[Suppl 5]:S537–S545.

45. Horowitz MA. Phagocytosis of microorganisms. *Rev Infect Dis* 1982;4:104–118.

46. Brown EJ, Hosea SW, Hammer CH, et al. A quantitative analysis of the interactions of antipneumococcal antibody and complement in experimental pneumococcal bacteremia. *J Clin Invest* 1982;69: 85–98.

47. Brown EJ, Joiner KA, Cole RM, et al. Localization of complement component 3 on *Streptococcus pneumoniae:* anti-capsular antibody causes complement deposition on the pneumococcal capsule. *Infect Immun* 1983;39:403–409.

48. Bruyn GAW, Zegers BJM, van Furth R. Mechanisms of host defense against infection with *Streptococcus pneumoniae*. *Clin Infect Dis* 1992;14:251–262.

49. Quinn PH, Crosson FJ, Winkelstein JA, et al. Activation of the alternative complement pathway by *Haemophilus influenzae* type b. *Infect Immun* 1977;16:400–402.

50. Corral CJ, Winkelstein JA, Moxon ER. Participation of complement in host defense against encapsulated *Haemophilus influenzae* types a, c, and d. *Infect Immun* 1982;35:759–763.

51. Crosson FA Jr, Winkelstein JA, Moxon ER. Participation of complement in the nonimmune host defense against experimental *Haemophilus influenzae* bacteremia and meningitis. *Infect Immun* 1976;14:882–887.

52. Zwahlen A, Winkelstein JA, Moxon ER. Surface determinants of *Haemophilus influenzae* pathogenicity: comparative virulence of capsular transformants in normal and complement depleted rats. *J Infect Dis* 1983;148:385–394.

53. Ross SC, Densen P. Complement deficiency states and infection: epidemiology, pathogenesis, and consequences of neisserial and other infections in an immune deficiency. *Medicine (Baltimore)* 1984;63:243–273.

54. Brandtzaeg P, Mollnes TE, Kierulf P. Complement activation and endotoxin levels in systemic meningococcal disease. *J Infect Dis* 1989;160:58–65.

55. Smith AL, Daum RS, Scheifele D, et al. Pathogenesis of *Haemophilus influenzae* meningitis. In: Sell SH, Wright PF, eds. Haemophilus influenzae: *epidemiology, immunology, and prevention of disease.* New York: Elsevier Science Publishing, 1982:89–109.

56. Ostrow PT, Moxon ER, Vernon N, et al. Pathogenesis of bacterial meningitis: studies on the route of meningeal invasion following *Haemophilus influenzae* inoculation in infant rats. *Lab Invest* 1979;40:678–685.

57. Parkkinen J, Korhonen TK, Pere A, et al. Binding sites in the rat brain for *Escherichia coli* S fimbriae associated with neonatal meningitis. *J Clin Invest* 1988;81:860–865.

58. Saukkonen KM, Nowicki B, Leinonen M. Role of type 1 and S fimbriae in the pathogenesis of *Escherichia coli* O18:K1 bacteremia and meningitis in the infant rat. *Infect Immun* 1988;56: 892–897.

59. Pron B, Taha MK, Rambaud C, et al. Interaction of *Neisseria meningitidis* with the components of the blood-brain barrier correlates with an increased expression of PilC. *J Infect Dis* 1997;176:1285–1292.

60. Meier C, Oelschlaeger TA, Merkert H, et al. Ability of *Escherichia coli* isolates that cause meningitis in newborns to invade epithelial and endothelial cells. *Infect Immun* 1996;64:2391–2399.

61. Wilson SL, Drevets DA. *Listeria monocytogenes* infection and activation of human brain microvascular endothelial cells. *J Infect Dis* 1998;178:1658–1666.

62. Huang SH, Wass C, Fu Q, et al. *Escherichia coli* invasion of brain microvascular endothelial cells *in vitro* and *in vivo*: molecular cloning and characterization of invasion gene *ibe10*. *Infect Immun* 1995;63:4470–4475.

63. Bingen E, Bonacorsi S, Brahimi N, et al. Virulence patterns of *Escherichia coli* K1 strains associated with neonatal meningitis. *J Clin Microbiol* 1997;35:2981–2982.

64. Hoffman JA, Zhang Y, Badger JL, et al. Identification of a novel gene locus contributing to *E. coli* invasion of the blood-brain barrier. In: *Program and abstracts of the 37th Interscience Conference on Antimicrobial Agents and Chemotherapy.* Washington, DC: American Society for Microbiology, 1998.

65. Bingen E, Picard B, Brahimi N, et al. Phylogenetic analysis of *Escherichia coli* strains causing neonatal meningitis suggests horizontal gene transfer from a predominant pool of highly virulent B2 group stains. *J Infect Dis* 1998;177:642–650.
66. Andersen BM, Solberg O. Endotoxin liberation and invasivity of *Neisseria meningitidis. Scand J Infect Dis* 1984;16:247–254.
67. Takala AK, Eskola J, Bol P, et al. *Haemophilus influenzae* type b strains of outer membrane subtypes 1 and 1c cause different types of invasive disease. *Lancet* 1987;2:647–650.
68. Williams AE, Blakemore WF. Pathogenesis of meningitis caused by *Streptococcus suis* type 2. *J Infect Dis* 1990;162:474–481.
69. Ring A, Weiser JN, Tuomanen EI. Pneumococcal trafficking across the blood-brain barrier: molecular analysis of a novel bidirectional pathway. *J Clin Invest* 1998;102:347–360.
70. Rahal JJ Jr, Simberkoff MS. Host defense and antimicrobial therapy in adult gram-negative bacillary meningitis. *Ann Intern Med* 1982;96:468–474.
71. Simberkoff MS, Moldover HN, Rahal JJ Jr. Absence of detectable bactericidal and opsonic activities in normal and infected cerebrospinal fluids: a regional host defense deficiency. *J Lab Clin Med* 1980;95:362–372.
72. Tofte RW, Peterson PK, Kim Y, et al. Opsonic activity of normal human cerebrospinal fluid for selected species. *Infect Immun* 1979;26:1093–1098.
73. Bernhardt LL, Simberkoff MS, Rahal JJ Jr. Deficient cerebrospinal fluid opsonization in experimental *Escherichia coli* meningitis. *Infect Immun* 1981;32:411–413.
74. Whittle HC, Greenwood BM. Cerebrospinal fluid immunoglobulins and complement in meningococcal meningitis. *J Clin Pathol* 1977;30:720–722.
75. Scheld WM, Keeley JM. Effect of cerebrospinal fluid antibody-complement on the course of experimental pneumococcal meningitis. *Clin Res* 1983;31:375A.
76. Zwahlen A, Nydegger UE, Vandaux P, et al. Complement-mediated opsonic activity in normal and infected human cerebrospinal fluid: early response during bacterial meningitis. *J Infect Dis* 1982;145:635–646.
77. Smith H, Bannister B, O'Shea MJ. Cerebrospinal fluid immunoglobulins in meningitis. *Lancet* 1973;1:591–593.
78. Gigliotti F, Lee D, Insel RA, et al. IgG penetration into the cerebrospinal fluid in a rabbit model of meningitis. *J Infect Dis* 1987;156:394–398.
79. Flexner S. The results of serum treatment in 1300 cases of epidemic meningitis. *J Exp Med* 1913;17:553–576.
80. Bradbury MWB. The structure and function of the blood-brain barrier. *Fed Proc* 1984;43:186–190.
81. Goldstein GW, Betz AL. The blood-brain barrier. *Sci Am* 1986;255:74–83.
82. Waggener JD. The pathophysiology of bacterial meningitis and cerebral abscesses: an anatomical interpretation. *Adv Neurol* 1974;6:1–17.
83. Lesse AJ, Moxon ER, Zwahlen A, et al. Role of cerebrospinal fluid pleocytosis and *Haemophilus influenzae* type b capsule on blood brain barrier permeability during experimental meningitis in the rat. *J Clin Invest* 1988;82:102–109.
84. Wispelwey B, Lesse AJ, Hansen EJ, et al. *Haemophilus influenzae* lipopolysaccharide-induced blood brain barrier permeability during experimental meningitis in the rat. *J Clin Invest* 1988;82: 1339–1346.
85. Wispelwey B, Hansen EJ, Scheld WM. *Haemophilus influenzae* outer membrane vesicle-induced blood-brain barrier permeability during experimental meningitis. *Infect Immun* 1989;57:2559–2562.
86. Roord JJ, Apicella M, Scheld WM. The induction of meningeal inflammation and blood-brain barrier permeability by *Haemophilus influenzae* type b peptidoglycan. *J Infect Dis* 1994;170:254–256.
87. Tunkel AR, Scheld WM. Alterations in the blood-brain barrier in bacterial meningitis: *in vivo* and *in vitro* models. *Pediatr Infect Dis J* 1989;8:911–913.
88. Tunkel AR, Rosser SW, Hansen EJ, et al. Blood-brain barrier alterations in bacterial meningitis: development of an *in vitro* model and observations on the effects of lipopolysaccharide. *In Vitro Cell Dev Biol* 1991;27A:113–120.
89. Patrick D, Betts J, Frey EA, et al. *Haemophilus influenzae* lipopolysaccharide disrupts confluent monolayers of bovine brain endothelial cells via a serum-dependent cytotoxic pathway. *J Infect Dis* 1992;165:865–872.
90. Quagliarello VJ, Ma A, Stukenbrok H, et al. Ultrastructural localization of albumin transport across the cerebral microvasculature during experimental meningitis in the rat. *J Exp Med* 1991;174: 657–672.

91. Quagliarello VJ, Wispelwey B, Long WJ Jr, et al. Recombinant human interleukin-1 induces meningitis and blood-brain barrier injury in the rat: characterization and comparison with tumor necrosis factor. *J Clin Invest* 1991;87:1360–1366.
92. Sharief MK, Ciardi M, Thompson EJ. Blood-brain barrier damage in patients with bacterial meningitis: association with tumor necrosis factor-α but not interleukin-1β. *J Infect Dis* 1992;166:350–358.
93. Paul R, Lorenzl S, Koedel U, et al. Matrix metalloproteinases contribute to the blood-brain barrier disruption during bacterial meningitis. *Ann Neurol* 1998;44:592–600.
94. Kieseier BC, Paul R, Koedel U, et al. Differential expression of matrix metalloproteinases in bacterial meningitis. *Brain* 1999;122:1579–1587.
95. Ernst JD, Hartiala KT, Goldstein IM, et al. Complement (C5)-derived chemotactic activity accounts for accumulation of polymorphonuclear leukocytes in cerebrospinal fluid of rabbits with pneumococcal meningitis. *Infect Immun* 1984;46:81–86.
96. Kadurugamuwa JL, Hengstler B, Zak O. Inhibition of complement-factor-5a-induced inflammatory reactions by prostaglandin E_2 in experimental meningitis. *J Infect Dis* 1989;160:715–719.
97. Stahel PF, Frei K, Fontana A, et al. Evidence for intrathecal synthesis of alternative pathway complement activation proteins in experimental meningitis. *Am J Pathol* 1997;151:897–904.
98. Stahel PF, Nadal D, Pfister HW, et al. Complement C3 and factor B cerebrospinal fluid concentrations in bacterial and aseptic meningitis. *Lancet* 1997;349:1886–1887.
99. Seebach J, Bartholdi D, Frei K, et al. Experimental *Listeria* meningoencephalitis: macrophage inflammatory protein-1α and -2 are produced intrathecally and mediate chemotactic activity in cerebrospinal fluid of infected mice. *J Immunol* 1995;155:4367–4375.
100. Inaba Y, Ishiguro A, Shimbo T. The production of macrophage inflammatory protein-1 in the cerebrospinal fluid at the initial stage of meningitis in children. *Pediatr Res* 1997;42:788–793.
101. Spanaus KS, Nadal D, Pfister HW, et al. C-X-C and C-C chemokines are expressed in the cerebrospinal fluid in bacterial meningitis and mediate chemotactic activity on peripheral blood-derived polymorphonuclear and mononuclear cells *in vitro*. *J Immunol* 1997;158:1956–1964.
102. Sprenger H, Rosler A, Tonn P, et al. Chemokines in the cerebrospinal fluid of patients with meningitis. *Clin Immunol Immunopathol* 1996;80:155–161.
103. Rodriguez AF, Kaplan SL, Hawkins EP, et al. Hematogenous meningitis in the infant rat: description of a model. *J Infect Dis* 1991;164:1207–1209.
104. Tuomanen E, Tomasz A, Hengstler B, et al. The relative role of bacterial cell wall and capsule in the induction of inflammation in pneumococcal meningitis. *J Infect Dis* 1985;151:535–540.
105. Tuomanen E, Liu H, Hengstler B, et al. The induction of meningeal inflammation by components of the pneumococcal cell wall. *J Infect Dis* 1985;151:859–868.
106. Tuomanen E, Hengstler B, Rich R, et al. Nonsteroidal antiinflammatory agents in the therapy for experimental pneumococcal meningitis. *J Infect Dis* 1987;155:985–990.
107. Friedland IR, Paris MM, Hickey S, et al. The limited role of pneumolysin in the pathogenesis of pneumococcal meningitis. *J Infect Dis* 1995;172:805–809.
108. Syrogiannopoulos GA, Hansen EJ, Erwin AL, et al. *Haemophilus influenzae* type b lipooligosaccharide induces meningeal inflammation. *J Infect Dis* 1988;157:237–244.
109. Mustafa MM, Ramilo O, Syrogiannopoulos GA, et al. Induction of meningeal inflammation by outer membrane vesicles of *Haemophilus influenzae* type b. *J Infect Dis* 1989;159:917–922.
110. Mustafa MM, Ramilo O, Olsen KD, et al. Tumor necrosis factor in mediating experimental *Haemophilus influenzae* type b meningitis. *J Clin Invest* 1989;84:1253–259.
111. Mustafa MM, Ramilo O, Mertsola J, et al. Modulation of inflammation and cachectin activity in relation to treatment of experimental *Haemophilus influenzae* type b meningitis. *J Infect Dis* 1989;160:818–825.
112. Moller B, Mogensen SC, Wendelboe P, et al. Bioactive and inactive forms of tumor necrosis factor-α in spinal fluid from patients with meningitis. *J Infect Dis* 1991;163:886–889.
113. Leist TP, Frei K, Kam-Hansen S, et al. Tumor necrosis factor in cerebrospinal fluid during bacterial, but not viral, meningitis: evaluation in murine model infections and in patients. *J Exp Med* 1988;167:1743–1748.
114. Nadal D, Leppert D, Frei K, et al. Tumor necrosis factor-α in infectious meningitis. *Arch Dis Child* 1989;64:1274–1279.
115. Glimaker M, Kragsbjerg P, Forsgren M, et al. Tumor necrosis factor-α (TNFα) in cerebrospinal fluid from patients with meningitis of different etiologies: high levels of TNFα indicate bacterial meningitis. *J Infect Dis* 1993;167:882–889.

116. Lopez-Cortes LF, Cruz-Ruiz M, Gomez-Mateos J, et al. Measurement of levels of tumor necrosis factor-α and interleukin-1β in the CSF of patients with meningitis of different etiologies: utility in the differential diagnosis. *Clin Infect Dis* 1993;16:534–9.

117. Mustafa MM, Ramilo O, Saez-Llorens X, et al. Cerebrospinal fluid prostaglandins, interleukin 1, and tumor necrosis factor in bacterial meningitis: clinical and laboratory correlations in placebo-treated and dexamethasone-treated patients. *Am J Dis Child* 1990;144:883–887.

118. Ramilo O, Saez-Llorens X, Mertsola J, et al. Tumor necrosis factor α/cachectin and interleukin 1β initiate meningeal inflammation. *J Exp Med* 1990;172:497–507.

119. Saukkonen K, Sande S, Cioffe C, et al. The role of cytokines in the generation of inflammation and tissue damage in experimental gram-positive meningitis. *J Exp Med* 1990;171:439–448.

120. Cabellos C, MacIntyre DE, Forrest M, et al. Differing roles for platelet-activating factor during inflammation of the lung and subarachnoid space: the special case of *Streptococcus pneumoniae*. *J Clin Invest* 1992;90:612–618.

121. Townsend GC, Scheld WM. Platelet-activating factor augments meningeal inflammation elicited by *Haemophilus influenzae* lipooligosaccharide in an animal model of meningitis. *Infect Immun* 1994;62:3739–3744.

122. McCracken GH Jr, Mustafa MM, Ramilo O, et al. Cerebrospinal fluid interleukin 1-beta and tumor necrosis factor concentrations and outcome from neonatal gram-negative enteric bacillary meningitis. *Pediatr Infect Dis J* 1989;8:155–159.

123. Arditi M, Ables L, Yogev R. Cerebrospinal fluid endotoxin levels in children with *H. influenzae* meningitis before and after administration of intravenous ceftriaxone. *J Infect Dis* 1989;160: 1005–1011.

124. Friedland IR, Jafari H, Ehrett S, et al. Comparison of endotoxin release by different antimicrobial agents and the effect on inflammation in experimental *Escherichia coli* meningitis. *J Infect Dis* 1993;168:657–662.

125. Mustafa MM, Mertsola J, Ramilo O, et al. Increased endotoxin and interleukin-1β concentrations in cerebrospinal fluid of infants with coliform meningitis and ventriculitis associated with intraventricular gentamicin therapy. *J Infect Dis* 1989;160:891–895.

126. Mustafa MM, Lebel MH, Ramilo O, et al. Correlation of interleukin-1 and cachectin concentrations in cerebrospinal fluid and outcome from bacterial meningitis. *J Pediatr* 1989;115:208–213.

127. Arditi M, Manogue KR, Caplan M, et al. Cerebrospinal fluid cachectin/tumor necrosis factor-α and platelet-activating factor concentrations and severity of bacterial meningitis in children. *J Infect Dis* 1990;162:139–147.

128. Ossege LM, Sindern E, Voss B, et al. Expression of tumor necrosis factor-α and transforming growth factor-β 1 in cerebrospinal fluid cells in meningitis. *J Neurol Sci* 1996;144:1–13.

129. Ichiyama T, Hayashi T, Furukawa S. Cerebrospinal fluid concentrations of soluble tumor necrosis factor receptor in bacterial and aseptic meningitis. *Neurology* 1996;46:837–838.

130. Saez-Llorens X, Ramilo O, Mustafa MM, et al. Pentoxifylline modulates meningeal inflammation in experimental bacterial meningitis. *Antimicrob Agents Chemother* 1990;34:837–843.

131. Burroughs MH, Tsenova-Berkova L, Sokol K, et al. Effect of thalidomide on the inflammatory response in cerebrospinal fluid in experimental bacterial meningitis. *Microb Pathog* 1995;19:245–255.

132. Kartalija M, Kim Y, White ML, et al. Effect of recombinant N-terminal fragment of bactericidal/permeability-increasing protein (rBPI$_{23}$) on cerebrospinal fluid inflammation induced by endotoxin. *J Infect Dis* 1990;65:684–707.

133. Paris MM, Friedland IR, Ehrett S, et al. Effect of interleukin-1 receptor antagonist and soluble tumor necrosis factor receptor in animal models of infection. *J Infect Dis* 1995;171:161–9.

134. Rusconi F, Parizzi F, Garlaschi L, et al. Interleukin 6 activity in infants and children with bacterial meningitis. *Pediatr Infect Dis J* 1991;10:117–121.

135. Waage A, Halstensen A, Shalaby R, et al. Local production of tumor necrosis factor α, interleukin 1, and interleukin 6 in meningococcal meningitis: relation to the inflammatory response. *J Exp Med* 1989;170:1859–1867.

136. Chavanet P, Bonnotte B, Guiguet M, et al. High concentrations of intrathecal interleukin-6 in human bacterial and nonbacterial meningitis. *J Infect Dis* 1992;166:428–431.

137. Azuma H, Tsuda N, Sasaki K, et al. Clinical significance of cytokine measurements for detection of meningitis. *J Pediatr* 1997;131:463–465.

138. Waage A, Brandtzaeg P, Halstensen A, et al. The complex pattern of cytokines in serum from patients with meningococcal septic shock: association between interleukin 6, interleukin 1, and fatal outcome. *J Exp Med* 1989;169:333–338.

139. Halstensen A, Ceska M, Brandtzaeg P, et al. Interleukin-8 in serum and cerebrospinal fluid from patients with meningococcal disease. *J Infect Dis* 1993;167:471–475.
140. Lopez-Cortes LF, Cruz-Ruiz M, Gomez-Mateous J, et al. Interleukin-8 in cerebrospinal fluid from patients with meningitis of different etiologies: its possible role as neutrophil chemotactic factor. *J Infect Dis* 1995;172:581–584.
141. Ostergaard C, Benfield TL, Sellebjerg F, et al. Interleukin-8 in cerebrospinal fluid from patients with septic and aseptic meningitis. *Eur J Clin Microbiol Infect Dis* 1996;15:166–169.
142. Frei K, Nadal D, Pfister HW, et al. *Listeria* meningitis: identification of a cerebrospinal fluid inhibitor of macrophage listericidal function as interleukin-10. *J Exp Med* 1993;178:1255–1261.
143. Van Furth AM, Seijmonsbergen EM, Langermans JAM, et al. High levels of interleukin-10 and tumor necrosis factor in cerebrospinal fluid during the onset of bacterial meningitis. *Clin Infect Dis* 1995;21:220–222.
144. Diab A, Zhu J, Lindquist L, et al. Cytokine mRNA profiles during the course of experimental *Haemophilus influenzae* bacterial meningitis. *Clin Immunol Immunopathol* 1997;85:236–245.
145. Kornelisse RF, Savelkoul HFJ, Mulder PHG, et al. Interleukin-10 and soluble tumor necrosis factor receptors in cerebrospinal fluid of children with bacterial meningitis. *J Infect Dis* 1996;173: 1498–1502.
146. Paris MM, Hickey SM, Trujillo M, et al. The effect of interleukin-10 on meningeal inflammation in experimental bacterial meningitis. *J Infect Dis* 1997;176:1239–1246.
147. Kornelisse RF, Hack CE, Savelkoul HFJ, et al. Intrathecal production of interleukin-12 and gamma interferon in patients with bacterial meningitis. *Infect Immun* 1997;65:877–881.
148. Schleimer RP, Rutledge BK. Cultured human vascular endothelial cells acquire adhesiveness for neutrophils after stimulation with interleukin 1, endotoxin, and tumor-promoting phorbol diesters. *J Immunol* 1986;136:649–654.
149. Thomas PD, Hampson FW, Casale JM, et al. Neutrophil adherence to human endothelial cells. *J Lab Clin Med* 1988;111:286–292.
150. Bevilacqua MP, Pober JS, Wheeler ME, et al. Interleukin 1 acts on cultured human vascular endothelium to increase the adhesion of polymorphonuclear leukocytes, monocytes, and related leukocyte cell lines. *J Clin Invest* 1985;76:2003–2011.
151. Varani J, Bendelow J, Sealey DE, et al. Tumor necrosis factor enhances susceptibility of vascular endothelial cells to neutrophil-mediated killing. *Lab Invest* 1988;59:292–295.
152. Moser R, Schleiffenbaum B, Groscurth P, et al. Interleukin 1 and tumor necrosis factor stimulate human vascular endothelial cells to promote transendothelial neutrophil passage. *J Clin Invest* 1989;83:444–455.
153. Springer TA. Adhesion receptors of the immune system. *Nature* 1990;346:425–434.
154. Bevilacqua MP, Stengelin S, Gimbrone MA Jr, et al. Endothelial leukocyte adhesion molecule 1: an inducible receptor for neutrophils related to complement regulatory proteins and lectins. *Science* 1989;243:1160–1165.
155. Tan TQ, Smith W, Hawkins EP, et al. Hematogenous bacterial meningitis in an intercellular adhesion molecule-1-deficient infant mouse model. *J Infect Dis* 1995;171:342–349.
156. Weber JR, Angstwurm K, Burger W, et al. Anti ICAM (CD 54) monoclonal antibody reduces inflammatory changes in experimental bacterial meningitis. *J Neuroimmunol* 1995;63:63–68.
157. Tuomanen EI, Saukkonen K, Sande S, et al. Reduction of inflammation, tissue damage, and mortality in bacterial meningitis in rabbits treated with monoclonal antibodies against adhesion-promoting receptors of leukocytes. *J Exp Med* 1989;170:959–968.
158. Saez-Llorens X, Jafari HS, Severien C, et al. Enhanced attenuation of meningeal inflammation and brain edema by concomitant administration of anti-CD18 monoclonal antibodies and dexamethasone in experimental *Haemophilus* meningitis. *J Clin Invest* 1991;88:2003–2011.
159. Rozdzinski E, Jones T, Burnette WN, et al. Antiinflammatory effects in experimental meningitis of prokaryotic peptides that mimic selectins. *J Infect Dis* 1993;168:1422–1428.
160. Tan TQ, Smith W, Hawkins EP, et al. Anti-CD11b monoclonal antibody in an infant rat model of *Haemophilus influenzae* type b sepsis and meningitis. *J Antimicrob Chemother* 1997;39: 209–216.
161. Tang T, Frenette PS, Hynes RO, et al. Cytokine-induced meningitis is dramatically attenuated in mice deficient in endothelial selectins. *J Clin Invest* 1996;97:2485–2490.
162. Granert C, Raud J, Xie I, et al. Inhibition of leukocyte rolling with polysaccharide fucoidin prevents pleocytosis in experimental meningitis in the rabbit. *J Clin Invest* 1994;93:929–936.
163. Tuomanen E. A spoonful of sugar to control inflammation? *J Clin Invest* 1994;93:917–918.

164. Lorenzl S, Loedel U, Dirnagl U, et al. Imaging of leukocyte-endothelium interaction using *in vivo* confocal laser scanning microscopy during the early phase of experimental pneumococcal meningitis. *J Infect Dis* 1993;168:927–933.
165. Weber JR, Angstwurm K, Rosenkranz T, et al. Heparin inhibits leukocyte rolling in pial vessels and attenuates inflammatory changes in a rat model of experimental bacterial meningitis. *J Cereb Blood Flow Metab* 1997;17:1221–1229.
166. Fishman RA. Brain edema. *N Engl J Med* 1975;293:706–711.
167. Scheld WM, Dacey RG, Winn HR, et al. Cerebrospinal fluid outflow resistance in rabbits with experimental meningitis: alterations with penicillin and methylprednisolone. *J Clin Invest* 1980;66: 243–253.
168. Täuber MG, Khayam-Bashi H, Sande MA. Effects of ampicillin and corticosteroids on brain water content, cerebrospinal fluid pressure, and cerebrospinal fluid lactate levels in experimental pneumococcal meningitis. *J Infect Dis* 1985;151:528–534.
169. Syrogiannopoulos GA, Olsen KD, Reisch JS, et al. Dexamethasone in the treatment of experimental *Haemophilus influenzae* type b meningitis. *J Infect Dis* 1987;155:213–219.
170. Tureen JH, Täuber MG, Sande MA. Effect of indomethacin on the pathophysiology of experimental meningitis in rabbits. *J Infect Dis* 1991;163:647–649.
171. Kadurugamuwa JL, Hengstler B, Zak O. Cerebrospinal fluid protein profile in experimental pneumococcal meningitis and its alteration by ampicillin and anti-inflammatory agents. *J Infect Dis* 1989;159:26–34.
172. Täuber MG, Shibl AM, Hackbarth CJ, et al. Antibiotic therapy, endotoxin concentrations in cerebrospinal fluid, and brain edema in experimental *Escherichia coli* meningitis in rabbits. *J Infect Dis* 1987;156:456–462.
173. Burroughs M, Prasad S, Cabellos C, et al. The biologic activities of peptido-glycan in experimental *Haemophilus influenzae* meningitis. *J Infect Dis* 1993;167:464–468.
174. Täuber MG, Borschberg U, Sande MA. Influence of granulocytes on brain edema, intracranial pressure, and cerebrospinal fluid concentrations of lactate and protein in experimental meningitis. *J Infect Dis* 1988;157:456–464.
175. Täuber MG, Burroughs M, Neimoller UM, et al. Differences of pathophysiology in experimental meningitis caused by three strains of *Streptococcus pneumoniae*. *J Infect Dis* 1991;163:806–811.
176. Engelhard D, Pomeranz S, Gallily R, et al. Serotype-related differences in inflammatory response to *Streptococcus pneumoniae* in experimental meningitis. *J Infect Dis* 1997;175:979–982.
177. Syrogiannopoulos GA, Olsen KD, McCracken GH Jr. Mannitol treatment in experimental *Haemophilus influenzae* type b meningitis. *Pediatr Res* 1987;22:118–122.
178. Lorenzl S, Koedel U, Pfister HW. Mannitol, but not allopurinol, modulates changes in cerebral blood flow, intracranial pressure, and brain water content during pneumococcal meningitis in the rat. *Crit Care Med* 1996;24:1874–1880.
179. Raimondi AJ, DiRocco C. The physiopathogenetic basis for the angiographic diagnosis of bacterial infection of the brain and its coverings in children. I. Leptomeningitis. *Child's Brain* 1979;5:398–413.
180. Igarashi M, Gilmartin RC, Gerald B, et al. Cerebral arteritis and bacterial meningitis. *Arch Neurol* 1984;41:531–535.
181. Yamashima T, Kashihara K, Ikeda K, et al. Three phases of cerebral arteriopathy in meningitis: vasospasm and vasodilatation followed by organic stenosis. *Neurosurgery* 1985;16:546–553.
182. Tureen JH, Dworkin SL, Kennedy SL, et al. Loss of cerebrovascular autoregulation in experimental meningitis in rabbits. *J Clin Invest* 1990;85:577–581.
183. Tureen JH, Täuber MG, Sande MA. Effect of hydration status on cerebral blood flow and cerebrospinal fluid lactic acidosis in rabbits with experimental meningitis. *J Clin Invest* 1992;89:947–953.
184. Tureen J, Liu Q, Chow L. Near-infrared spectroscopy in experimental pneumococcal meningitis in the rabbit: cerebral hemodynamics and metabolism. *Pediatr Res* 1996;40:759–763.
185. Slater AJ, Berkowitz ID, Wilson DA, et al. Role of leukocytes in cerebral autoregulation and hyperemia in bacterial meningitis in rabbits. *Am J Physiol* 1997;42:H380–H386.
186. Koedel U, Lorenzl S, Gorriz C, et al. Endothelin B receptor-mediated increase of cerebral blood flow in experimental pneumococcal meningitis. *J Cereb Blood Flow Metab* 1998;18:67–74.
187. Koedel U, Gorriz C, Lorenzl S, et al. Increased endothelin levels in cerebrospinal fluid samples from adults with bacterial meningitis. *Clin Infect Dis* 1997;25:329–330.
188. Paulson OB, Brodersen P, Hansen EL, et al. Regional cerebral blood flow, cerebral metabolic rate of oxygen, and cerebrospinal fluid acid-base variables in patients with acute meningitis and with acute encephalitis. *Acta Med Scand* 1974;196:191–205.

189. McMenamin JB, Volpe JJ. Bacterial meningitis in infancy: effects on intracranial pressure and cerebral blood flow velocity. *Neurology* 1984;34:500–504.
190. Goh D, Minns RA. Cerebral blood flow velocity monitoring in pyogenic meningitis. *Arch Dis Child* 1993;68:111–119.
191. Ashwal S, Stringer W, Tomasi L, et al. Cerebral blood flow and carbon dioxide reactivity in children with bacterial meningitis. *J Pediatr* 1990;117:523–530.
192. Ashwal S, Tomasi L, Schneider S, et al. Bacterial meningitis in children: pathophysiology and treatment. *Neurology* 1992;42:739–748.
193. Pfister HW, Borasio GD, Dirnagl U, et al. Cerebrovascular complications of bacterial meningitis in adults. *Neurology* 1992;42:1497–504.
194. Guerra-Romero L, Täuber MG, Fournier MA, et al. Lactate and glucose concentrations in brain interstitial fluid, cerebrospinal fluid, and serum during experimental pneumococcal meningitis. *J Infect Dis* 1992;166:546–550.
195. Park WS, Chang YS, Lee M. Effect of induced hyperglycemia on brain cell membrane function and energy metabolism during the early phase of experimental meningitis in newborn piglets. *Brain Res* 1998;798:195–203.
196. Pfister HW, Koedel U, Lorenzl S, et al. Antioxidants attenuate microvascular changes in the early phase of experimental pneumococcal meningitis in rats. *Stroke* 1992;23:1798–1804.
197. Pfister HW, Ködel U, Dirnagl U, et al. Effect of catalase on regional cerebral blood flow and brain edema during the early phase of experimental pneumococcal meningitis. *J Infect Dis* 1992;166:1442–1445.
198. Leib SL, Kim YS, Chow LL, et al. Reactive oxygen intermediates contribute to necrotic and apoptotic neuronal injury in an infant rat model of bacterial meningitis due to group B streptococci. *J Clin Invest* 1996;98:2632–2639.
199. Bogdan I, Leib SL, Bergeron M, et al. Tumor necrosis factor-α contributes to apoptosis in hippocampal neurons during experimental group B streptococcal meningitis. *J Infect Dis* 1997;176:693–697.
200. Tsao N, Kanakamma PP, Luh TY, et al. Inhibition of *Escherichia coli*-induced meningitis by carboxyfullerence. *Antimicrob Agents Chemother* 1999;43:2273–2277.
201. Bottcher T, Gerber J, Wellmer A, et al. Rifampin reduces production of reactive oxygen species of cerebrospinal fluid phagocytes and hippocampal neuronal apoptosis in experimental *Streptococcus pneumoniae* meningitis. *J Infect Dis* 2000;181:2095–2098.
202. Auer M, Pfister LA, Leppert D, et al. Effects of clinically used antioxidants in experimental pneumococcal meningitis. *J Infect Dis* 2000;182:347–350.
203. Shenep JL, Tuomanen E. Perspective: targeting nitric oxide in the adjuvant therapy of sepsis and meningitis. *J Infect Dis* 1998;177:766–769.
204. Kortytko PJ, Boje KMK. Pharmacological characterization of nitric oxide production in a rat model of meningitis. *Neuropharmacology* 1996,35.231=237.
205. Koedel U, Bernatowicz A, Paul R, et al. Experimental pneumococcal meningitis: cerebrovascular alterations, brain edema, and meningeal inflammation are linked to the production of nitric oxide. *Ann Neurol* 1995;37:313–323.
206. Paul R, Koedel U, Pfister HW. 7-Nitroindazole inhibits pial vasodilation in a rat model of pneumococcal meningitis. *J Cereb Blood Flow Metab* 1997;17:985–991.
207. Buster BL, Weintrob AC, Townsend GC, et al. Potential role of nitric oxide in the pathophysiology of experimental bacterial meningitis in the rat. *Infect Immun* 1995;63:3835–3839.
208. Boje KMK. Inhibition of nitric oxide synthase attenuates blood-brain barrier disruption during experimental meningitis. *Brain Res* 1996;720:75–83.
209. Leib SL, Kim YS, Black SM, et al. Inducible nitric oxide synthase and the effect of aminoguanidine in experimental neonatal meningitis. *J Infect Dis* 1998;177:692–700.
210. Lorenzl S, Koedel U, Frei K, et al. Effect of the bradykinin B_2 receptor antagonist Hoe140 in experimental pneumococcal meningitis in the rat. *Eur J Pharmacol* 1996;308:335–341.
211. Koedel U, Bernatowicz A, Frei K, et al. Systemically (but not intrathecally) administered IL-10 attenuates pathophysiologic alterations in experimental pneumococcal meningitis. *J Immunol* 1996;157:5185–5191.
212. Kornelisse RF, Hoekman K, Visser JJ, et al. The role of nitric oxide in bacterial meningitis in children. *J Infect Dis* 1996;174:120–126.
213. Van Furth AM, Seijmonsbergen EM, Groeneveld PHP, et al. Levels of nitric oxide correlate with high levels of tumor necrosis factor in cerebrospinal fluid samples from children with bacterial meningitis. *Clin Infect Dis* 1996;22:876–878.

214. Kastenbauer S, Koedel U, Pfister HW. Role of peroxynitrite as a mediator of pathophysiological alterations in experimental pneumococcal meningitis. *J Infect Dis* 1999;180:1164–1170.
215. Guerra-Romero L, Tureen JH, Gournier MA, et al. Amino acids in cerebrospinal and brain interstitial fluid in experimental pneumococcal meningitis. *Pediatr Res* 1993;33:510–513.
216. Leib SL, Kim YS, Ferriero DM, et al. Neuroprotective effect of excitatory amino acid antagonist kynurenic acid in experimental bacterial meningitis. *J Infect Dis* 1996;173:166–171.
217. Spranger M, Krempien S, Schwab S, et al. Excess glutamate in the cerebrospinal fluid in bacterial meningitis. *J Neurol Sci* 1996;143:126–131.
218. Spranger M, Schwab S, Krempien S, et al. Excess glutamate levels in the cerebrospinal fluid predict clinical outcome of bacterial meningitis. *Arch Neurol* 1996;53:992–996.

4

Clinical Presentation

The clinical features of patients with acute bacterial meningitis are critical for clinicians to recognize because earlier suspicion of this disorder leads to prompt initiation of appropriate therapy that may improve outcome. Many of the clinical features of bacterial meningitis can be correlated to the pathogenic and pathophysiologic mechanisms operable in this disorder (Table 4.1). In the review by Swartz and Dodge of 207 patients with bacterial meningitis who presented to the Massachusetts General Hospital from 1956 to 1962, headache, lethargy or confusion, vomiting, irritability, and fever were noted in the majority of patients (1). More than 80% of patients had nuchal rigidity, a finding absent most often in young infants with bacterial meningitis. The initial clinical findings of patients in this study could be divided into two groups based on rapidity of onset of symptoms and signs: (a) a rapidly progressive clinical course that developed over the first 24 hours of illness and (b) progression of symptomatology over several days.

In another study of 209 patients with bacterial meningitis who presented to King County Hospital in Seattle, Washington (2), most patients also reported fever, lethargy, confusion, headache, vomiting, and/or stiff neck to support the diagnosis of bacterial meningitis; in addition, some degree of confusion was evident in the majority of patients at the time of presentation. The initial clinical presentation followed one of three patterns: (a) rapid onset of headache, confusion, lethargy, and loss of consciousness; (b) slowly progressive symptoms of meningitis for 1 to 7 days prior to admission; and (c) an infection in the respiratory tract that developed 1 to 3 weeks before the first "meningeal" symptoms appeared. In this study, 81% of patients presented with stiff neck, Kernig's sign, or Brudzinski's sign, the classic signs of meningeal irritation (3). Kernig's sign is elicited with the patient in the supine position, in which the thigh is flexed on the abdomen with the knee flexed. The leg is then passively extended, and, in the presence of meningeal irritation, the patient resists leg extension. This differs somewhat from the maneuver as initially described by Kernig, in which the patient was initially placed in the seated position; in this position, knee extension was resisted so that a "contracture of the extremities" was maintained. Several signs were described by Brudzinski, although the best known is the nape-of-the-neck sign, in which passive flexion of the neck results in flexion of the

TABLE 4.1. *Correlation of pathogenesis and pathophysiology to clinical presentation in patients with bacterial meningitis*

Pathogenic or pathophysiologic parameter	Potential clinical findings
Bacteremia and sepsis	Hyperthermia, hypothermia, myalgias, arthralgias, gastrointestinal dysfunction, respiratory distress, petechiae or purpura, shock
Subarachnoid space inflammation	Nuchal rigidity, Kernig's sign, Brudzinski's sign, cranial nerve palsies, ataxia, hearing loss, headache
Increased intracranial pressure	Altered mental status, headache, cranial nerve palsies, focal neurologic deficits, seizures, bulging fontanelle, nausea, vomiting, hyperreflexia, bradycardia and hypertension (Cushing's reflex)
Alteration in cerebral blood flow	Focal neurologic deficits, seizures, altered mental status, encephalopathy

hips and knees. The identical contralateral reflex sign is elicited with the patient in the supine position by passively flexing the hip and the knee on one side; the sign is positive when the contralateral leg flexes. The reciprocal contralateral reflex sign is elicited when the leg that has flexed in response to passive flexion of the other leg begins to extend spontaneously, resembling a "little kick." However, these signs may not be elicited in the very young, very old, or severely obtunded patient with acute bacterial meningitis.

The severity and rapidity of progression of clinical findings prior to initial presentation was recently reviewed in an analysis of 22 studies consisting of 4,707 patients with bacterial meningitis (4); these studies were heterogeneous with regard to study numbers, ages of patients, and causative microorganisms. Three basic patterns of illness prior to clinical presentation were described. The most common presentation was an insidious one with nonspecific symptoms (e.g., fever, malaise, irritability, vomiting) that progressed over less than 3 to 5 days before bacterial meningitis was diagnosed. A second presentation (seen in a small number of patients) was a fulminant course with rapid deterioration early in the course of illness. A third group had clinically recognizable evidence of meningitis that was not fulminant and progressed over the course of a day or so. Recognition of these patterns may be helpful in determining the need for emergent antimicrobial therapy in patients with bacterial meningitis. This is discussed in detail in Chapter 7.

Despite the clinical features of bacterial meningitis documented in these reviews, the clinical presentation may vary based on a number of factors, including patient age, presence of underlying conditions, severity of illness at presentation, and the specific microorganism isolated. The following sections will review the importance of these parameters in the clinical presentation of acute bacterial meningitis.

AGE

Neonates

The clinical manifestations of bacterial meningitis in the neonate are shown in Table 4.2 (5–10). As a rule, the clinical findings of bacterial meningitis in neonates are minimal and often subtle, making an early diagnosis difficult to establish clinically. In this patient population, the classic signs of meningeal irritation (nuchal rigidity, Kernig's or Brudzinski's signs) are less common, and a bulging fontanelle usually occurs late in the course of disease. Therefore it is critical to maintain a high index of suspicion in this patient population to make an early diagnosis of bacterial meningitis.

The clinical presentation of bacterial meningitis in neonates can be divided into two groups based on age: (a) those with early-onset disease (less than 48 hours of age) and (b) those with late-onset disease (from 7 days after birth up to 6 weeks of age) (9). In neonates with early-onset disease, the clinical picture is one of sepsis without specific symptoms referable to the central nervous system (CNS). In this group, symptoms of gastrointestinal dysfunction and respiratory distress predominate; CNS dysfunction is observed in only one-third of patients. Typically, these neonates have fever with subsequent temperature instability, respiratory distress, abdominal distention, vomiting, poor feeding, weak suck, diarrhea, poor muscle tone, and lethargy.

TABLE 4.2. *Clinical findings in neonatal bacterial meningitis*

Clinical finding	Relative frequency (%)
Temperature instability[a]	60–65
Lethargy	60
Irritability	30–60
Gastrointestinal dysfunction[b]	50
Respiratory distress	30–35
Seizures	20–50
Bulging fontanelle	20–25
Nuchal rigidity	10–15

[a] Hypothermia or hyperthermia.
[b] Abdominal distention, anorexia, vomiting, diarrhea.
Data from Saez-Llorens X, McCracken GH Jr. Bacterial meningitis in neonates and children. *Infect Dis Clin North Am* 1990;4:623–644; Baumgartner ET, Augustine RA, Steele RW. Bacterial meningitis in older neonates. *Am J Dis Child* 1983;137:1052–1054; Shattuck K, Chonmaitree T. The changing spectrum of neonatal meningitis over a fifteen-year period. *Clin Pediatr* 1992;31:130–136; Adhikari M, Coovadia YM, Singh D. A 4-year study of neonatal meningitis: clinical and microbiologic findings. *J Trop Pediatr* 1995;41:81–85; Smith AL. Neonatal bacterial meningitis. In: Scheld WM, Whitley RJ, Durack DT, eds. *Infections of the central nervous system*, 2nd ed. New York: Lippincott-Raven Publishers; 1997:313–334; and Pong A, Bradley JS. Bacterial meningitis and the newborn infant. *Infect Dis Clin North Am* 1999;13: 711–733, with permission.

In contrast, neonates with late-onset disease have more specific CNS findings, with seizures reported in approximately 50% of cases, although subtle seizures may be missed. Fever is a more prominent finding in this patient group.

Children

Bacterial meningitis in children may present insidiously with development of progressive symptoms over 1 or more days, or acutely and fulminantly with clinical manifestations over a few hours followed by rapid progression to cerebral edema and transtentorial herniation. The usual initial complaints in children with bacterial meningitis are fever, headache, photophobia, anorexia, nausea and vomiting, mental confusion and lethargy, restlessness, somnolence, and excessive irritability (5,11,12). A change in the child's affect and/or state of alertness is among the most important signs of bacterial meningitis. Meningeal signs are usually present later in the course of illness. In one review of bacterial meningitis in children 1 to 4 years of age, fever (94%), vomiting (82%), and nuchal rigidity (77%) were the most common presenting symptoms (13). Although fever is an expected finding in children with bacterial meningitis, one study found that 44% of older children (>6 years of age) were afebrile at the time of initial presentation (14).

The clinical presentation of bacterial meningitis in children may also include seizures (20% to 40% of cases), focal neurologic findings (approximately 15% of cases), ataxia, and hearing deficits (5,11,12). Seizures usually occur within the first 2 or 3 days of illness. Although seizures may be associated with fever in young children (generally those between 3 months and 5 years of age), when seizures occur with any clinical signs of meningitis, a lumbar puncture is indicated. In addition, all children with new onset of febrile seizures should be reexamined within 1 to 4 hours of initial evaluation to be certain that serious disease is not present. Focal neurologic deficits (e.g., hemiparesis, quadriparesis, facial palsy, endophthalmitis, visual field defects) may occur early or late in the course of disease and may be related to several pathophysiologic processes. Cranial nerve palsies may result as the nerve becomes ensheathed in purulent exudate in the subarachnoid sheath as it exits the base of brain, or may occur secondary to increased intracranial pressure. Hemiparesis may be caused by alterations in cerebral blood flow (from vasculitis and cerebral infarction) or may be a sign of a large subdural effusion, which develops when the infection in the adjacent subarachnoid space leads to increased permeability of thin-walled capillaries and veins in the inner layer of the dura. This process is usually self-limited, although an enlarging effusion may cause mass effect. The majority (84%) of subdural effusions occur in patients between 1 and 24 months of age (5). The concomitant presence of fever suggests the possibility of an infected subdural effusion. Ataxia may result from vestibular dysfunction and is associated with hearing loss in children with bacterial meningitis. The hearing loss is likely related to damage to the inner ear or cranial nerve VIII and is independent of damage to the CNS.

Children with bacterial meningitis may also present with a more rapidly progressive illness with symptoms and signs of increased intracranial pressure, manifesting as an altered level of consciousness, dilated, poorly reactive or nonreactive pupils, abnormalities of ocular motility, pathologically brisk lower-extremity reflexes, and bradycardia and hypertension (Cushing's reflex). It is important to note that the absence of papilledema at initial presentation does not exclude the presence of increased intracranial pressure in any patient with bacterial meningitis.

Adults

Adult patients with bacterial meningitis classically present with fever, headache, nuchal rigidity, and signs of cerebral dysfunction (i.e., confusion, delirium, or a declining level of consciousness ranging from lethargy to coma) (1,2,11). Two recent reviews of bacterial meningitis in adults have attempted to define the relative frequency of certain clinical findings (Table 4.3) (15,16). In one review of 279 episodes of acute community-acquired bacterial meningitis in adults (16 years of age and older) (15), the classic triad of fever, nuchal rigidity, and change in mental status was found in only two-thirds of patients, but all patients had at least one of these findings. Fever was present in 95% of patients at presentation and in an additional 4% of patients during the next 24 hours. Neck stiffness and altered mental status were observed in 88% and 78% of patients, respectively. Papilledema was documented in only 4% of episodes, although funduscopic examinations were not recorded for many patients. Seizures (focal, generalized, or those not characterized) occurred in 23% of episodes, in contrast to other studies that reported seizures in 0 to 12% of adult patients with bacterial meningitis. Similar clinical findings were observed in a recent 20-year review of 119 episodes of bacterial meningitis in adults in Iceland (Table 4.3) (16). The most common findings were fever, neck stiffness, and altered mental status, with all three findings observed in 51% of cases.

TABLE 4.3. *Clinical findings in adults with bacterial meningitis*

	Relative frequency	
Clinical finding	Massachusetts General Hospital (1962–1988) ($N = 279$ episodes)	University of Iceland (1975–1994) ($N = 119$ episodes)
Fever	95	97
Neck stiffness	88	82
Altered mental status	78	66
Triad of fever, neck stiffness, and altered mental status	66	51
Focal neurologic findings	29	10
Seizures	23	10
Rash	11	52
Papilledema	4	—

Data from Durand ML, Calderwood SB, Weber DL, et al. Acute bacterial meningitis in adults: a review of 493 episodes. *N Engl J Med* 1993;328:21–28; and Sigurdardottir B, Bjornsson OM, Jonsdottir KE, et al. Acute bacterial meningitis in adults: A 20-year overview. *Arch Intern Med* 1997;157:425–430, with permission.

TABLE 4.4. *Sensitivity of physical examination findings in the diagnosis of acute meningitis*

Physical examination finding	Percentage of pooled sensitivity (confidence interval)
Fever	85 (78–91)
Neck stiffness	70 (58–82)
Altered mental status	67 (52–82)
Triad of fever, neck stiffness, and altered mental status	46 (22–69)
Focal neurologic findings	23 (15–31)
Rash	22 (1–43)

Data from Attia J, Hatala R, Cook DJ, et al. Does this adult patient have acute meningitis? *JAMA* 1999;282: 175–181, with permission.

To further characterize the accuracy and precision of the clinical examination in adult patients with acute meningitis, a recent study reviewed previously published data on 845 patient episodes of acute meningitis (confirmed by lumbar puncture or autopsy) in patients aged 16 to 95 years and determined the sensitivity of the clinical history and physical examination in the diagnosis of acute meningitis (17). Although the majority of patients in this review had acute bacterial meningitis, 62 of the patients had tuberculous or "aseptic" meningitis. The results indicated that individual items of the clinical history (i.e., headache, nausea, and vomiting) had a low accuracy for the diagnosis of acute meningitis in adults. However, on review of the accuracy of physical examination findings (Table 4.4), the absence of fever, neck stiffness, and altered mental status effectively eliminated the likelihood of acute meningitis. The sensitivity was 99% to 100% for the presence of one of these findings in the diagnosis of acute meningitis. However, despite these findings and given the serious nature of this disease, physicians should have a low threshold for lumbar puncture in patients at high risk for bacterial meningitis.

Elderly

Bacterial meningitis in elderly patients, especially those with underlying conditions (e.g., diabetes mellitus or cardiopulmonary disease), may present insidiously with lethargy or obtundation and variable signs of meningeal irritation.

In one review of 54 elderly patients (aged 50 years and older) with bacterial meningitis (18), confusion was very common on initial presentation, occurring in 92% and 78% of those with pneumococcal and gram-negative bacillary meningitis, respectively. Overall, 89% of patients presented with altered mental status. In another review of 28 episodes of bacterial meningitis in patients 65 years of age and older (19), fever and altered mental status at presentation were observed in 100% and 96% of patients, respectively, although neck stiffness was found in only 57% of cases. Therefore the diagnosis of acute bacterial meningitis must be considered in all febrile elderly patients who are either disoriented, stuporous, or comatose. In addition, the elderly patient with bacterial meningitis may also present with an antecedent or concurrent bronchitis, pneumonia, or paranasal sinusitis.

UNDERLYING CONDITIONS

Head Trauma

The symptoms and signs of posttraumatic bacterial meningitis are similar to those seen in acute bacterial meningitis due to other causes. However, since the patient has sustained head trauma, the clinical detection of meningitis may be difficult because nearly all the conventional symptoms and signs are already present (20,21). The only indication of posttraumatic bacterial meningitis may be deterioration in the patient's level of consciousness. Other symptoms include headache, confusion, inappropriate behavior, fever, chills, myalgias, stiff neck, vomiting, and seizures. Therefore an altered or changed mental status in this patient group should not be ascribed to other causes until bacterial meningitis has been excluded by cerebrospinal fluid (CSF) examination.

In patients who have suffered a basilar skull fracture in which a dural fistula is produced between the subarachnoid space and nasal cavity, paranasal sinuses, or middle ear, a common presentation is rhinorrhea or otorrhea due to a CSF leak; meningitis may be recurrent in these patients. The most frequent site for a dural fistula is the anterior cranial fossa in the area of the cribriform plate, where the bone is very thin and the dura is tightly adherent to bone; a fracture in this area allows CSF to leak through torn arachnoid and dura and into the nasal cavity, resulting in CSF rhinorrhea. CSF rhinorrhea can be distinguished from nasal secretions by testing the fluid for glucose using Dextrostix (22), although this test may be falsely negative during acute bacterial meningitis when the CSF glucose concentration is decreased.

Postneurosurgery

The clinical presentation of bacterial meningitis following a neurosurgical procedure (e.g., craniotomy) is usually insidious in onset and difficult to distinguish from other neurologic abnormalities in the postoperative period (11,21). These patients may experience altered mental status and signs of meningeal irritation postoperatively, since many postcraniotomy patients develop an aseptic or chemical meningitis several days after surgery that cannot be reliably distinguished from bacterial meningitis (23). In addition, postoperative neurosurgical patients are usually at increased risk of nosocomial infections at sites outside of the CNS, and the symptoms and signs of CNS infection may be difficult to distinguish from encephalopathy related to fever caused by infections at these sites (24). However, the presence of continued fever or prolonged mental status changes should prompt examination of CSF for a definitive diagnosis. Although the incubation period for postoperative meningitis extends to a month, most cases begin within 10 days of neurosurgery.

Cerebrospinal Fluid Shunts

The clinical presentation of CSF shunt infection can be quite variable and depends on the pathogenesis of infection, organism virulence, and type of shunt (25–27). Clinical features at presentation may occur as a result of shunt malfunction, systemic infection, or focal infection. The most frequent symptoms are headache, nausea, lethargy, and/or change in mental status (up to 65% of cases); these occur as a result of shunt malfunction with increased intracranial pressure. Fever, the most sensitive sign of systemic infection, is usually present but has been reported in as few as 14% to as many as 92% of cases, so its absence cannot be interpreted as a factor against infection. Other findings of systemic disease include anorexia, lethargy, and malaise.

Symptoms and signs of CSF shunt infection may also be referable to either the proximal or distal portions of the shunt. Infection beginning in the proximal portion of the shunt (i.e., the catheter within the CSF space) results in a meningitis or ventriculitis in about 30% of cases. However, meningeal symptoms should not be expected with infected ventricular shunts, since there is usually a lack of communication between the infected ventricles and the CSF in contact with the meninges.

Infections presenting with symptoms referable to the distal portion of the shunt are more specific to terminus location. Infected vascular shunts (e.g., those terminating in the right atrium) lead to bacteremia, with the clinical presentation of fever and malaise; bacteremia may also result from an infected thrombus at the end of the vascular catheter. Complications include septic pulmonary embolism, tricuspid valve endocarditis, and mycotic aneurysm of the pulmonic valve. With chronic vascular shunt infection, there may be development of nephritis with deposition of IgM and IgG antigen-antibody complexes in the glomerular basement membrane and consumption of complement factors C3 and C4; this complication has been observed in less than 4% and up to 14% of cases (25,28). When the shunt terminates in the peritoneal or pleural space, there is an inflammatory response in the absorbing tissue (i.e., peritonitis or pleuritis), leading to a reduction in drainage of CSF followed by an insidious increase in CSF pressure. Peritonitis is the usual manifestation of a distal infection in the peritoneum, although intestinal perforation, intestinal obstruction, and intraabdominal abscess have been reported. Frank peritonitis may also develop if there is leakage of CSF that has been encysted in the peritoneum. Empyema is the usual distal infection associated with ventriculopleural shunts. Pain, often related to infection at the peritoneal or pleural endings of the shunt, may be absent in up to 60% of infections. Furthermore, some shunt infections are insidious, causing few or no symptoms in which an intermittent low-grade fever or general malaise may be the only clinical findings.

Immunocompromised State

The clinical presentation of bacterial meningitis in an immunocompromised patient depends on the underlying disease and its treatment, and the type of immune abnormality (29). In neutropenic patients, consideration of the diagnosis of bacterial meningitis requires a high index of suspicion because symptoms and signs may initially be subtle, because of the impaired ability of the patient to mount a subarachnoid space inflammatory response. Low-grade fever, lethargy, and/or a change in pattern of headache may be the only findings. Patients with defective humoral immunity or who have undergone splenectomy are at increased risk for systemic infection caused by encapsulated bacteria; the clinical presentation of meningitis in these patients is often fulminant, with death occurring within several hours. In patients with deficiencies in cell-mediated immunity, intracellular microorganisms, such as *Listeria monocytogenes,* may cause meningitis. The clinical presentation of infection caused by this bacterium will be discussed later.

SPECIFIC MICROORGANISMS

Regardless of the microorganism isolated from the patient with acute bacterial meningitis, the clinical presentation is generally similar to that described earlier. However, some patients may present with clinical features that suggest a particular bacterial pathogen as the etiologic agent of meningitis.

Streptococcus pneumoniae

Patients with pneumococcal meningitis often have clinical evidence of contiguous or distant foci of pneumococcal infection (11). These include pneumonia, otitis media, mastoiditis, sinusitis, or endocarditis. In the study by Carpenter and Petersdorf (2), 35 (56%) of 63 patients with pneumococcal meningitis had pneumonia at the time of admission, although most other studies have found coexisting pneumonia in only 10% to 25% of patients with pneumococcal meningitis. In another series of 178 patients with pneumococcal meningitis (30), acute otitis media was the most common associated infection, being present in 33% of cases. In patients with pneumococcal meningitis in whom none of the preceding foci are identified, the possibility of a dural defect (as a result of head trauma with basilar skull fracture) or a structural defect (either traumatic or congenital in origin) should be considered (20,21).

Neisseria meningitidis

About 50% to 75% of patients with meningococcal meningitis present with a prominent rash, located principally on the extremities (1,11). Early in the course of illness, the rash is typically erythematous and macular, and may blanch upon pressure, but it quickly evolves into a petechial phase with further coalescence into a purpuric form (Fig. 4.1). The rash often matures rapidly, with new petechial lesions appearing during the physical examination. In severe cases complicated by meningococcemia and septic shock, peripheral vasoconstriction with gangrene and necrosis may also occur. In one recent review of the clinical features of 255 patients with acute meningococcal meningitis (Table 4.5) (31), a petechial rash was observed in three-quarters of the

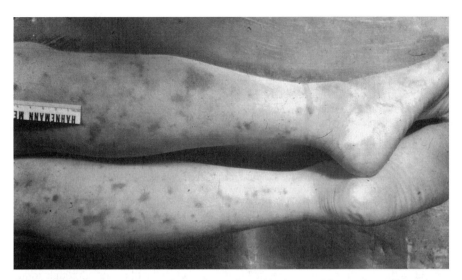

FIG. 4.1. Massive intracutaneous hemorrhages (petechiae/purpura) in a patient with meningococcal meningitis. (Courtesy of Cheryl A. Hanau, M.D.)

patients. The rash was more commonly seen in children and young adults less than 30 years of age (81%) than in patients 30 years of age and older (62%). A similar rash may also be seen in patients who have previously undergone splenectomy and who develop rapidly overwhelming sepsis caused by *Streptococcus pneumoniae* or *Haemophilus influenzae* type b, or in patients with *Staphylococcus aureus* endocarditis, Rocky Mountain spotted fever, epidemic typhus, or viral meningitis caused by echovirus 9.

TABLE 4.5. *Selected clinical findings in 255 patients with meningococcal meningitis*

Clinical finding	Relative frequency (%)
Fever on admission	99
Neck stiffness	98
Conscious mental state[a]	89
Petechial rash	75
Vomiting	51
Seizures[b]	6

[a] A depressed level of consciousness (reaction to painful stimuli or coma) was significantly ($P < 0.01$) more common in patients ≥ 50 yr of age (32% of cases) than in younger patients.

[b] Primarily observed in children.

Data from Anderson J, Backer V, Voldsgaard P, et al. Acute meningococcal meningitis: analysis of features of the disease according to the age of 255 patients. *J Infect* 1997;34:227–235, with permission.

TABLE 4.6. *Clinical findings in 367 episodes of meningitis/meningoencephalitis caused by Listeria monocytogenes*

Clinical finding	Relative frequency (%)
Fever	92
Altered sensorium	65
Headache	46
Gastrointestinal symptoms	22
Focal neurologic findings	18
Seizures	5
Photophobia	3

Data from Myolonakis E, Hohmann EL, Calderwood SB. Central nervous system infection with *Listeria monocytogenes*: 33 years' experience at a general hospital and review of 776 episodes from the literature. *Medicine (Baltimore)* 1998;77:313-336, with permission.

Listeria monocytogenes

Patients with meningitis caused by *L. monocytogenes* have a clinical presentation similar to those with meningitis caused by other bacterial pathogens, although some features are seen more commonly in patients with listerial meningitis (32, 33). These patients have an increased tendency to have seizures (at least 25% of cases in some series), focal neurologic deficits, and movement disorders (ataxia, tremors, myoclonus) early in the course of infection. Fluctuating mental status is common, although nuchal rigidity is absent in 15% to 20% of adults with *Listeria* meningitis. Some patients may present with an unusual form of listerial encephalitis characterized by the abrupt onset of asymmetric cranial nerve palsies, cerebellar signs, hemiparesis, and/or hemisensory deficits as a result of rhombencephalitis (33). This illness usually occurs in healthy adults. In a large review of CNS infections caused by *L. monocytogenes,* the clinical features of 367 episodes of meningitis/meningoencephalitis caused by this organism were described (34) (Table 4.6). Given the high morbidity and mortality associated with CNS infection caused by this organism, the presence of certain underlying conditions and the clinical presentation may provide helpful diagnostic clues in consideration of this microorganism as the cause of meningitis, leading to emergent initiation of appropriate antimicrobial therapy.

REFERENCES

1. Swartz MN, Dodge PR. Bacterial meningitis: a review of selected aspects. I. General clinical features, special problems and unusual meningeal reactions mimicking bacterial meningitis. *N Engl J Med* 1965;272:725–731.
2. Carpenter RR, Petersdorf RG. The clinical spectrum of bacterial meningitis. *Am J Med* 1962;33: 262–275.
3. Verghese A, Gallemore G. Kernig's and Brudzinski's signs revisited. *Rev Infect Dis* 1987;9:1187–1192.
4. Radetsky M. Duration of symptoms and outcome in bacterial meningitis: an analysis of causation and the implications of a delay in diagnosis. *Pediatr Infect Dis J* 1992;11:694–698.
5. Saez-Llorens X, McCracken GH Jr. Bacterial meningitis in neonates and children. *Infect Dis Clin North Am* 1990;4:623–644.
6. Baumgartner ET, Augustine RA, Steele RW. Bacterial meningitis in older neonates. *Am J Dis Child* 1983;137:1052–1054.

7. Shattuck K, Chonmaitree T. The changing spectrum of neonatal meningitis over a fifteen-year period. *Clin Pediatr* 1992;31:130–136.
8. Adhikari M, Coovadia YM, Singh D. A 4-year study of neonatal meningitis: clinical and microbiologic findings. *J Trop Pediatr* 1995;41:81–85.
9. Smith AL. Neonatal bacterial meningitis. In: Scheld WM, Whitley RJ, Durack DT, eds. *Infections of the central nervous system,* 2nd ed. Philadelphia: Lippincott-Raven, 1997:313–334.
10. Pong A, Bradley JS. Bacterial meningitis and the newborn infant. *Infect Dis Clin North Am* 1999; 13:711–733.
11. Roos KL, Tunkel AR, Scheld WM. Acute bacterial meningitis in children and adults. In: Scheld WM, Whitley RJ, Durack DT, eds. *Infections of the central nervous system,* 2nd ed. Philadelphia: Lippincott-Raven, 1997:335–401.
12. Feigin RD, McCracken GH Jr. Diagnosis and management of meningitis. *Pediatr Infect Dis J* 1992;11:785–814.
13. Ashwal S, Perkin RM, Thompson JR, et al. Bacterial meningitis in children: current concepts of neurologic management. *Curr Prob Pediatr* 1994;24:267–284.
14. Bonadio WA, Mannenbach M, Krippendorf R. Bacterial meningitis in older children. *Am J Dis Child* 1990;144:463–465.
15. Durand ML, Calderwood SB, Weber DL, et al. Acute bacterial meningitis in adults: a review of 493 episodes. *N Engl J Med* 1993;328:21–28.
16. Sigurdottir B, Bjornsson OM, Jonsdottir KE, et al. Acute bacterial meningitis in adults: a 20-year overview. *Arch Intern Med* 1997;157:425–430.
17. Attia J, Hatala R, Cook DJ, et al. Does this adult patient have acute meningitis? *JAMA* 1999;282: 175–181.
18. Gorse GJ, Thrupp LD, Nudleman KL, et al. Bacterial meningitis in the elderly. *Arch Intern Med* 1989;149:1603–1606.
19. Behrman RE, Meyers BR, Mendelson MH, et al. Central nervous system infections in the elderly. *Arch Intern Med* 1989;149:1596–1599.
20. Tunkel AR, Scheld WM. Acute infectious complications of head trauma. In: Braakman R, ed. *Handbook of clinical neurology: head injury.* Amsterdam: Elsevier Science Publishing, 1990: 317–326.
21. Kaufman BA, Tunkel AR, Pryor JC, et al. Meningitis in the neurosurgical patient. *Infect Dis Clin North Am* 1990;4:677–701.
22. Hyslop NE, Montgomery WW. Diagnosis and management of meningitis associated with cerebrospinal fluid leaks. In: Remington JS, Swartz MN, eds. *Current clinical topics in infectious diseases,* vol. 3. New York: McGraw-Hill, 1982:254–285.
23. Ross D, Rosegay H, Pons V. Differentiation of aseptic and bacterial meningitis in postoperative neurosurgical patients. *J Neurosurg* 1988;69:669–674.
24. Tenney JH. Bacterial infections of the central nervous system in neurosurgery. *Neurol Clin* 1986;4: 91–114.
25. Schoenbaum SC, Gardner P, Shillito J. Infections of cerebrospinal fluid shunts: epidemiology, clinical manifestations, and therapy. *J Infect Dis* 1975;131:543–552.
26. Kaufman BA. Infections of cerebrospinal fluid shunts. In: Scheld WM, Whitley RJ, Durack DT, eds. *Infections of the central nervous system,* 2nd ed. Philadelphia: Lippincott-Raven, 1997:555–577.
27. Morris A, Low DE. Nosocomial bacterial meningitis, including central nervous system shunt infections. *Infect Dis Clin North Am* 1999;13:735–750.
28. Kontny U, Hofling B, Gutjahr P, et al. CSF shunt infections in children. *Infection* 1993;21:89–92.
29. Tunkel AR, Scheld WM. Central nervous system infection in the compromised host. In: Rubin RH, Young LS, eds. *Clinical approach to infection in the compromised host,* 3rd ed. New York: Plenum, 1994:163–210.
30. Geiseler PJ, Nelson KE, Levin S, et al. Community-acquired purulent meningitis: a review of 1,316 cases during the antibiotic era, 1954–1976. *Rev Infect Dis* 1980;2:725–745.
31. Anderson J, Backer V, Voldsgaard P, et al. Acute meningococcal meningitis: analysis of features of the disease according to the age of 255 patients. *J Infect* 1997;34:227–235.
32. Gellin BG, Broome CV. Listeriosis. *JAMA* 1989;261:1313–1320.
33. Lorber B. Listeriosis. *Clin Infect Dis* 1997;24:1–11.
34. Myolonakis E, Hohmann EL, Calderwood SB. Central nervous system infection with *Listeria monocytogenes.* 33 years' experience at a general hospital and review of 776 episodes from the literature. *Medicine (Baltimore)* 1998;77:313–36.

5

Diagnosis

The diagnosis of bacterial meningitis rests on examination of cerebrospinal fluid (CSF) obtained after lumbar puncture. Prior to lumbar puncture, however, certain blood specimens that may assist in confirming the suspicion of acute bacterial infection must be obtained. A complete blood count may demonstrate leukocytosis or leukopenia, with elevated immature forms, and evidence of thrombocytopenia. Leukopenia and thrombocytopenia have correlated with poor outcome in patients with bacterial meningitis (1,2). In one study of children with pneumococcal meningitis, the mortality rate was higher in children with peripheral white blood cell counts of less than 5,000/mm^3 than in those with white blood cell counts of more than 5,000/mm^3 (63% versus 11%; $P = 0.0023$) (3). In another study of patients with meningococcal meningitis, the mortality rate was 25% in patients with platelet counts of less than 100,000/mm^3 versus 6% in those with counts of more than 100,000/mm^3 ($P < 0.01$) (4). In addition, coagulation studies, which may be consistent with disseminated intravascular coagulation, and serum chemistries, which may reveal hyponatremia or an anion gap metabolic acidosis, must be obtained. A serum sodium of less than 135 mEq/L suggests the possibility of concurrent adrenal insufficiency or the syndrome of inappropriate secretion of antidiuretic hormone (5). Patients should also be evaluated for evidence of renal insufficiency and hypo- or hyperglycemia.

Several acute-phase reactants have been examined for their usefulness in the diagnosis of acute bacterial infection. These include the erythrocyte sedimentation rate, C-reactive protein, fibrinogen, haptoglobin, and α_1 acid glycoprotein (6). However, none of these tests, utilized either alone or in combination, is diagnostic for acute bacterial infection and should not be used to determine whether an individual patient should receive antimicrobial therapy. Recently, elevated serum concentrations of procalcitonin, a polypeptide that increases in patients with severe bacterial infection, were shown to be a useful marker in differentiating between bacterial and viral meningitis (7,8). A serum procalcitonin concentration of more than 0.2 ng/mL had a sensitivity and specificity of up to 100% in the diagnosis of bacterial meningitis (8). Confirmation of these results in additional studies will determine the usefulness of this polypeptide in the differential diagnosis of bacterial meningitis.

Blood cultures, obtained prior to administration of antimicrobial therapy, are also imperative and may occasionally be positive when CSF cultures are negative. In one large study of patients with bacterial meningitis not previously treated with antimicrobial therapy, blood cultures were positive in 90%, 80%, and 90% of patients with meningitis caused by *Haemophilus influenzae* type b, *Streptococcus pneumoniae,* and *Neisseria meningitidis,* respectively (9). In another study of 169 patients with bacterial meningitis who had blood cultures performed, 86% had the organism responsible for meningitis recovered in the blood (10). Blood cultures were positive in 94% of patients with *H. influenzae* meningitis, and the yield increased to 100% in those not previously treated with antimicrobial therapy. Gram stain and culture of other body fluids (e.g., petechial lesions, middle ear effusions) and cultures of mucosal surfaces may also aid in the etiologic diagnosis of meningitis. For example, meningococci can be isolated from the nasopharynx of up to 50% of patients with invasive meningococcal disease, regardless of whether a dose of benzylpenicillin has been previously given (11), leading to the recent recommendation of obtaining a swab of the posterior pharyngeal wall if meningococcal sepsis is suspected (12). However, cultures of mucosal surfaces are neither sensitive (the bacterium causing meningitis may not be present) nor specific (other microorganisms may be isolated) for the diagnosis of bacterial meningitis and generally are not routinely helpful in identification of the etiologic agent (1).

LUMBAR PUNCTURE

Lumbar puncture is an essential procedure in the diagnosis of bacterial meningitis. Although controversy exists in the performance of lumbar puncture, several points should be emphasized (13). First, maximize reassurance to the patient by discussing the procedure. Second, position the patient and needle properly to obtain adequate amounts of cerebrospinal fluid (CSF). The patient is usually placed curled in the lateral recumbent position on a firm surface with the back at the edge of the table and perpendicular to the table surface. Third, the needle (preferably 20-gauge or smaller) should be inserted in the midline (generally in the space between the third and fourth lumbar vertebrae) and perpendicular to the back. Frequent removal of the stylet allows the physician to determine quickly if the subarachnoid space has been reached. As soon as CSF is observed in the hub of the needle, a manometer is attached for measurement of the opening pressure.

Complications associated with performance of the lumbar puncture are variable (Table 5.1), ranging from mild alterations in comfort (e.g., pain with insertion of the needle) to life-threatening (i.e., brain herniation) (13,14). The most common complication is headache (10% to 25% of cases). Characteristically, the headache is absent when the patient is recumbent and appears rapidly when the patient stands upright. The headache is believed to be caused by low CSF pressure as a result of continued leakage of CSF at the site of the lumbar puncture. The risk of headache may be modified by using 20-gauge needles or smaller or by placing the patient in the prone position for several hours after the procedure. In one study, the incidence of headache

TABLE 5.1. *Complications of lumbar puncture*

Headache
Painful paresthesias
Persistent pain or paresthesias
Local bleeding
Spinal subdural or epidural hematoma with or without
    compression of the cauda equina
Local infection
Meningitis
Brain herniation
Cortical blindness
Cervical spinal cord infarction
Intraspinal epidermoid tumor

after lumbar puncture was 36.5% in patients kept supine versus 0.5% in those who were placed in the prone position (15). The headache usually resolves spontaneously within hours to days. Persistent headache can be treated by use of a "blood patch," in which some of the patient's own venous blood is injected outside the meninges at the site of the lumbar puncture. This technique seals the site of CSF leakage.

Infection is a more significant complication of lumbar puncture, although the overall incidence of local infection or development of meningitis is exceedingly low, even in patients with concomitant bacteremia. In one study of 1,089 patients with sepsis of whom 200 underwent lumbar puncture, the incidence of possible lumbar puncture–associated meningitis was no different than would have been expected by chance alone (16). This contrasts with another study utilizing an experimental dog model in which 81% of animals undergoing cisternal puncture in the presence of severe bacteremia ($>10^3$ organisms/mL of blood) developed meningitis, whereas meningitis did not develop in bacteremic dogs that did not undergo cisternal puncture (17). Despite these conflicting results, the importance of performing a diagnostic lumbar puncture greatly outweighs any minor risk that the procedure itself might induce meningitis in a bacteremic patient. Lumbar puncture should not be performed if there is established infection (i.e., spinal epidural abscess or subdural empyema, or superficial or deep paraspinal infection) in the area that the needle will traverse to obtain CSF. In these instances, CSF should be obtained under fluoroscopic guidance via high cervical or cisternal puncture.

Local bleeding is more common after lumbar puncture (13,14), with as many as 20% of patients having a so-called traumatic tap (18). Bleeding may occur as a result of inadvertent puncture of the venous plexuses located dorsally and ventrally to the spinal sack or from injury to the vessels that accompany the cauda equina. This bleeding rarely does harm to the patient, although lumbar puncture in patients with coagulation deficits or who are receiving anticoagulants may be complicated by continued bleeding and the development of spinal subdural or epidural hematomas that may compress the cauda equina and produce permanent neurologic injury.

Despite the complications discussed earlier and listed in Table 5.1, the most feared complication following lumbar puncture is tonsillar herniation in the patient with elevated intracranial pressure (13,14). Following lumbar puncture, there is normally a mild, transient lowering of lumbar CSF pressure that is rapidly communicated throughout the subarachnoid space. In patients with intracranial space-occupying lesions, there is a relative pressure gradient (with downward displacement of the cerebrum and brainstem) that can be increased by lumbar puncture, thereby precipitating brain herniation. The incidence of this complication is unknown, although one study, which examined the outcome of the lumbar puncture in 129 patients with elevated intracranial pressure, found that 1.2% of patients with papilledema and 12% of those without papilledema had unfavorable outcomes within 48 hours after the procedure (19). From these data and from a review of 418 patients with papilledema, the authors concluded that the actual risk of serious complications from lumbar puncture in the presence of papilledema was "much less than 1.2%." In two other studies, 30 instances of brain herniation were identified during a 1-year period (total number of punctures not indicated), and severe deterioration occurred in seven of 55 patients with subarachnoid hemorrhage who underwent lumbar puncture. Both of these reports suggested an incidence of brain herniation of more than 1% (13). In addition, another study of 302 infants and children with bacterial meningitis found that brain herniation developed in 6% of patients (20), with herniation occurring in all patients within 8 hours of lumbar puncture.

These data offer no definitive conclusions but suggest that patients selected for lumbar puncture should be carefully chosen because of the significant frequency of fatal outcome in the setting of elevated intracranial pressure. If the patient has a severely depressed sensorium or papilledema or if there is some suspicion of an intracranial mass lesion, neuroimaging should be performed prior to attempting the lumbar puncture (see later). Lumbar puncture should also be approached with caution in patients with bacterial meningitis and suspected intracranial hypertension or impending herniation (manifested clinically as a dilated, nonreactive pupil; drowsiness; abnormalities of ocular motility; and bradycardia and hypertension) (14). Some authorities would also delay lumbar puncture for 30 minutes in patients with short, convulsive seizures, or not perform the lumbar puncture at all in those with prolonged seizures because the seizure may be associated with transient increases in intracranial pressure (21). However, in patients with suspected bacterial meningitis in whom performance of a diagnostic lumbar puncture is delayed, empiric antimicrobial therapy must be initiated in a timely manner because of the potential for increased morbidity and mortality when initiation of therapy is delayed (see Chapter 7).

Once CSF is obtained, the fluid is sent to the laboratory for analysis (Table 5.2). Typical results of routine and commonly utilized tests in patients suspected of having acute bacterial meningitis are shown in Table 5.3 and are discussed in detail later.

Opening Pressure

CSF opening pressure should be measured with an air–water manometer with the patient in the lateral recumbent position (14). In adult patients, the normal opening pressure ranges from 50 to 195 mm H_2O. In virtually all adult patients with bacterial

TABLE 5.2. *Recommended tests of cerebrospinal fluid in patients with suspected meningitis*

Routine
  Cell count
  White blood cell differential count
  Glucose concentration
  Protein concentration
  Gram stain
  Bacterial culture
When indicated
  Latex agglutination for bacterial antigens
  Viral culture
  Smear for acid-fast bacilli
  Mycobacterium tuberculosis culture
  VDRL
  India ink prep
  Cryptococcal polysaccharide antigen
  Fungal culture
  Cytology and flow cytometry
Specialized tests
  Polymerase chain reaction
  Limulus lysate assay

meningitis, the opening pressure is elevated, generally in the range of 200 to 500 mm H_2O, with values of more than 600 mm H_2O suggesting the presence of cerebral edema, intracranial suppurative foci, or communicating hydrocephalus. In one recent review of 296 cases of community-acquired bacterial meningitis in adults, 39% of patients had a CSF opening pressure of 300 mm H_2O or more (22). In term neonates, normal CSF lumbar pressures are significantly lower, with a mean value of 100 mm H_2O. In one published series of infants and children with bacterial meningitis, the mean CSF opening pressure at the time of diagnosis was 180 mm H_2O (23), a value more than twice the upper limit of normal in this age group (24).

TABLE 5.3. *Typical cerebrospinal fluid (CSF) findings in children and adults with bacterial meningitis*

Cerebrospinal fluid parameter	Typical findings
Opening pressure	200–500 mm H_2O
Appearance	Turbid and/or discolored
White blood cell count	1,000–5,000/mm^3 (range <100 to >10,000)
Percentage of neutrophils	≥80%
Protein	100–500 mg/dL
Glucose	<40 mg/dL
CSF:serum glucose	≤0.4
Gram stain	Positive in 60% to 90%
Culture	Positive in 70% to 85%
Bacterial antigen detection	Positive in 50% to 100%

See text for in-depth discussion of each CSF finding.

Appearance

Normally, the CSF is clear and colorless, but it may appear cloudy or turbid with increased concentrations of white blood cells (>200/mm^3), red blood cells (>400/mm^3), bacteria ($>10^5$ CFU/mL), and/or protein (14,25,26). In cases of a "traumatic tap," an initially bloody CSF sample should clear as flow continues; CSF will appear grossly bloody when there are at least 6,000 red blood cells/mm^3. Xanthochromia, a yellow or yellow-orange color in the supernatant of centrifuged spinal fluid, distinguishes CSF that is bloody secondary to subarachnoid hemorrhage from CSF that is bloody secondary to a traumatic lumbar puncture in which the supernatant of centrifuged CSF is clear. In most cases, xanthochromia is a result of red blood cell lysis and the presence of oxyhemoglobin, methemoglobin, and bilirubin. It characteristically appears about 2 to 4 hours after red blood cells have entered the subarachnoid space, although occasionally may not be seen for as long as 12 hours. Xanthochromia has also been observed with elevated CSF protein concentrations of more than 150 mg/dL or as a consequence of systemic hyperbilirubinemia (above 10 to 15 mg/dL).

Cell Count

The normal CSF white blood cell count in children and adults is 0 to 5/mm^3. CSF white cell counts up to 32/mm^3 (mean of 8 to 9/mm^3) may be normal in term neonates (27), although by 1 month of age normal CSF has fewer than 10 white blood cells/mm^3 (14). In untreated bacterial meningitis, the white blood cell count is elevated, usually from 1,000 to 5,000/mm^3 (range of less than 100 to more than 10,000/mm^3). In one large series of 1,316 patients with community-acquired meningitis, more than 100 white blood cells/mm^3 were seen in more than 90% of patients and in excess of 1,000 cells/mm^3 were seen in 68% of cases (28). In another review of 493 episodes of bacterial meningitis in adults, 60% to 65% of patients had between 100 and 4,999 cells/mm^3 (22). However, the absence of a CSF pleocytosis can characterize up to 4% of cases of bacterial meningitis overall (26), most commonly in premature neonates (up to 15% of cases) and infants younger than 4 weeks of age (17% of cases). In addition, normal CSF white blood cell counts have been seen in patients with meningococcal meningitis (29, 30), accounting for almost 10% of cases of in one study (29). The reason for the absence of a CSF pleocytosis may be secondary to collection of CSF during the early stages of bacterial meningitis before white blood cells have entered the subarachnoid space. Therefore a Gram stain and culture should be performed on all spinal fluid specimens even if the white blood cell count is normal. Patients with very low CSF white cell counts (0 to 20/mm^3) despite high CSF bacterial concentrations tend to have a poor prognosis. One study of 291 evaluable children with invasive meningococcal disease demonstrated a frequency of adverse outcome (defined as death during hospitalization, limb amputation, or loss of all five digits on an extremity) of 40% if the CSF culture was positive without evidence of CSF pleocytosis. This compared with 3.4% for patients with positive CSF cultures and pleocytosis ($P < 0.001$) and 9.6% for patients with bacteremia alone ($P = 0.001$) (31). In addition, in a study of children with pneumococcal meningitis, there was a trend to increased mortality (25% versus 6%; $P = 0.06$) in those patients with CSF white blood cell counts of less than $1,000/mm^3$ (3).

False-positive elevations of CSF white cells can be seen following traumatic lumbar puncture or in patients with intracerebral or subarachnoid hemorrhage during which red blood cells (RBCs) and white blood cells (WBCs) are introduced into the subarachnoid space. In these instances, the following formula should be used as a correction factor for the white blood cell count in the presence of blood in CSF (32):

$$\text{True WBC in CSF} = \text{Actual WBC in CSF} - \frac{\text{WBC in Blood} \times \text{RBC in CSF}}{\text{RBC in Blood}}$$

Another useful method to interpret the CSF findings associated with traumatic lumbar puncture is to calculate the ratio of the observed to predicted CSF white blood cell count (O:P ratio). The predicted white blood cell count is determined by the following formula (26):

$$\text{Predicted WBC in CSF} = \text{CSF RBC} \times \frac{\text{WBC in Blood}}{\text{RBC in Blood}}$$

In a study of 92 previously healthy children (30 with bacterial meningitis and 62 with negative CSF cultures) more than 1 month of age (18), all 30 patients with bacterial meningitis had a O:P ratio of 1 or more and 93% had ratios of more than 10. Only two patients (3%) with culture-negative CSF had an O:P ratio of more than 10.

Generalized seizures may also induce a transient CSF pleocytosis, primarily neutrophilic, although the total CSF white blood cell count should not exceed 80 cells/mm^3. The pleocytosis should not be ascribed to seizure activity alone unless the fluid is clear and colorless, the opening pressure and CSF glucose are normal, the Gram stain is negative, and the patient has no clinical evidence of bacterial meningitis (33). In addition, other infectious etiologies may produce a predominance of CSF neutrophils and produce seizures, and may also need to be excluded (see Chapter 6). Falsely low CSF white blood cell counts may be observed as a result of a delay (after 30 to 60 minutes) in measurement of the CSF white blood cell count (14,26). This occurs secondary to white blood cell lysis or from adherence of the white blood cells to the glass or plastic walls of the collecting tube. One study demonstrated a significant degradation of neutrophils after obtaining CSF, with counts decreasing to 68% of initial values after 1 hour and to 50% of initial values after 2 hours (34).

Bacterial meningitis usually leads to a neutrophilic predominance in CSF, with the range typically between 80% and 95% (22,26,28). In one series, more than 80% neutrophils were observed in 85% of cases and more than 70% neutrophils in 98% of cases (35). Although "normal" CSF does not contain any neutrophils, an occasional neutrophil may be seen following centrifugation (14). In addition, most CSF differential counts are performed on cytocentrifuged specimens in hospital laboratories, in which a few neutrophils may be seen even in the absence of disease or in association with high peripheral leukocyte counts. In normal term neonates, differential CSF white blood cell counts demonstrating up to 60% neutrophils have been reported (27). Approximately 10% of patients with acute bacterial meningitis present with a lymphocytic predominance (defined as more than 50% lymphocytes or mononuclear cells) in spinal fluid. This is more common in patients with meningitis caused by *Listeria monocytogenes* (about one-third of cases). A predominance of lymphocytes may also be seen following initiation of appropriate antimicrobial therapy. In one study, 14% of cases were associated with conversion from a neutrophilic to a lymphocytic predominance in CSF after 48 hours of adequate antimicrobial therapy (36).

Glucose

A decreased CSF glucose concentration less than 40 mg/dL (hypoglycorrhachia) is found in about 50% to 60% of patients with bacterial meningitis (22,37). In one large series, 30% of patients had a CSF glucose concentration of less than 15 mg/dL (28). The pathogenesis of hypoglycorrhachia is multifactorial and may include an increased rate of macrovescicular glucose transport across arachnoid villi, increased glycolysis by leukocytes and bacteria, increased metabolic rate of the brain and spinal cord, and/or inhibition of glucose entry into the subarachnoid space caused by alterations in the membrane carrier system responsible for glucose transfer from blood to CSF (26). In addition, there is cerebral vasculitis and a decrease in cerebral blood flow (as a result of increased intracranial pressure), resulting in less delivery of glucose to the brain and glucose utilization via anaerobic glycolysis (see Chapter 3) (38). The CSF glucose may be falsely low in the presence of hypoglycemia or be incorrectly interpreted as normal when the serum glucose is elevated (e.g., severe hyperglycemia in diabetic patients). Therefore measurement of the CSF glucose should always be compared with a simultaneous serum glucose (drawn prior to the lumbar puncture); the CSF:serum glucose ratio can then be utilized as a more accurate interpretation of the CSF glucose meaning. The normal CSF:serum glucose ratio is 0.6, with a ratio of less than 0.5 considered abnormal. A CSF:serum glucose ratio of less than 0.31 is seen in about 70% of patients with bacterial meningitis (37). One study demonstrated that a CSF:serum glucose ratio of 0.4 or less was 80% sensitive and 98% specific for the diagnosis of bacterial meningitis in children older than 2 months of age (39). Of note, the normal CSF:serum glucose ratio is higher in term neonates, so a ratio of 0.6 or less is considered abnormal in this patient group (27). Low CSF glucose concentrations at presentation have been shown to be predictive of unilateral or bilateral hearing loss in children with bacterial meningitis (40,41).

Protein

The CSF protein concentration is elevated in virtually all patients with bacterial meningitis (22,28), presumably due to disruption of the blood-brain barrier manifested morphologically as increased numbers of pinocytotic vesicles and separation of intercellular tight junctions in cerebral microvascular endothelial cells (see

Chapter 3) (42). Lumbar CSF protein concentrations above 50 mg/dL and ventricular CSF protein concentrations above 15 mg/dL are considered abnormal; in full-term neonates, the mean normal lumbar CSF protein concentration is 90 mg/dL (range of 20 to 170 mg/dL) (27). However, elevated CSF concentrations of protein are among the most common and least specific of all CSF parameters and may be seen in a variety of infectious and noninfectious neurologic disorders (14). In cases of a traumatic lumbar puncture with blood in CSF, the true CSF protein concentration is determined by subtracting 1 mg/dL of protein for every 1,000 red blood cells/mm^3 in CSF (32). Furthermore, a normal CSF protein concentration may be seen in specimens obtained at the onset of meningitis, in some cases of neonatal meningitis, and in severely immunocompromised patients. One study demonstrated a significantly higher mortality rate in patients whose CSF protein concentration was 250 mg/dL or more (32% versus 4%; $P = 0.0021$) (3), although this finding has not been confirmed in other studies (2).

Combination of Cell Count, Glucose, and Protein

Although the tests described earlier are utilized on all CSF specimens to determine the likelihood of the diagnosis of bacterial meningitis, in the absence of a positive CSF Gram stain, culture, or bacterial antigen test (see later), none is definitive evidence for or against the diagnosis. However, a combination of test results may permit an accurate prediction of the likelihood of bacterial versus other causes of acute meningitis. An analysis of the records of 422 patients with acute bacterial or viral meningitis found that a CSF glucose concentration of less than 34 mg/dL, a CSF:blood glucose ratio of less than 0.23, a CSF protein concentration of more than 220 mg/dL, more than 2,000/mm^3 CSF leukocytes, or more than 1,180/mm^3 CSF neutrophils individually predicted bacterial, rather than viral, meningitis, with 99% certainty or better (43). This model was validated in one retrospective review of adult patients with bacterial or viral meningitis (44), although proof of the clinical utility of this model will require a prospective application. Furthermore, this model has only been evaluated to distinguish between acute bacterial and viral meningitis, and cannot be applied in acute or chronic meningitides caused by other etiologic agents. At present, this model should not be utilized to make decisions regarding the initiation of antimicrobial therapy in patients with meningitis, but it may be useful in confirming the clinical diagnosis or by suggesting a reconsideration of the diagnosis in doubtful cases.

Lactate

Elevated CSF lactate concentrations may be useful in differentiating bacterial from nonbacterial meningitis in patients who have not received prior antimicrobial therapy. In one study of 50 patients with acute bacterial meningitis, 92% had CSF lactate concentrations of 35 mg/dL or more (45). CSF lactate concentrations were also found to be superior to the CSF:blood glucose ratio in the diagnosis of bacterial meningitis in postneurosurgical patients, in which a CSF lactate concentration of 4.0 mg/dL was used as a cutoff value for the diagnosis (46). The authors suggested that the CSF lactate may be particularly useful as a diagnostic test for bacterial meningitis in patients with meningeal symptoms after neurosurgery. However, despite the high sensitivity of the CSF lactate concentration in the diagnosis of acute bacterial meningitis, the results are generally nonspecific and provide little additional diagnostic information (47). Cerebral hypoxia/ischemia, anaerobic glycolysis, vascular compromise, and/or metabolism of CSF leukocytes are all potentially important factors in the elevation of CSF lactate concentrations during bacterial meningitis.

Gram Stain

Gram stain examination of CSF permits a rapid, accurate identification of the causative bacterium in 60% to 90% of patients with community-acquired bacterial meningitis and has a specificity of 97% or more (13,22,28). The likelihood of detecting the organism by Gram stain correlates with the concentration of bacteria in CSF. Concentrations of 10^3 or fewer colony-forming units (CFU) per milliliter are associated with positive Gram stains about 25% of the time, 10^3 to 10^5 CFU/mL yield positive Gram stains in 60% of patients, and CSF concentrations of bacteria in excess of 10^5 CFU/mL lead to positive microscopy in up to 97% of cases (48). The probability of observing bacteria on Gram stain can be increased up to 100-fold by utilizing Cytospin centrifugation (Shandon Southern Products, Cheshire, England) of CSF specimens (49,50). The clinical utility of the Gram stain also depends on the bacterial pathogen causing meningitis (14,51). Bacteria have been observed in 90% of cases of meningitis caused by *S. pneumoniae,* 86% of cases caused by *H. influenzae,* 75% of cases caused by *N. meningitidis,* and 50% of cases caused by gram-negative bacilli; the CSF Gram stain is positive in only one-third of patients with *L. monocytogenes* meningitis (52). False-positive CSF Gram stains may result from observer misinterpretation, reagent contamination, or use of an unoccluded needle for lumbar puncture in which an excised skin fragment is contaminated with bacteria (1,14). The yield of Gram stain is about 20% lower in patients who have received prior antimicrobial therapy (14).

Culture

The CSF culture is positive in 70% to 85% of patients with acute bacterial meningitis (22,25); cultures may take up to 48 hours for organism identification. In one series of 1,316 patients with community-acquired bacterial meningitis, 75% of patients had positive cultures of CSF and/or blood (28). The media routinely used for CSF bacterial culture are 5% sheep blood agar, enriched chocolate agar, and an enrichment broth (e.g., thioglycolate, Columbia, *Brucella,* supplemented peptone, or eugonic) (51); cultures should be incubated for at least 72 hours at 37 degrees Celsius in an atmosphere containing 5% to 10% CO_2.

Bacterial Antigen Tests

Several rapid diagnostic tests have been developed to aid in the etiologic diagnosis of bacterial meningitis (51,53). These tests use serum containing bacterial antibodies or commercially available antisera directed against the capsular polysaccharides of meningeal pathogens; available techniques are counterimmunoelectrophoresis (CIE), coagglutination (COAG), and latex agglutination (LA). The advantage of these tests is that they may be positive in the absence of viable organisms, and when the CSF Gram stain and culture are negative. CIE may detect specific antigens in CSF when meningitis is caused by meningococci (serogroups A, C, Y, or W135), *H. influenzae* type b, pneumococci (83 serotypes), type III group B streptococci, and *Escherichia coli* K1. The sensitivity ranges from 67% to 85% for *H. influenzae* type b, 50% to 100% for *S. pneumoniae,* and 50% to 90% for *N. meningitidis,* although the test is highly specific (25). However, CIE is only rarely used today because it requires high-quality antisera, stringent quality control, special equipment, and an experienced technician for optimal sensitivity (51). COAG and LA are simpler to perform, do not require special equipment, are more rapid (results in 15 minutes or less), and are 10-fold more sensitive than CIE in the detection of bacterial antigens (Table 5.4). Currently available LA techniques detect the antigens of *H. influenzae* type b, *S. pneumoniae, N. meningitidis, E. coli* K1, and group B streptococci. However, many of the kits do not include tests for group B meningococci, and other kits are probably poor because of the limited immunogenicity of group B meningococcal polysaccharide. In addition, it must be emphasized that a negative bacterial antigen test does not rule out infection caused by a specific meningeal pathogen. Although false-positive CSF results are uncommon with LA, they have been reported in some patients without bacterial meningitis.

Recently, the routine use of CSF bacterial antigen tests for the etiologic diagnosis of bacterial meningitis has been questioned (54–56). In one study of 901 CSF bacterial antigen tests performed over a 37-month period, no modification of therapy occurred

TABLE 5.4. *Sensitivity of assays for detection of bacterial antigens in cerebrospinal fluid from patients with culture-proven bacterial meningitis*

Organism	Percentage of sensitivity		
	Counterimmuno-electrophoresis (CIE)	Coagglutination (COAG)[a]	Latex agglutination (LA)[b]
Haemophilus influenzae type b	67–85	66–100	78–100
Neisseria meningitidis	50–90	50–78	50–93
Streptococcus pneumoniae	50–100	59–93	67–100
Streptococcus agalactiae	62–82	62–87	69–100

[a] Range of values obtained with the Phadebact CSF Test.
[b] Range of values obtained with the Bactigen, Directigen, and Wellcogen bacterial antigen detection kits.
Data from Bonadio WA. The cerebrospinal fluid: physiologic aspects and alterations associated with bacterial meningitis. *Pediatr Infect Dis J* 1992;11:423–432; and Gray LD, Fedorko DP. Laboratory diagnosis of bacterial meningitis. *Clin Microbiol Rev* 1992;5:130–145, with permission.

in 22 of 26 patients with positive results (54). Furthermore, false-positive results have occasionally resulted in unnecessary treatment and prolonged hospitalization (57). A recent study of 344 CSF specimens submitted for bacterial antigen assays found that 10 specimens represented true infections (by culture criteria), for a sensitivity and specificity of 70% and 99.4%, respectively (58). A positive CSF antigen test did not affect clinical therapy or hospital course. In addition, there were three false-negative and two false-positive test results. Therefore the bacterial antigen test is most effectively utilized when the clinical presentation and CSF findings are consistent with the diagnosis of bacterial meningitis and the CSF Gram stain is negative. Furthermore, some authors have advocated holding CSF specimens for 24 to 48 hours awaiting positive culture results before performing antigen testing (51,54). LA may be most efficacious in those patients who have received antimicrobial therapy prior to lumbar puncture, thereby decreasing the yield of Gram stain and culture in making an etiologic diagnosis (59).

Limulus Lysate Assay

Lysate prepared from the amebocytes of the horseshoe crab *Limulus polyphemus* may be useful in suspected cases of gram-negative meningitis in which a positive test indicates the presence of endotoxin (51,60). A correctly performed *Limulus* lysate assay can detect about 10^3 gram-negative bacteria/mL of CSF and as little as 0.1 ng/mL of endotoxin. Compared with cultures for gram-negative bacteria, the sensitivity and specificity of this assay are 93% and 99.4%, respectively (51), although other investigators have demonstrated a sensitivity of only 71% in neonates with gram-negative meningitis (61). The *Limulus* lysate assay is most often employed in the setting of an abnormal CSF following neurosurgery or head trauma when the CSF Gram stain and cultures are negative. However, this test does not distinguish between specific gram-negative organisms, and a negative test does not rule out the diagnosis of gram-negative meningitis. Therefore the test result rarely influences patient management and should not be routinely utilized.

Polymerase Chain Reaction

Polymerase chain reaction (PCR) has been utilized to amplify DNA from patients with meningitis caused by the common meningeal pathogens, including *N. meningitidis, S. pneumoniae, H. influenzae* type b, *Streptococcus agalactiae,* and *L. monocytogenes* (62–71). In one study of CSF samples from 54 patients with meningococcal disease or from controls, the sensitivity and specificity of PCR for the diagnosis of meningococcal meningitis were both 91% (64). In another study utilizing a seminested PCR strategy for simultaneous detection of *N. meningitidis, H. influenzae,* and streptococci in 304 clinical CSF samples (including 125 samples from patients with bacterial meningitis), the diagnostic sensitivity and specificity were 94% and 96%, respectively, although some false-positive results were obtained (65). By use of a seminested PCR based on the amplification of the pneumococcal penicillin-binding protein 2B gene to detect pneumococci in CSF, PCR detected pneumococci in all 18 samples that were culture-positive, including those isolates nonsusceptible to penicillin, and there were no false-positive results (72). The test was performed in a few hours and required only 15 μL of CSF, indicating that it may be promising in the diagnosis of pneumococcal meningitis.

However, there may be problems with false-positive results when utilizing PCR, although further refinements in this technique may demonstrate its usefulness in the etiologic diagnosis of bacterial meningitis, particularly when the CSF Gram stain, bacterial antigen tests, and cultures are negative. Furthermore, PCR may prove valuable in identifying the etiology of meningitis caused by other pathogens (e.g., viruses, *Mycobacterium tuberculosis,* and fungi), which may decrease the need for hospitalization and continued antimicrobial therapy (see Chapter 6).

Miscellaneous Cerebrospinal Fluid Tests

Several other tests of CSF have been evaluated in an attempt to determine their usefulness in distinguishing between acute bacterial and viral meningitis. C-reactive protein, an acute-phase reactant associated with tissue injury, has been shown to be quite sensitive in distinguishing bacterial from viral meningitis when CSF concentrations are more than 100 ng/mL (25). Some studies have demonstrated that when CSF indices are consistent with meningitis, a negative CSF C-reactive protein excludes the diagnosis of bacterial meningitis with 99% certainty (73,74). Elevated CSF concentrations of various enzymes (e.g., lactate dehydrogenase and creatine phosphokinase), fibrin degradation products, and fibronectin have also been found in patients with bacterial meningitis (25,75–77), although the elevations were nonspecific. These tests are not routinely performed by clinical laboratories to aid in the diagnosis of bacterial meningitis.

Partially Treated Meningitis

Some patients with acute bacterial meningitis may have received antimicrobial therapy (either oral or intravenous) prior to obtaining CSF for analysis. Prior antimicrobial therapy can generally be expected to reduce the yield of Gram stain and culture by 20% and 30%, respectively (14,78), although there may be variability in these percentages based on the duration of therapy prior to CSF analysis and the route of antimicrobial administration. In 98% of cases of *H. influenzae* type b meningitis, a previously positive Gram stain converts to no organisms visualized on repeat CSF analysis after 24 to 48 hours of adequate antimicrobial therapy (36). In other studies of infants and children with bacterial meningitis, initially positive CSF cultures became sterile in 90% to 100% of patients within 24 to 36 hours of administration of "appropriate" antimicrobial therapy (26). However, in most patients with bacterial meningitis who have received prior antimicrobial therapy, no significant differences in the CSF formula occur (28), although some studies have disputed this conclusion. In one study of 272 untreated and 202 partially treated patients with culture-proven

H. influenzae type b meningitis, children who had been partially treated had lower CSF protein concentrations and a lower percentage of positive CSF Gram stains than the untreated children (79). In another series describing two prospective studies of 281 children with *H. influenzae* type b meningitis, there were significant decreases in percentage of neutrophils ($P < 0.03$), CSF protein concentrations ($P < 0.001$), and rates of CSF Gram stain or culture positivity ($P < 0.05$) in children who received preadmission oral antimicrobial therapy (80). When adjusted for duration of illness prior to hospitalization, only the CSF protein concentration remained significantly different ($P < 0.01$). Other parameters (i.e., CSF white blood cell count, CSF glucose, CSF:serum glucose ratio, and results of bacterial antigen tests and blood cultures) were not statistically altered by prior administration of antimicrobial agents.

Based on these data, initial management decisions must be based on analysis of CSF findings whether or not the patient has previously received antimicrobial therapy. Since the results of cultures of CSF and blood may be negative in these patients, a complete course of parenteral antimicrobial therapy may need to be administered if the clinical findings are consistent with the diagnosis of bacterial meningitis (see Chapter 4). Bacterial antigen tests or molecular techniques (e.g., PCR) may provide evidence confirming the diagnosis of bacterial meningitis, although none of these tests is 100% sensitive, so a negative test does not exclude the diagnosis (81).

Cerebrospinal Fluid Shunts

The diagnosis of CSF shunt infection requires appropriate bacterial cultures. Blood cultures generally have a poor ability to identify CSF shunt infection (negative cultures approaching 80%) (82,83), with the exception of infected vascular shunts in which blood cultures are positive in more than 90% of patients (84). Direct culture of the shunt, or any fluid in contact with it, is the most accurate diagnostic test for infection (83–86). CSF is obtained from ventricular shunts via a reservoir that is typically located in an easily accessible subcutaneous location. Elevated CSF white blood cell counts are highly correlated with the presence of infection, although infection may still be present in patients with normal counts. In addition, recent shunt surgery may produce a CSF inflammatory response in the absence of infection. CSF Gram stain should be performed, although the yield is greater with infections caused by gram-negative bacteria (90% positivity) than with those caused by gram-positive bacteria (87). Cultures of CSF may be positive even when the CSF white blood cell count, glucose, and protein are normal. Because of the often "benign" clinical presentation of CSF shunt infection, all positive CSF cultures must be taken seriously (84).

NEUROIMAGING STUDIES

Cranial computed tomography (CT scan) or magnetic resonance (MR) imaging does not aid in the diagnosis of acute bacterial meningitis (21,88). However, one of these modalities should be considered during the course of illness in patients who have persistent or prolonged fever, clinical evidence of increased intracranial pressure,

TABLE 5.5. *Abnormalities of neuroimaging studies in patients with bacterial meningitis*

Subdural effusion
Subdural empyema
Cerebral edema
Transient dilatation of ventricles
Meningeal enhancement
Ventriculitis
Communicating hydrocephalus
Obstructive hydrocephalus
Cerebral infarction
Hemorrhagic infarction
Spinal cord infarction
Brain abscess
Venous sinus thrombosis

focal neurologic findings, new or recurrent seizures, enlarging head circumference (in neonates), persistent neurologic dysfunction, or persistently abnormal CSF parameters or cultures (1,25,89). Cranial CT or MR has been recommended at the end of antimicrobial therapy in newborn infants to be certain that no intracranial complications have occurred. In one review of 107 children with bacterial meningitis who underwent CT scanning (90), one or more abnormalities were found in 52% of cases, although the majority of findings did not require specific intervention.

Of the intracranial abnormalities that may complicate bacterial meningitis (Table 5.5), subdural effusions were relatively common, being reported in 20% to 50% of children with bacterial meningitis (25,91). In most of these cases, the fluid is sterile and reabsorbed as inflammation subsides. However, children with prolonged fever and subdural collections detected by CT may require a drainage procedure because of the possibility of the development of a subdural empyema. This may be suggested on CT by increased density or significant enhancement after administration of intravenous contrast (Fig. 5.1), or by higher signal intensity than CSF on T_2-weighted MR imaging (Fig. 5.2).

Raised intracranial pressure may be secondary to cerebral edema, or obstructive or communicating hydrocephalus. Cerebral edema is manifested on CT or MR by loss of differentiation between gray and white matter, compression of the ventricles, loss of sulcal markings, and lack of visualization of the perimesencephalic, suprasellar, or quadrigeminal cisterns (Fig. 5.3) (25). Communicating hydrocephalus is diagnosed by enlargement of the entire ventricular system, including the fourth ventricle, with periventricular lucencies surrounding the frontal horns (Fig. 5.4). In contrast, the development of obstructive hydrocephalus has the appearance of dilation of the lateral and third ventricles, with nonvisualization of the fourth ventricle.

Other neuroradiographic findings in patients with bacterial meningitis include cortical infarctions as a result of vasculitis (Fig. 5.5), hemorrhagic infarctions, and leptomeningeal enhancement. MR imaging is superior to CT in demonstrating these abnormalities (92). With the advent of MR angiography, it may also be possible to demonstrate major vessel vasculitis associated with bacterial meningitis.

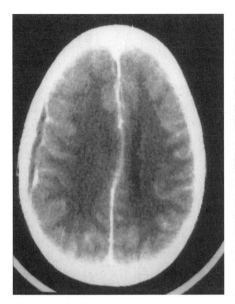

FIG. 5.1. Contrast-enhanced CT scan of the head (axial view) demonstrating a subdural empyema over the right cerebral hemisphere; note the low density of the empyema with evidence of medial enhancement. There is also a small interhemispheric empyema and contralateral bowing of the falx. (Courtesy of Eric N. Faerber, M.D.)

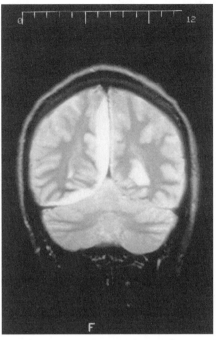

FIG. 5.2. T_2-weighted MR imaging study (coronal view) revealing high signal intensity of a right parafalcine subdural empyema.

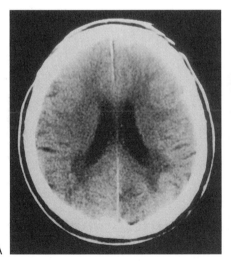

A

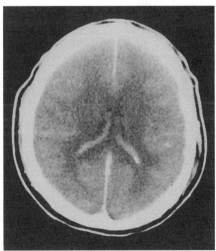

B

FIG. 5.3. CT scans of the head (axial view) in a patient with pneumococcal meningitis. A: CT scan on presentation, revealing moderate cortical atrophy. B: CT scan 3 days later, revealing diffuse swelling of the cerebral hemispheres bilaterally with effacement of the ventricular system.

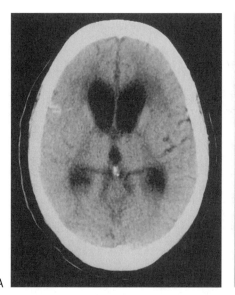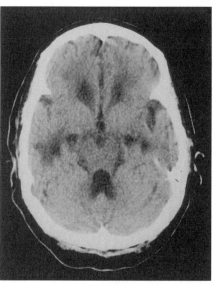

A   B

FIG. 5.4. CT scans of the head (axial view) in a patient with pneumococcal meningitis and communicating hydrocephalus revealing enlargement of the entire ventricular system. **A:** Enlargement of the lateral and third ventricles. **B:** Enlargement of the fourth ventricle.

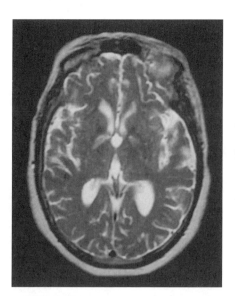

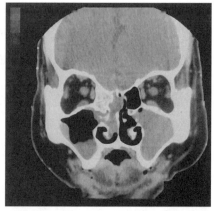

FIG. 5.5. T_2-weighted MR imaging scan of the head (axial view) in a patient with pneumococcal meningitis revealing high signal intensity areas in the basal ganglia bilaterally consistent with cortical infarction. (Courtesy of Arun Khazanchi, M.D.)

FIG. 5.6. CT scan of the head (coronal view) revealing extensive bilateral sinusitis most prominently involving the left maxillary and the right ethmoid sinuses. (Courtesy of Arun Khazanchi, M.D.)

Radiographic studies may also be useful in the subset of patients with meningitis as a result of a basilar skull fracture with CSF leak (93, 94). CT scanning may detect air/fluid levels or opacification of the paranasal sinuses (Fig. 5.6), or intracranial air. CT scanning with sagittal reconstruction can also be used to document or localize fracture sites. Radioisotope cisternography, with cottonoid pledgets placed at the outlet of the sinuses within the nasal passage, can be used to document a CSF leak, although high-resolution CT scanning with water-soluble contrast enhancement of the CSF (metrizamide cisternography) is the best test for defining the site of leakage.

REFERENCES

1. Feigin RD, McCracken GH Jr, Klein JO. Diagnosis and management of meningitis. *Pediatr Infect Dis J* 1992;11:785–814.
2. Kaplan SL. Clinical presentations, diagnosis, and prognostic factors of bacterial meningitis. *Infect Dis Clin North Am* 1999;13:579–594.
3. Kornelisse RF, Westerbeek CML, Spoor AB, et al. Pneumococcal meningitis in children: prognostic indicators and outcome. *Clin Infect Dis* 1995;21:1390–1397.
4. Andersen J, Backer V, Voldsgaard P, et al. Acute meningococcal meningitis: analysis of features of the disease according to the age of 255 patients. *J Infect* 1997;34:227–235.
5. Kaplan SL, Feigin RD. The syndrome of inappropriate secretion of antidiuretic hormone in children with bacterial meningitis. *J Pediatr* 1978;92:758–761.
6. Smith AL. Neonatal bacterial meningitis. In: Scheld WM, Whitley RJ, Durack DT, eds. *Infections of the central nervous system,* 2nd ed. Philadelphia: Lippincott-Raven, 1997:313–334.
7. Gendrel D, Raymond J, Assicot M, et al. Measurement of procalcitonin levels in children with bacterial or viral meningitis. *Clin Infect Dis* 1997;24:1240–1242.
8. Viallon A, Zeni F, Lambert C, et al. High sensitivity and specificity of serum procalcitonin levels in adults with bacterial meningitis. *Clin Infect Dis* 1999;28:1313–1316.
9. Bohr V, Rasmussen N, Hansen B, et al. Eight hundred seventy-five cases of bacterial meningitis: diagnostic procedures and the impact of preadmission oral antibiotic therapy. *J Infect* 1983;7:193–202.
10. Coant PN, Kornberg AE, Duffy LC, et al. Blood culture results as determinants in the organism identification of bacterial meningitis. *Pediatr Emerg Care* 1992;8:200–205.
11. Cartwright KAV, Reilly S, White D, et al. Early treatment with parenteral penicillin in meningococcal disease. *Br Med J* 1992;305:143–147.
12. Begg N, Cartwright KAV, Cohen J, et al. Consensus statement on diagnosis, investigation, treatment and prevention of acute bacterial meningitis in immunocompetent adults. *J Infect* 1999;39:1–15.
13. Marton KI, Gean AD. The spinal tap: a new look at an old test. *Ann Intern Med* 1986;104:840–848.
14. Greenlee JE, Carroll KC. Cerebrospinal fluid in CNS infections. In: Scheld WM, Whitley RJ, Durack DT, eds. *Infections of the central nervous system,* 2nd ed. Philadelphia: Lippincott-Raven, 1997:899–922.
15. Brocker RJ. Technique to avoid spinal tap headache. *JAMA* 1958;68:261–263.
16. Eng RHK, Seligman SJ. Lumbar puncture-induced meningitis. *JAMA* 1981;245:1456–1459.
17. Petersdorf RG, Swarner DR, Garcia M. Studies on the pathogenesis of meningitis. II. Development of meningitis during pneumococcal bacteremia. *J Clin Invest* 1962;41:320–327.
18. Bonadio WA, Smith D, Goddard S, et al. Distinguishing cerebrospinal fluid abnormalities in children with bacterial meningitis and traumatic lumbar puncture. *J Infect Dis* 1990;162:251–254.
19. Korein J, Cravisto H, Leicach M. Reevaluation of lumbar puncture: a study of 129 patients with papilledema or intracranial hypertension. *Neurology* 1959;9:290–297.
20. Horwitz SJ, Boxerbaum B, O'Bell J. Cerebral herniation in bacterial meningitis in childhood. *Ann Neurol* 1980;7:524–528.
21. Mellor DH. The place of computed tomography and lumbar puncture in suspected bacterial meningitis. *Arch Dis Child* 1992;67:1417–1419.
22. Durand ML, Calderwood SB, Weber DJ, et al. Acute bacterial meningitis in adults: a review of 493 episodes. *N Engl J Med* 1993;328:21–28.

23. Odio CM, Faingezicht I, Paris M, et al. The beneficial effects of early dexamethasone administration in infants and children with bacterial meningitis. *N Engl J Med* 1991;324:1525–1531.
24. Minns RA, Engleman HM, Stirling H. Cerebrospinal fluid measure in pyogenic meningitis. *Arch Dis Child* 1989;64:814–820.
25. Roos KL, Tunkel AR, Scheld WM. Acute bacterial meningitis in children and adults. In: Scheld WM, Whitley RJ, Durack DT, eds. *Infections of the central nervous system,* 2nd ed. Philadelphia: Lippincott-Raven, 1997:335–401.
26. Bonadio WA. The cerebrospinal fluid: physiologic aspects and alterations associated with bacterial meningitis. *Pediatr Infect Dis J* 1992;11:423–432.
27. Sarff LD, Platt LH, McCracken GH Jr. Cerebrospinal fluid evaluation in neonates: comparison of high-risk infants with and without meningitis. *J Pediatr* 1976;88:473–477.
28. Geiseler PJ, Nelson KE, Levin S, et al. Community-acquired purulent meningitis: a review of 1,316 cases during the antibiotic era, 1954–1976. *Rev Infect Dis* 1980;2:725–745.
29. Coll MT, Uriz MS, Pineda V, et al. Meningococcal meningitis with "normal" cerebrospinal fluid. *J Infect* 1994;29:289–294.
30. Sivakmaran M. Meningococcal meningitis revisited: normocellular CSF. *Clin Pediatr* 1997;36:351–355.
31. Malley R, Inkelis SH, Coelho P, et al. Cerebrospinal fluid pleocytosis and prognosis in invasive meningococcal disease in children. *Pediatr Infect Dis J* 1998;17:855–859.
32. Conly JM, Ronald AR. Cerebrospinal fluid as a diagnostic body fluid. *Am J Med* 1983;75:102–107.
33. Schmidley JW, Simon RP. Postictal pleocytosis. *Ann Neurol* 1981;9:81–84.
34. Steele R, Marmer D, O'Brien M, et al. Leukocyte survival in cerebrospinal fluid. *J Clin Microbiol* 1986;23:965–966.
35. Bonadio WA. Acute bacterial meningitis: cerebrospinal fluid differential count. *Clin Pediatr* 1988; 27:445–447.
36. Bonadio WA. Cerebrospinal fluid changes after 48 hours of effective therapy for *Haemophilus influenzae* type b meningitis. *Am J Clin Pathol* 1990;94:426–428.
37. Powers WJ. Cerebrospinal fluid to serum glucose ratios in diabetes mellitus and bacterial meningitis. *Am J Med* 1981;71:217–220.
38. Tunkel AR, Scheld WM. Pathogenesis and pathophysiology of bacterial meningitis. *Clin Microbiol Rev* 1993;6:118–136.
39. Donald P, Malan C, van der Walt A. Simultaneous determination of cerebrospinal fluid glucose and blood glucose concentrations in the diagnosis of bacterial meningitis. *J Pediatr* 1983;103:413–415.
40. Wald ER, Kaplan SL, Mason EO Jr, et al. Dexamethasone therapy for children with bacterial meningitis. *Pediatrics* 1996;95:21–28.
41. Arditi M, Mason EO Jr, Bradley JS, et al. Three-year multicenter surveillance of pneumococcal meningitis in children: clinical characteristics and outcome related to penicillin susceptibility and dexamethasone use. *Pediatrics* 1998;102;538–545.
42. Quagliarello VJ, Long WJ, Scheld WM. Morphologic alterations of the blood-brain barrier with experimental meningitis in the rat: temporal sequence and role of encapsulation. *J Clin Invest* 1986;77:1084–1095.
43. Spanos A, Harrell FE Jr, Durack DT. Differential diagnosis of acute meningitis: an analysis of the predictive value of initial observation. *JAMA* 1989;262:2700–2707.
44. McKinney WP, Heudebert GR, Harper SA, et al. Validation of a clinical prediction rule for the differential diagnosis of acute meningitis. *J Gen Intern Med* 1994;9:8–12.
45. Genton B, Berger JP. Cerebrospinal fluid lactate in 78 cases of adult meningitis. *Intensive Care Med* 1990;16:196–200.
46. Leib SL, Boscacci R, Gratzl O, et al. Predictive value of cerebrospinal fluid (CSF) lactate level versus CSF/blood glucose ratio for the diagnosis of bacterial meningitis following neurosurgery. *Clin Infect Dis* 1999;29:69–74.
47. Lannigan R, MacDonald MA, Marrie TJ, et al. Evaluation of cerebrospinal fluid lactic acid levels as an aid in differential diagnosis of bacterial and viral meningitis in adults. *J Clin Microbiol* 1980;11:324–327.
48. La Scolea LJ Jr, Dryja D. Quantitation of bacteria in cerebrospinal fluid and blood of children with meningitis and its diagnostic significance. *J Clin Microbiol* 1984;19:187–190.
49. Shanholtzer CJ, Schaper PJ, Peterson LR. Concentrated gram-stained smears prepared with a cytospin centrifuge. *J Clin Microbiol* 1982;16:1052–1056.

50. Chapin-Robertson K, Dahlberg SE, Edberg SC. Clinical and laboratory analyses of cytospin-prepared Gram stains for recovery and diagnosis of bacteria from sterile body fluids. *J Clin Microbiol* 1992;30:377–380.
51. Gray LD, Fedorko DP. Laboratory diagnosis of bacterial meningitis. *Clin Microbiol Rev* 1992;5:130–145.
52. Mylonakis E, Hohmann EL, Calderwood SB. Central nervous system infection with *Listeria monocytogenes*: 33 years' experience at a general hospital and review of 776 episodes from the literature. *Medicine (Baltimore)* 1998;77:313–336.
53. Hoban DJ, Witwicki E, Hammond GW. Bacterial antigen detection in cerebrospinal fluid of patients with meningitis. *Diagn Microbiol Infect Dis* 1985;3:373–379.
54. Maxson S, Lewno MJ, Schutze GE. Clinical usefulness of cerebrospinal fluid bacterial antigen studies. *J Pediatr* 1994;125:235–238.
55. Feuerborn SA, Capps WI, Jones JC. Use of latex agglutination testing in diagnosing pediatric meningitis. *J Fam Pract* 1992;34:176–179.
56. Finlay FO, Witheerow H, Rudd PT. Latex agglutination testing in bacterial meningitis. *Arch Dis Child* 1995;73:160–161.
57. Perkins MD, Mirrett S, Reller LB. Rapid bacterial antigen detection is not clinically useful. *J Clin Microbiol* 1995;33:1486–1491.
58. Hayden RT, Frenkel LD. More laboratory testing: greater cost but not necessarily better. *Pediatr Infect Dis J* 2000;19:290–292.
59. Bhisitkul DM, Hogan AE, Tanz RR. The role of bacterial antigen detection tests in the diagnosis of bacterial meningitis. *Pediatr Emerg Care* 1994;10:67–71.
60. Saubolle MA, Jorgensen JH. Use of the *Limulus* amebocyte lysate test as a cost-effective screen for gram-negative agents of meningitis. *Diagn Microbiol Infect Dis* 1987;7:177–183.
61. McCracken GH Jr, Sarff LD. Endotoxin in cerebrospinal fluid: detection in neonates with bacterial meningitis. *JAMA* 1976;235:617–620.
62. Kristiansen BE, Ask E, Jenkins A, et al. Rapid diagnosis of meningococcal meningitis by polymerase chain reaction. *Lancet* 1991;337:1568–1569.
63. Jaton K, Sahli R, Bille J. Development of polymerase chain reaction assays for detection of *Listeria monocytogenes* in clinical cerebrospinal fluid samples. *J Clin Microbiol* 1992;30:1931–1936.
64. Ni H, Knight AI, Cartwright K, et al. Polymerase chain reaction for diagnosis of meningococcal meningitis. *Lancet* 1992;340:1432–1434.
65. Radstrom P, Backman A, Qian N, et al. Detection of bacterial DNA in cerebrospinal fluid by an assay for simultaneous detection of *Neisseria meningitidis, Haemophilus influenzae,* and streptococci using a seminested PCR strategy. *J Clin Microbiol* 1994;32:2738–2744.
66. Isaacman DJ, Zhang Y, Rydquist-White J, et al. Identification of a patient with *Streptococcus pneumoniae* bacteremia and meningitis by the polymerase chain reaction (PCR). *Mol Cell Probes* 1995;9:157–160.
67. Olcen P, Lantz PG, Backman A, et al. Rapid diagnosis of bacterial meningitis by a seminested PCR strategy. *Scand J Infect Dis* 1995;27:537–539.
68. Hall LMC, Duke B, Urwin G. An approach to the identification of the pathogens of bacterial meningitis by polymerase chain reaction. *Eur J Clin Microbiol Infect Dis* 1995;14:1090–1094.
69. Caugant DA, Hoiby EA, Froholm LO, et al. Polymerase chain reaction for case ascertainment of meningococcal meningitis: application to the cerebrospinal fluids collected in the course of the Norwegian meningococcal serogroup B protection trial. *Scand J Infect Dis* 1996;28:149–153.
70. Saunders NB, Shoemaker DR, Brandt BL, et al. Confirmation of suspicious cases of meningococcal meningitis by PCR and enzyme-linked immunosorbent assay. *J Clin Microbiol* 1997;35:3215–3219.
71. Kotilainen P, Jalava J, Meurman O, et al. Diagnosis of meningococcal meningitis by broad-range bacterial PCR with cerebrospinal fluid. *J Clin Microbiol* 1998;36:2205–2209.
72. Du Plessis M, Smith AM, Klugman KP. Rapid detection of penicillin-resistant *Streptococcus pneumoniae* in cerebrospinal fluid by a seminested-PCR strategy. *J Clin Microbiol* 1998;36:453–457.
73. Gray BM, Simmons DR, Mason H, et al. Quantitative levels of C-reactive protein in cerebrospinal fluid in patients with bacterial meningitis and other conditions. *J Pediatr* 1986;108:665–670.
74. Abramson JS, Hampton KD, Babu S, et al. The use of C-reactive protein from cerebrospinal fluid for differentiating meningitis from other central nervous system diseases. *J Infect Dis* 1985;151:854–858.
75. Martin WJ. Rapid and reliable techniques for the laboratory detection of bacterial meningitis. *Am J Med* 1983;75:119–123.

76. Nussinovitch M, Klinger G, Soen G, et al. Increased creatine kinase brain isoenzyme concentration in cerebrospinal fluid with meningitis. *Clin Pediatr* 1996;349–351.
77. Torre D, Zeroli C, Issi M, et al. Cerebrospinal fluid concentration of fibronectin in meningitis. *J Clin Pathol* 1991;44:183–184.
78. Blazer S, Berant M, Alon U. Bacterial meningitis: effect of antibiotic treatment on cerebrospinal fluid. *Am J Clin Pathol* 1983;80:386–387.
79. Davis SD, Hill HR, Feigl P, et al. Partial antibiotic therapy in *Haemophilus influenzae* meningitis: its effect on cerebrospinal fluid abnormalities. *Am J Dis Child* 1975;129:802–807.
80. Kaplan SL, O'Brian Smith E, Willis C, et al. Association between preadmission oral antibiotic therapy and cerebrospinal fluid findings and sequelae caused by *Haemophilus influenzae* type b meningitis. *Pediatr Infect Dis J* 1986;5:626–632.
81. Ashkenazi S, Mor M. Partially treated meningitis in children: room for clinical judgement. *Is J Med Sci* 1995;31:638–639.
82. Schoenbaum SC, Gardner P, Shillito J. Infections of cerebrospinal fluid shunts: epidemiology, clinical manifestations, and therapy. *J Infect Dis* 1975;131:543–552.
83. Forward KR, Fewer HD, Stiver HG. Cerebrospinal fluid shunt infections: a review of 35 infections in 32 patients. *J Neurosurg* 1983;59:389–394.
84. Kaufman BA. Infections of cerebrospinal fluid shunts. In: Scheld WM, Whitley RJ, Durack DT, eds. *Infections of the central nervous system,* 2nd ed. Philadelphia: Lippincott-Raven, 1997:555–577.
85. Myers MG. Schoenbaum SC. Shunt fluid aspiration. *Am J Dis Child* 1975;129:220–222.
86. Gardner P, Leipzig T, Phillips P. Infections of central nervous system shunts. *Med Clin North Am* 1985;69:297–314.
87. Yogev R. Cerebrospinal fluid shunt infections: a personal view. *Pediatr Infect Dis J* 1985;4:113–118.
88. Haslam RHA. Role of computed tomography in the early management of bacterial meningitis. *J Pediatr* 1991;119:157–159.
89. Kline MW, Kaplan SL. Computed tomography in bacterial meningitis of childhood. *Pediatr Infect Dis J* 1988;7:855–857.
90. Friedland IR, Paris MM, Rinderknecht S, et al. Cranial computed tomographic scans have little impact on management of bacterial meningitis. *Am J Dis Child* 1992;146:1484–1487.
91. Syrogiannopoulos GA, Nelson JD, McCracken GH Jr. Subdural collections of fluid in acute bacterial meningitis: a review of 136 cases. *Pediatr Infect Dis* 1986;5:343–352.
92. Zimmerman RA, Girard NJ. Imaging of intracranial infections. In: Scheld WM, Whitley RJ, Durack DT, eds. *Infections of the central nervous system,* 2nd ed. Philadelphia: Lippincott-Raven, 1997:923–944.
93. Tunkel AR, Scheld WM. Acute infectious complications of head trauma. In: Braakman R, ed. *Handbook of clinical neurology, head injury.* Amsterdam: Elsevier Science Publishing, 1990:317–326.
94. Kaufman BA, Tunkel AR, Pryor JC, et al. Meningitis in the neurosurgical patient. *Infect Dis Clin North Am* 1990;4:677–701.

6

Differential Diagnosis

The clinical syndromes of meningitis and meningoencephalitis may be caused by a variety of infectious agents, as well as by many diseases of noninfectious or unknown etiology (Table 6.1) (1–4). It is beyond the scope of this chapter to review all the etiologies to be considered in the differential diagnosis of bacterial meningitis. Here I will concentrate on the common and/or clinically important etiologies that are most often considered in the differential diagnosis, emphasizing the epidemiology, clinical features, and diagnostic approach to these infectious agents of the central nervous system.

VIRUSES

Enteroviruses

Enteroviruses are currently the leading recognizable cause of the "aseptic meningitis syndrome, " a term used to define any meningitis (infectious or noninfectious), particularly one with a cerebrospinal fluid (CSF) lymphocytic pleocytosis, for which a cause is not apparent after initial evaluation and routine stains and cultures of CSF (1,5). With use of viral culture techniques, enteroviruses are isolated in 85% to 95% of cases of aseptic meningitis for which an etiology is found. More than 75,000 cases occur each year in the United States. Enteroviruses are worldwide in distribution. In temperate climates they appear during the summer and fall seasons, although in tropical and subtropical areas there is a high year-round incidence. Spread is believed to occur via the fecal/oral and perhaps respiratory routes. In one study in the United States during the years 1970 to 1983, the predominant enteroviruses isolated from patients with meningitis were (in decreasing order) echovirus 11; echovirus 9; coxsackievirus B5; echoviruses 30, 4, and 6; coxsackieviruses B2, B4, B3, and A9; echoviruses 3, 7, 5, and 21; and coxsackievirus B1 (6). In addition, the newly numbered enteroviruses 70 and 71 have been reported to commonly cause central nervous system (CNS) disease (5,7–9). Infants and young children are the primary victims of enteroviral meningitis because they are the most susceptible host population (i.e., there is absence of previous exposure and immunity) within the community, although the enteroviruses are also the most common causes of aseptic meningitis among adults (10). Persons

119

TABLE 6.1. *Reported etiologies in the differential diagnosis of meningitis and meningoencephalitis*

Major Infectious Etiologies
  Viruses
    Nonpolio enteroviruses[a]
    Mumps virus
    Arboviruses[b]
    Herpesviruses[c]
    Lymphocytic choriomeningitis virus
    Human immunodeficiency virus type 1
    JC virus (progressive multifocal leukoencephalopathy)
    Adenovirus
    Parainfluenza virus type 3
    Influenza virus
    Measles virus
    Rubella
    Poliovirus[d]
    Rotavirus
    Encephalomyocarditis virus
    Vaccinia virus
    Rabies virus
    Parvovirus B19
    Sandfly fever virus serotype Toscana
  Rickettsiae
    Rickettsia rickettsii (Rocky Mountain spotted fever)
    Rickettsia conorii
    Rickettsia prowazekii (epidemic or louse-borne typhus)
    Rickettsia typhi (endemic or murine typhus)
    Rickettsia tsutsugamushi (scrub typhus)
    Ehrlichia sp (monocytic and granulocytic)
  Mycobacteria
    Mycobacterium tuberculosis
    Nontuberculous mycobacteria[e]
  Spirochetes
    Treponema pallidum (syphilis)
    Borrelia burgdorferi (Lyme disease)
    Leptospira sp
    Borrelia recurrentis (relapsing fever)
    Spirillum minor (rat bite fever)
  Mycoplasmae
    Mycoplasma pneumoniae
    Mycoplasma hominis
    Ureaplasma urealyticum
  Chlamydiae
    Chlamydia psittaci
    Chlamydia trachomatis
  Other bacteria
    Tropheryma whippelii
    Bartonella sp [f]
  Fungi
    Cryptococcus neoformans
    Coccidioides immitis
    Histoplasma capsulatum
    Candida sp
    Aspergillus sp
    Blastomyces dermatitidis

TABLE 6.1. *Continued.*

Sporothrix schenckii
Paracoccidioides brasiliensis
Pseudallescheria boydii
Cladosporium sp
Zygomycetes
Pneumocystis carinii
Protozoa and helminths
  Naegleria fowleri
  Acanthamoeba
  Angiostrongylus cantonensis
  Strongyloides stercoralis (hyperinfection syndrome)
  Toxoplasma gondii
  Plasmodium falciparum
  Taenia solium
  Trichinella spiralis
  Trypanosoma sp
  Paragonimus sp
  Echinococcus granulosus
  Schistosoma sp
  Entamoeba histolytica
  Gnathostoma spinigerum
  Multiceps multiceps
Algae
  Prototheca wickerhamii
Other infectious syndromes
  Parameningeal foci of infection[g]
  Infective endocarditis
  Viral postinfectious syndromes
  Postvaccination[h]
  Bacterial toxin-mediated diseases[i]
Noninfectious and Diseases of Unknown Etiology
Neoplastic diseases
  Lymphomatous meningitis
  Carcinomatous meningitis
  Leukemia
Intracranial tumors and cysts
  Craniopharyngioma
  Dermoid/epidermoid cyst
  Teratoma
  Pituitary adenoma
  Astrocytoma
  Glioblastoma multiforme
  Medulloblastoma
  Pinealoma
  Ependymoma
Medications
  Antimicrobial agents[j]
  Nonsteroidal antiinflammatory agents[k]
  Muromonab-CD3 (OKT3)
  Azathioprine
  Cytosine arabinoside (high dose)
  Carbamazepine[l]
  Immune globulin
  Ranitidine
  Phenazopyridine

TABLE 6.1. *Continued.*

Systemic illnesses
  Systemic lupus erythematosus
  Vogt-Koyanagi-Harada syndrome
  Sarcoidosis
  Behcet's disease
  Sjogren's syndrome
  Mixed connective-tissue disease
  Rheumatoid arthritis
  Polymyositis
  Wegener's granulomatosis
  Polyarteritis nodosa
  Lymphomatoid granulomatosis
  Granulomatous angiitis
  Other cerebral vasculitides
  Familial Mediterranean fever
  Kawasaki's syndrome
Procedure related
  Postneurosurgery
  Spinal anesthesia
  Intrathecal injections[m]
  Chymopapain injection
  Teflon implantation
Miscellaneous
  Seizures
  Migraine or migraine-like syndromes
  Mollaret's meningitis[n]
  Serum sickness
  Heavy metal poisoning[o]

[a] Primarily echoviruses and coxsackieviruses.

[b] The etiologic agents include the mosquito-borne California, St. Louis, Eastern equine, Western equine, Venezuelan equine, LaCrosse, Japanese, and West Nile encephalitis viruses; and the tick-borne Colorado tick fever and Powassan virus.

[c] Primarily herpes simplex virus types 1 and 2, but also varicella-zoster virus, cytomegalovirus, Epstein-Barr virus, human herpesvirus-6, and herpes B virus.

[d] A common cause in areas where vaccination is not used or not available.

[e] *Mycobacterium avium* complex, *Mycobacterium kansasii, Mycobacterium fortuitum, Mycobacterium gordonae, Mycobacterium genavense, Mycobacterium terrae* complex.

[f] *Bartonella henselae, Bartonella bacilliformis.*

[g] Brain abscess, sinusitis, otitis, mastoiditis, subdural abscess, epidural abscess, venous sinus thrombophlebitis, pituitary abscess, cranial osteomyelitis.

[h] Mumps, measles, polio, pertussis, rabies, vaccinia.

[i] Scarlet fever, streptococcal pharyngitis, toxic shock syndrome, pertussis, diphtheria.

[j] Trimethoprim-sulfamethoxazole, trimethoprim, sulfamethoxazole, sulfisoxazole, ciprofloxacin, penicillin, cephalosporin, metronidazole, isoniazid, pyrazinamide.

[k] Ibuprofen, sulindac, naproxen, tolmetin, diclofenac sodium, ketoprofen.

[l] In patients with connective-tissue diseases.

[m] Air, isotopes, antimicrobial agents, antineoplastic agents, steroids, radiographic contrast media.

[n] Most cases may be caused by herpes simplex virus type 2.

[o] Lead, arsenic.

Data from Connolly KJ, Hammer SM. The acute aseptic meningitis syndrome. *Infect Dis Clin North Am* 1990;4:599–622; Tunkel AR, Scheld WM. Central nervous system infections. In: Reese RE, Betts RF, eds. *A practical approach to infectious diseases*, 4th ed. Boston: Little, Brown, and Company, 1996:133–183; Moris G, Garcia-Monco JC. The challenge of drug-induced aseptic meningitis. *Arch Intern Med* 1999;159:1185–1194; and Scheld WM, Whitley RJ, Durack DT, eds. *Infections of the central nervous system*, 2nd ed. Philadelphia: Lippincott-Raven Publishers, 1997, with permission.

may develop more than one episode of enteroviral meningitis, although the same enteroviral serotype has not been implicated more than once in any immunocompetent patient (5).

The clinical manifestations of enteroviral meningitis are dependent upon host age and immune status (5). In neonates (2 weeks of age or younger) with proven enteroviral meningitis, the usual findings are fever, vomiting, anorexia, rash, and/or upper respiratory symptoms and signs. Neurologic involvement may include a bulging anterior fontanelle and altered mental status, whereas focal neurologic and meningeal signs are uncommon. A more severe meningoencephalitis may be seen in neonates, in which the morbidity and mortality may be as high as 74% and 10%, respectively (11), particularly when symptoms and signs develop during the first day of life, likely through transplacental transmission of the virus; lack of humoral antibody may contribute to the severity of neonatal infection. However, beyond the neonatal period (older than 2 weeks), severe disease and poor outcome from enteroviral meningitis are rare. The onset of illness is usually sudden, with fever (76% to 100% of patients) and nuchal rigidity (>50% of patients) (12). Headache (often severe and frontal in location) is nearly always present in adults; photophobia is also common. Nonspecific symptoms and signs include vomiting, anorexia, rash, diarrhea, cough, upper respiratory findings (especially pharyngitis), and myalgias. The presence of exanthems, myopericarditis, conjunctivitis, and specifically recognizable enteroviral syndromes such as pleurodynia, herpangina, and hand-foot-and-mouth disease may suggest the presence of enteroviral disease (10). The duration of illness in enteroviral meningitis is usually less than 1 week, with many patients reporting improvement after the lumbar puncture (13), presumably as a result of reduction of intracranial pressure. In contrast, during a recent outbreak of enterovirus 71 infection in Taiwan in patients 3 months to 8.2 years of age, the chief neurologic complaint was rhombencephalitis (seen in 90% of children), which carried a case fatality rate of 14% (8). Persons who are agammaglobulinemic may also develop chronic enteroviral meningitis or meningoencephalitis lasting several years, often with a fatal outcome (14).

The typical CSF findings in enteroviral meningitis are shown in Table 6.2. CSF pleocytosis is almost always present in enteroviral meningitis (1,5), with counts in the several thousands reported in association with a greater likelihood of isolating the causative enterovirus (15). Early in infection, neutrophils may dominate the CSF profile, although this quickly gives way to a lymphocytic predominance over the first 6 to 48 hours. However, in a recent retrospective chart review of 158 cases of meningitis

TABLE 6.2. *Cerebrospinal fluid findings in bacterial versus viral meningitis*

Parameter	Bacterial	Viral
Opening pressure	200–500 mm H_2O	≤250 mm H_2O
White blood cell count	1,000–5,000/mm^3	50–1,000/mm^3
White blood cell differential	Neutrophilic	Lymphocytic[a]
Glucose	<40 mg/dL	>45 mg/dL
Protein	100–500 mg/dL	<200 mg/dL

[a] May find a neutrophilic pleocytosis early in infection.

(138 aseptic and 20 bacterial), 51% of the 53 patients with aseptic meningitis and duration of illness of more than 24 hours had a neutrophil predominance in CSF (16), suggesting that a CSF neutrophil predominance is not useful as a sole criterion in distinguishing between aseptic and bacterial meningitis. An elevated CSF protein and decreased CSF glucose, if present, are usually mild, although extreme degrees of both have been reported. Specific virologic diagnosis of enteroviral meningitis depends upon isolation of the virus from the CSF in tissue culture (17), although the sensitivity is only 65% to 75%, largely a result of low CSF titers of enteroviruses and the inability to grow many coxsackievirus A serotypes that require suckling mouse inoculations. Although isolation of a nonpolio enterovirus from the throat or rectum of a patient with aseptic meningitis is suggestive of an etiologic diagnosis, the mean shedding periods from those sites following infection are 1 week and several weeks, respectively, and viral shedding can occur in 7.5% of healthy controls during enterovirus epidemics (10). Therefore shedding from a past infection cannot be ruled out. Rapid diagnosis of enterovirus infections by immunoassay techniques has been hampered by the lack of a common antigen among the various serotypes and the low concentrations of virus in body fluids (1,5). Polymerase chain reaction (PCR) is the most promising alternative to viral culture for the diagnosis of enteroviral meningitis. All the primers are directed at highly conserved regions of the 5′ noncoding region of the viral genome and designed for reverse transcription combined with PCR (RT-PCR). Enteroviral RT-PCR has been tested in clinical settings by numerous investigators and found to be more sensitive than culture and 94% to 100% specific for the diagnosis of enteroviral meningitis (5,18–22).

Mumps Virus

Mumps is one of the most common causes of aseptic meningitis and encephalitis in unimmunized populations (5,23). Meningitis is the most common neurologic manifestation of infection with mumps virus and is estimated to occur in 10% to 30% of mumps patients overall. Males are affected two to five times more often than females, and the peak incidence is in children 5 to 9 years of age. Cases of vaccine-associated mumps meningitis have also been reported (24).

In patients with mumps, symptoms of high fever, vomiting, and headache usually follow the onset of parotitis by about 5 days, although 40% to 50% of patients with mumps meningitis have no evidence of salivary gland enlargement (25). Other findings include neck stiffness, lethargy or somnolence, and abdominal pain. Most patients have signs of meningitis but no evidence of cortical dysfunction. In uncomplicated cases, the total duration of illness is 7 to 10 days. Rarely, mumps may cause encephalitis, seizures, polyradiculitis, polyneuritis, cranial nerve palsies, myelitis, Guillain-Barré syndrome, and fatality.

CSF examination reveals a pleocytosis (usually less than 500 cells/mm^3) that is primarily mononuclear cells, with more than 80% lymphocytes seen in 80% to 90% of patients (23,25). The CSF protein is reported to be normal in more than 50% of patients in some series. The CSF glucose is normal in most patients, although it may be depressed in up to 25% of cases. Complement fixation and hemagglutination inhibition tests on acute and convalescent serum specimens are the most reliable serologic tests for the diagnosis of mumps, demonstrating a diagnostic fourfold rise in mumps antibody titer. Mumps virus can be grown from CSF in tissue culture for at least 1 week following the onset of disease, but the sensitivity of this technique is only 30% to 50% if collected from CSF early during the course of mumps CNS infection (25). Use of molecular diagnostic techniques, such as PCR, may have applicability in diagnosis of mumps meningitis in the future.

Lymphocytic Choriomeningitis Virus

Lymphocytic choriomeningitis virus was previously one of the earliest and seemingly most significant viruses to be associated with human aseptic meningitis (1,5), although this virus is now rarely reported as an etiologic agent. Lymphocytic choriomeningitis virus is transmitted to humans by contact with rodents (e.g., hamsters, rats, mice) or their excreta (26–28). Infection has been documented in pet owners, persons living in impoverished and nonhygienic situations, and laboratory workers. One outbreak was described in laboratory workers who were caring for nude mice that had been injected with lymphocytic choriomeningitis virus–infected tumor cell lines (29). Presumed routes of transmission include ingestion of food contaminated with animal urine and exposure of open wounds to dirt; there is no evidence for human-to-human transmission.

Infection with lymphocytic choriomeningitis virus begins with nonspecific viral symptoms. After a brief period of improvement, approximately 15% of patients develop severe headache, photophobia, lightheadedness, lumbar myalgias, and pharyngitis (1). Orchitis, arthritis, myopericarditis, and alopecia are also occasionally seen, usually as late manifestations.

The CSF of patients with meningitis caused by lymphocytic choriomeningitis virus typically shows a lymphocytic pleocytosis (usually less than 750 cells/mm^3, although cell counts up to several thousand may be seen) (1,30). Up to 25% of patients have hypoglycorrhachia. The etiologic diagnosis may be difficult, as no rapid detection method for lymphocytic choriomeningitis virus is available; the diagnosis is usually made by a fourfold rise between acute and convalescent sera. The virus may be cultured from blood and CSF early in infection and later from urine.

Herpes Simplex Viruses

Meningitis

Herpes simplex viruses account for approximately 0.5% to 3% of all cases of aseptic meningitis (31). Most cases are associated with primary genital infection with herpes simplex virus type 2 (32–34). In one study, 36% of women and 13% of men developed an aseptic meningitis syndrome concomitant with primary infection (34). Primary genital infection with herpes simplex virus type 1 and nonprimary genital infection with herpes simplex virus of either type rarely result in meningitis (34,35). Cases of

Mollaret's recurrent meningitis have been associated with herpes simplex virus type 1 (36,37) and herpes simplex virus type 2 (38,39).

Meningitis associated with herpes simplex virus type 2 infection is usually characterized by stiff neck, headache, and fever (34). In one review of 27 patients with herpes simplex virus type 2 meningitis (35), neurologic complications were found in 37% of cases, consisting of urinary retention, dysesthesias, paresthesias, neuralgia, motor weakness, paraparesis, concentration difficulties of about 3 months' duration, and impaired hearing. All complications, however, subsided within 6 months in all patients. Recurrent meningitis was also documented in five patients.

CSF examination in patients with herpes simplex virus type 2 meningitis typically reveals a lymphocytic meningitis (<500 cells/mm^3) and a normal glucose (1). The virus has been cultured from the CSF and buffy coat of some patients. PCR of CSF appears promising for the diagnosis. Using PCR, herpes simplex virus type 2 was strongly associated with typical cases of Mollaret's meningitis in patients without symptoms or signs of genital infection (38).

Encephalitis

Herpes simplex encephalitis is among the most severe of all human viral infections of the brain and is associated with significant morbidity and mortality ($>70\%$ mortality in patients receiving no or ineffective therapy) (40). In the United States, herpes simplex encephalitis is thought to account for about 10% to 20% of encephalitic viral infections of the CNS (31); the majority of cases (94% to 96%) are caused by herpes simplex virus type 1. Herpes simplex encephalitis occurs throughout the year and in patients of all age groups (41). Whites account for 95% of patients with biopsy-proven disease.

The majority of patients with herpes simplex encephalitis present with a focal encephalopathic process characterized by altered mentation, a decreasing level of consciousness, and focal neurologic findings (Table 6.3) (e.g., dysphasia, weakness, paresthesias) (41,42). These patients nearly always present with fever and personality changes; seizures, either focal or generalized, occur in approximately two-thirds of patients with proven disease. The clinical course may evolve slowly or with alarming rapidity; progressive loss of consciousness leading to coma is common in patients with herpes simplex encephalitis. Although clinical evidence of a localized temporal lobe lesion is often thought to be herpes simplex encephalitis, a variety of other diseases can be shown to mimic this condition (43). Immunocompromised patients with herpes simplex encephalitis may develop a more diffuse nonnecrotizing encephalitis involving the cerebral hemispheres and brain stem (44).

Noninvasive neurodiagnostic studies may support a diagnosis of herpes simplex encephalitis. Electroencephalography (EEG) appears to be the most sensitive (about 84%) for diagnosis, exhibiting characteristic spike-and-slow-wave activity and periodic lateralized epileptiform discharges (PLEDs), arising predominantly over the temporal and frontotemporal regions (45,46); however, the specificity of EEG is only 32.5%. CT scans initially show low-density areas with mass effect localized to the temporal lobe, which can progress to radiolucent and/or hemorrhagic areas (47,48);

TABLE 6.3. *Clinical findings in patients with herpes simplex encephalitis*

Findings	Percentage of patients with finding	
	Brain biopsy positive	Brain biopsy negative
Symptoms		
Alteration of consciousness	97	98
Fever	90	78
Headache	81	77
Personality change	71	68
Seizures	67	59
Vomiting	46	46
Hemiparesis	33	26
Memory loss	24	19
Signs at presentation		
Fever	92	81
Personality change	85	74
Dysphasia	76	67
Autonomic dysfunction	60	56
Ataxia	40	40
Hemiparesis	38	30
Seizures	38	47
Cranial nerve deficits	32	33
Visual field loss	14	12
Papilledema	14	11

Data from Whitley RJ. Herpes simplex virus. In: Scheld WM, Whitley RJ, Durack DT, eds. *Infections of the central nervous system*, 2nd ed. Philadelphia: Lippincott-Raven, 1997:73–89; and Whitley RJ, Tilles J, Linneman C, et al. Herpes simplex encephalitis: clinical assessment. *JAMA* 1982;247:317–320, with permission.

these areas are seen in 50% to 75% of patients at some time during the illness. Magnetic resonance (MR) imaging (with enhancement) demonstrates lesions earlier and is superior to CT in localizing these lesions to the orbital-frontal and temporal lobes (Fig. 6.1) (49,50).

The definitive diagnosis of herpes simplex encephalitis is established by brain biopsy, which currently remains the most specific means of diagnosis. Early during infection, congestion of capillaries and other small vessels in the cortex and subcortical white matter is evident, as are petechiae (51,52). Perivascular cuffing becomes prominent in the second and third weeks of infection, followed by evidence of necrosis and inflammation, with widespread areas of hemorrhagic necrosis. The presence of intranuclear inclusions (Cowdry type A) supports the diagnosis of viral infection but is found in only about 50% of patients. Immunofluorescent studies of brain tissue provide a rapid, sensitive, and reliable method for detecting herpes antigen, if sufficient antigen is present in the specimen and nonspecific immunofluorescence can be minimized (53); virus can also be isolated from brain biopsy specimens (54). Currently, brain biopsy is reserved for patients who do not respond to appropriate antiviral therapy (i.e., acyclovir) or who have an unknown abnormality on CT or MR imaging (55).

Routine studies of CSF in patients with herpes simplex encephalitis are nondiagnostic (41,55), revealing an elevated white cell count (mean of 100 cells/mm^3, predominantly lymphocytic) in 97% of patients with brain-biopsy-proven disease.

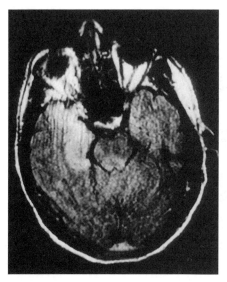

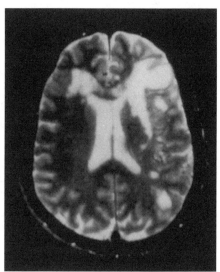

FIG. 6.1. T_1-weighted MR imaging study of the brain (axial view) in a patient with herpes simplex virus encephalitis, revealing abnormal signal intensity within the temporal lobes bilaterally (right greater than left). There is also mass effect with effacement of the cortical sulci. (Courtesy of Melanie Koscelnick, M.D.)

FIG. 6.2. T_2-weighted MR imaging study (axial view) of the brain in an AIDS patient with progressive multifocal leukoencephalopathy, revealing increased signal intensity in the left frontoparietal region with several smaller lesions in the right frontal and left occipital lobes.

The presence of red blood cells in CSF is not diagnostic for herpes simplex encephalitis but suggests the diagnosis in the appropriate clinical setting. The CSF protein is similarly elevated, averaging 100 mg/dL. About 5% to 10% of patients with herpes simplex encephalitis have completely normal CSF on first evaluation. Routine attempts to isolate the virus from CSF are rarely successful (approximately 4% positive). An assay technique for the detection of herpes simplex virus antigen in the CSF of patients with herpes simplex encephalitis has been developed and is 80% sensitive and 90% specific if performed within 3 days of the onset of illness (56). Recent studies suggest that detection of herpes simplex virus DNA within CSF cells by PCR is highly efficacious in the diagnosis of herpes simplex encephalitis (57), with a sensitivity and specificity of 91% and 92%, respectively, in one study of patients with biopsy-proven disease (58). The specificity would have been higher except that some tissue specimens were fixed in formalin, which killed infectious virus. PCR detection of herpes simplex virus DNA in CSF has become the diagnostic procedure of choice in patients with herpes simplex encephalitis (41).

Varicella Zoster Virus

Varicella zoster virus causes two clinically distinct diseases. The first is varicella, which is characterized by a generalized vesicular rash that occurs in epidemics (59).

The incidence of CNS complications during active varicella infection is unknown, although the observed incidence ranges from 0.1% to 0.75% in some series (60). The second is herpes zoster, which is a consequence of reactivation of latent varicella zoster virus; persons at greatest risk for developing herpes zoster, as well as those at increased risk for complications, are individuals with deficiencies in cell-mediated immunity (59). A direct correlation exists between cutaneous dissemination and the appearance of visceral complications, including meningoencephalitis (61,62). In general, the CNS complications of herpes zoster are associated with a higher morbidity and mortality than are those of acute varicella, possibly due, in part, to the patient's advanced age and underlying disease status (57). Acute aseptic meningitis has also been associated with herpes zoster in patients with or without typical skin lesions (63–65); the latter are known as zoster sine herpete. In addition, a variety of varicella zoster virus–induced neurologic disorders have also been described in patients with the acquired immunodeficiency syndrome (AIDS), including multifocal leukoencephalitis, ventriculitis, myelitis, myeloradiculitis, and focal brain stem lesions (59).

Several categories of CNS infection are seen in patients with varicella. Cerebellar ataxia is the most common neurologic abnormality, with a frequency of cerebellar dysfunction of approximately 1 in 4,000 cases (59). Symptoms include nausea, vomiting, headache, nuchal rigidity, and ataxia. These manifestations are usually self-limited, generally resolving within several weeks. Meningoencephalitis or cerebritis is a less common, but frequently more severe, CNS complication of varicella. Headache, fever, and vomiting are often accompanied by an altered sensorium, with seizures occurring in 29% to 52% of cases. Focal neurologic abnormalities include cranial nerve dysfunction, aphasia, and hemiplegia (61). These neurologic symptoms may occur from 11 days before to several weeks after the onset of the varicella rash.

Encephalitis is the most common CNS abnormality associated with herpes zoster, seen most commonly in patients of advanced age, patients who have experienced immunosuppression, and those with disseminated cutaneous zoster (59,66). Altered mentation without other explanation in patients with either localized or disseminated herpes zoster may be the sole clinical manifestation. Other symptoms and signs include hallucinations, meningismus, ataxia, seizures, and motor paralysis. Contralateral hemiplegia in patients with ophthalmic zoster accounts for up to one-third of cases of CNS abnormalities in herpes zoster (59). In typical cases, zoster ophthalmicus precedes the appearance of hemiplegia by several weeks or more (67), although the onset of hemiplegia may be as late as 6 months after the rash has resolved (68).

In varicella-associated cerebritis, the CSF is often abnormal, with a mild to moderate lymphocytic pleocytosis and elevated protein (59). The EEG is usually diffusely abnormal, although focal abnormalities may occur even without clinical seizure activity. In herpes zoster–associated encephalitis, lumbar puncture frequently yields an abnormal CSF formula, with a lymphocytic pleocytosis, elevated protein, and normal glucose. However, as many as 40% to 50% of patients with uncomplicated herpes zoster without CNS symptoms have a mild CSF pleocytosis or elevated CSF protein concentration (59). Varicella zoster virus has been cultured from brain and CSF in a number of cases of herpes zoster–associated encephalitis (69–71). Varicella zoster virus antibodies and lymphocyte–associated varicella zoster virus antigens have also been demonstrated in the CSF of these patients (70,72,73). In zoster ophthalmicus with contralateral hemiplegia, cerebral angiography often demonstrates unilateral arteritis or thrombosis of individual vessels (67,68). CT may show evidence of cerebral infarction in some cases (74). PCR has also been used to confirm the presence of varicella zoster viral DNA in the CSF of patients with herpes zoster meningitis (75,76).

Cytomegalovirus

The most common form of CNS disease caused by cytomegalovirus is cytomegalic inclusion disease, which occurs early in life as a consequence of intrauterine infection. Only 1% of newborns excrete cytomegalovirus at birth, 10% of whom develop clinical evidence of disease. Immunocompromised patients (e.g., patients with AIDS or those who have had bone marrow or organ transplantation) represent a common group that can present with life- and sight-threatening disease due to cytomegalovirus (77–79).

CNS complications due solely to cytomegalovirus infection are uncommon and usually manifest as meningitis, encephalitis, or meningoencephalitis. A form of CNS disease caused by cytomegalovirus also occurs in the immunocompromised host following organ transplantation (usually documented on postmortem examination of brain tissue) (80,81) and in patients with AIDS (82,83). Cytomegalovirus encephalitis in AIDS usually presents in a subacute or chronic course, with cortical dysfunction leading to confusion, disorientation, and perhaps seizures (84). If present, brain stem lesions may produce focal signs. In patients with necrotizing ventriculoencephalitis, a rapidly fatal form of CMV encephalitis, cranial nerve defects, nystagmus, and cognitive disturbances (mental slowness and memory deficit) are often observed (85,86). Cytomegalovirus may also cause aseptic meningitis in association with a mononucleosis syndrome (87), particularly in the immunocompromised host.

The gold standard for the diagnosis of cytomegalovirus disease in any site is isolation of the organism, although it may take as long as 2 to 4 weeks before evidence of cytopathic effect is observed in cell culture systems. Even if brain biopsy specimens are obtained, they may not reveal typical cytomegalovirus histopathology or a positive culture. Focal abnormalities on CT have also been described in CNS infections caused by cytomegalovirus (88), including one patient with a ring-enhancing lesion that proved to be a cytomegalovirus abscess (89). Diagnosis of CNS infection caused by cytomegalovirus is best made by PCR of CSF, which has a high sensitivity and specificity for CNS involvement (90–93).

Other Herpesviruses

CNS involvement in patients with infectious mononucleosis caused by Epstein-Barr virus is more common than generally appreciated and may occur shortly before, during, or after the onset of illness (94). The most common neurologic complication of Epstein-Barr virus infection is aseptic meningitis, which usually has a good prognosis and resolves without significant sequelae. Encephalitis has also been reported following Epstein-Barr virus infection, most frequently of the cerebellum, although any area of the brain may be involved; patients may present with seizures, coma, personality changes, disorders of perception, cerebellar ataxia, or focal cerebral or brain stem findings (95).

Human herpesvirus 6 has been associated with meningitis in conjunction with roseola infantum (96), encephalitis (97), recurrent seizures in children (98), and CNS disease after allogeneic bone marrow transplantation (99). The diagnosis of primary infection with human herpesvirus 6 is by isolation of the virus in culture coupled with seroconversion. However, this virus can exhibit persistence in the CNS and has been demonstrated in the CSF of asymptomatic persons (100). Initial studies utilizing PCR of CSF have shown promise as a diagnostic tool (101), but large-scale studies and further refinements are needed before this technique is routinely used.

Herpes B virus has also been reported to cause cases of severe or fatal encephalitis (55). The disease is transmitted by a monkey bite. The incubation period is generally 3 to 5 days, with the onset of neurologic symptoms 3 to 7 days after appearance of a vesicular rash (102). Mortality is 75% in patients who develop encephalitis.

Human Immunodeficiency Virus Type 1

Involvement of the CNS is a common manifestation of infection with human immuno-deficiency virus type 1 (HIV-1) (103–105). The virus enters the CNS early in the course of infection and has been shown to be present in all stages of disease, irrespective of neurologic symptoms, although most CNS diseases complicating HIV-1 infection occur in its late, or AIDS, phase. Prominent neurologic symptoms are observed in 40% to 70% of patients with AIDS or symptomatic HIV-1 infection, and as many as 90% of patients with AIDS have abnormalities of the nervous system identified at autopsy (106–109). The CNS syndromes associated with HIV-1 infection may result directly from HIV-1 infection or from specific opportunistic infections. The following sections review the neurologic manifestations directly related to HIV-1; specific CNS opportunistic infections are reviewed in other parts of this chapter.

HIV-1 may directly cause a variety of neurologic manifestations, either early after infection or related to persistence in the CNS after initial infection. Following initial infection, there are generally no CNS symptoms or signs, although approximately 5% to 10% of those newly infected with HIV-1 develop an acute aseptic menin-goencephalitis syndrome (110,111), occurring just before seroconversion and during or after the "mononucleosis-like syndrome." Patients may manifest headache, fever, meningismus, cranial neuropathies (most often involving cranial nerves V, VII, and VIII), altered mental status, and focal or generalized seizures.

AIDS dementia complex (also called HIV-1 encephalitis, HIV-1 encephalopathy, or HIV-1-associated cognitive/motor complex) occurs almost exclusively during the AIDS phase of infection and is characterized by the triad of cognitive, motor, and behavioral dysfunction (103,105,112,113). Recent prospective data from the Multicenter AIDS Cohort Study demonstrated an incidence rate, over a 5-year period, of AIDS dementia complex of 7.3 cases per 100 person-years for individuals with

CD4 lymphocyte counts of $\leq 100/mm^3$, 3.0 cases in those with counts of 101 to $200/mm^3$, 1.3 to 1.7 cases for counts of 201 to $500/mm^3$, and 0.5 cases with counts $>500/mm^3$ (114). AIDS dementia complex is a dementia of the subcortical type, with a predilection for frontal white matter, in which patients initially present with behavioral symptoms of apathy, inattention, forgetfulness, impaired concentration, mental slowing, and social withdrawal. Difficulty in reading is common and is usually due to problems in concentration rather than to failure to understand the printed word. Other presentations include acute confusion, hallucinations, and psychosis. Seizures occur as an early symptom in about 10% of cases and eventually in 20% to 50% of patients with more advanced illness. Motor disturbances (including loss of coordination, tremors, and unsteady gait) are seen in nearly 50% of patients and usually lag behind intellectual impairment. This syndrome may progress gradually over a period of several months to more than 1 year, or it may fluctuate with sudden deterioration, sometimes in association with systemic illness.

At least 75% of HIV-1-infected children have abnormal neurologic development (115–117). Two recent longitudinal studies of 172 and 766 children estimated that 23% of perinatally infected children with AIDS developed progressive encephalopathy (104), manifested clinically as seizures and lethargy, followed by spastic paraparesis or quadriparesis, neurologic deterioration, and dementia with loss of previously attained developmental milestones.

In persons with asymptomatic HIV-1 infection, electrophysiologic tests (electroencephalography, multimodal evoked-potential tests, and otoneurologic tests) may be the most sensitive indicators of subclinical neurologic impairment (118), with abnormalities tending to progress over time. CSF examination can be normal, although at least 40% of HIV-1-infected patients have nonspecific CSF abnormalities (111,119–121). There is usually a mild lymphocytic pleocytosis (20% of patients) with cell counts ranging from 5 to 50 cells/mm^3, increased protein from 50 to 100 mg/dL (60% of patients), and a normal glucose. HIV-1 is grown from approximately 20% to more than 60% of CSF cultures and can be recovered from CSF in all stages of virus infection independent of the degree of clinically apparent immune suppression (122,123); however, the value of CSF virus isolation in predicting neurologic involvement is poor (103). High titers of anti-HIV-1 antibodies may also be detected in CSF (112,124). Calculation of relative CSF and serum titers may indicate the presence of anti-HIV-1 antibody synthesis within the CNS. However, neither culture of HIV-1 from CSF nor the finding of intrathecal synthesis of antibodies to HIV-1 is specific for AIDS dementia complex. Both findings may be present in the absence of neurologic symptoms, although they are more common in patients with full-blown AIDS. CSF p24 antigen may also be detected (125), with CSF concentrations often higher than those found in serum. Increased CSF concentrations of β_2-microglobulin (126) and quinolinic acid (127) have also been reported in HIV-1-infected patients. High CSF concentrations of β-microglobulin correlate with the severity of symptoms attributable to the AIDS dementia complex. Recently, a number of investigators have measured CSF concentrations of HIV-1 RNA (the "viral load") and have found a correlation between CSF viral load and severity of AIDS dementia (128,129). However, there was considerable overlap in CSF values of HIV-1 RNA in relation to clinical neurologic severity, so that CSF viral load cannot be used in isolation as a diagnostic marker for AIDS dementia complex or even as an independent predictor of its severity (130). Another study found no significant differences in CSF concentrations of HIV-1 RNA in patients with or without HIV encephalitis, although CSF concentrations of HIV-1 RNA correlated with concentrations of HIV-1 RNA found in plasma (131). Further studies are needed to determine the importance of CSF viral load as a marker for neurologic disease in HIV-1-infected patients.

JC Virus

JC virus is a member of the polyoma subgroup of the genus *Papovaviridae* and causes a syndrome known as progressive multifocal leukoencephalopathy (PML), a demyelinating condition that occurs exclusively in immunocompromised patients (132,133). The designation JC virus is taken from the initials of the patient from whom it was recovered. The virus is ubiquitous and acquisition of antibody to JC virus begins in infancy. By late adult life, the prevalence of antibody in the general population is more than 70%. Urinary excretion of JC virus, believed to represent reactivated JC virus infection, is common under conditions of immunosuppression. The virus has been detected in the urine of 13% of patients with leukemia, 7% of bone marrow transplant patients, and 18% of renal transplant recipients at some time during the period of immunosuppression. Urinary excretion also occurs in 0.4% of pregnant women. Infection is known to occur in patients with defects in cell-mediated immunity, most often with lymphoproliferative disorders, but also in patients receiving antineoplastic chemotherapy for myeloproliferative disorders and malignancies, bone marrow transplantation, renal transplantation, autoimmune diseases, sarcoidosis, tuberculosis, Whipple's disease, nontropical sprue, hypogammaglobulinemia, and idiopathic $CD4^+$ T lymphocytopenia (133–136). Within the last decade, however, it has become apparent that infection with HIV-1 greatly increases the risk of PML (133,137–139), which occurs in up to 4% of patients with AIDS. PML may be the presenting manifestation of this immunodeficient state.

PML usually begins insidiously with alterations in personality, followed by blunting of intellect and frank dementia as the disease progresses (132). Involvement of the dominant hemisphere may produce expressive and/or receptive aphasia; visual abnormalities (e.g., quadrantanopsias or hemianopsias) occur in approximately 50% of patients. Ataxic gait, limb dysmetria, and dysarthria often indicate cerebellar involvement (140). In AIDS patients, limb weakness, gait abnormalities (typically ataxia), visual loss, and altered mental status are the most common initial complaints. Brain stem and cerebellar involvement are uncommon as initial presentations. In the majority of patients with PML, death occurs within 1 year, although the disease may be rapidly progressive, with death occurring within 2 months, or more prolonged, with reported survivals of 8 to 10 years. In AIDS patients, the clinical course of PML is similar to that seen in PML in other immunocompromised persons and is characteristically steadily and rapidly progressive, with an average survival previously reported of 4 months (range, 0.3 to 18 months) (137). However, these data were obtained before availability of highly active antiretroviral therapy, which has been reported to lead to prolonged survival in AIDS patients with PML (141–144).

PML should be considered in any immunocompromised patient who develops neurologic findings. CSF is usually normal or contains increased protein. CT scanning shows demyelination in most cases, manifested as hypodense, nonenhancing white matter lesions without mass effect or evidence of edema (145). MR imaging is the diagnostic method of choice because it is more sensitive than CT and can detect injury to myelin (145–147). Abnormalities noted on MR imaging are chiefly high-intensity-signal lesions located in the centrum semiovale, periventricular areas, and cerebellum on T_2-weighted images (Fig. 6.2). Confirmation of the diagnosis of PML during life requires brain biopsy (132,148). Pathologically, there is virus-induced lysis of oligodendrocytes with resultant loss of myelin; nuclei of infected oligodendrocytes contain JC viral nucleic acids, express early and late viral proteins, and contain typical polyomavirus virions. The diagnostic sensitivity of brain biopsy may be increased by use of immunocytochemical or *in situ* nucleic acid hybridization methods (149,150). Recently, PCR has been utilized as a diagnostic test for detection of JC virus DNA in CSF samples from patients with PML (151–153), with a sensitivity and specificity of 82% and 100%, respectively, in one study (151). Pending further studies, PCR is likely to prove to be a sensitive and highly specific diagnostic test for confirming the diagnosis of PML and may reduce the need for brain biopsy to establish the diagnosis.

MYCOBACTERIA

Mycobacterium tuberculosis

Virtually all tuberculous infections of the CNS are caused by the human tubercle bacillus *Mycobacterium tuberculosis*. Factors such as advanced age, immunosuppressive drug therapy, transplantation, lymphoma, gastrectomy, pregnancy, diabetes mellitus, and alcoholism are known to compromise the immune response in patients with smoldering chronic organ tuberculosis, leading to reactivation of latent foci and progression to the clinical syndrome of late generalized tuberculosis (154,155), which may include involvement of the CNS. The advent of HIV-1 infection has influenced the epidemiology of tuberculosis in the United States, with an estimated 6,000 to 9,000 new cases annually (156). Extrapulmonary tuberculosis (including CNS disease) occurs in more than 70% of patients with AIDS or AIDS discovered soon after the diagnosis of tuberculosis, but in only 24% to 45% of patients with tuberculosis and less advanced HIV-1 infection (157). CNS tuberculosis is also particularly common in less developed areas of the world (e.g., India and Africa) (158).

The specific clinical syndromes of CNS tuberculosis are quite variable and depend upon the original location of the tubercle (159). Foci located on the surface of the brain or ependyma rupture into the subarachnoid space or ventricle, causing meningitis, and foci deep within the brain or spinal cord parenchyma enlarge to form tuberculomas or, more rarely, tuberculous abscesses. Children with tuberculous meningitis commonly develop nausea, vomiting, and behavioral changes (159); headache is seen in fewer than 25% of cases. Seizures are infrequent (seen in 10% to 20% of children prior to hospitalization), although more than 50% of patients may develop seizures during hospitalization. An encephalitic course has also been described in children characterized by stupor, coma, and convulsions without signs of meningitis. In adults, the clinical presentation of tuberculous meningitis tends to be more indolent, with an insidious prodrome characterized by malaise, lassitude, low-grade fever, intermittent headache, and changing personality (159–161). This is followed by development of a meningitis phase within 2 or 3 weeks manifested as protracted headache, meningismus, vomiting, and confusion. In contrast, some adult patients may present with a rapidly progressive meningitis syndrome indistinguishable from bacterial meningitis, or the meningitis may take the form of a slowly progressive dementia over several months or years characterized by personality changes, social withdrawal, and memory deficits (154). On physical examination, children and adults present with more uniform findings, although considerable variation does exist (154,159–167). Fever is observed in 50% to 98% of patients, whereas meningismus and signs of meningeal irritation are absent in 25% to 80% of children and adults with tuberculous meningitis. Focal neurologic signs most frequently consist of unilateral or, less commonly, bilateral cranial nerve palsies (seen in up to 30% of patients on presentation); the most frequently affected is cranial nerve VI, followed by cranial nerves III, IV, and VIII. Hemiparesis may result from ischemic infarction in the anterior cerebral circulation, most commonly in the territory of the middle cerebral artery (168). The clinical manifestations of tuberculous meningitis do not seem to be modified by HIV-1 infection (169,170). Most patients present with fever, headache, and altered mentation. Meningeal signs are absent in up to 50% of patients, although in a recent review of patients with tuberculous meningitis admitted to an intensive care unit, 88% had meningeal findings (167).

Symptoms of tuberculomas are often limited to seizures and correlates of increased intracranial pressure (159); fever and signs of systemic infection are rarely present. Papilledema is seen in most cases, accompanied by neurologic deficits reflecting the location of the lesions. The mean duration of symptoms is weeks to months, and some observers note that the patient's symptoms are less dramatic than would be expected from the radiologic or surgical size of the lesion. Only about 30% of patients with tuberculomas have evidence of tuberculous infection outside the CNS (154).

CSF abnormalities are traditionally seen in tuberculous meningitis (Table 6.4) (154,159). The fluid is typically clear or opalescent, but when the CSF is allowed to stand at room temperature or in the refrigerator for a short time, there may form a cobweblike clot that is the classic "pellicle" of tuberculosis; it occurs secondary to the high fibrinogen concentration in the fluid along with the presence of inflammatory cells. A moderate pleocytosis is characteristic of tuberculous meningitis, with 90% to 100% of patients having more than 5 cells/mm.^{3} The number of cells seldom exceeds 300/mm^3, although exceptions do occur (between 500 and 1,500 cells/mm^3 in about 20% of patients) (166). Initially, both lymphocytes and neutrophils predominate, with rapid conversion into a lymphocytic predominance over several weeks. The converse

TABLE 6.4. *Cerebrospinal fluid findings in tuberculous meningitis*

Parameter	Typical findings
Opening pressure	180–300 mm H_2O
White blood cell count[a]	50–300/mm^3
Mononuclear cells[b]	60–100%
Glucose	<45 mg/dL
Protein[c]	50–300 mg/dL
Acid-fast smears[d]	Positive in 8% to 86%
Culture	Positive in 25% to 86%
Radiolabeled bromide partition	Positive in 90% to 94%
Adenosine deaminase	Positive in 73% to 100%
Tuberculostearic acid	Positive in 95%
Mycobacterial antigen	Positive in 79% to 94%
Mycobacterial antibody	Positive in 27% to 100%
Polymerase chain reaction	Positive in 83% to 100%

[a] White cell counts range from 500 to 1500/mm^3 in 20% of patients.
[b] Following initiation of antituberculous chemotherapy, there may be a neutrophil predominance on subsequent CSF examination.
[c] Values are in excess of 1–2 g/dL in patients with spinal block.
[d] Most series report a rate of smear positivity of <25%.
Data from Leonard JM, Des Prez RM. Tuberculous meningitis. *Infect Dis Clin North Am* 1990;4:769–787; and Zugar A, Lowy FD. Tuberculosis of the central nervous system. In: Scheld WM, Whitley RJ, Durack DT, eds. *Infections of the central nervous system*, 2nd ed. Philadelphia: Lippincott-Raven, 1997:417–443, with permission.

can be seen following the introduction of antituberculous chemotherapy, in which an initial lymphocytic predominance shifts to a neutrophilic predominance on subsequent CSF examinations, the so-called therapeutic paradox. There is usually a modest depression of CSF glucose, with a median of 40 mg/dL reported in most series; hypoglycorrhachia has correlated with more advanced stages of clinical disease (159). CSF protein is elevated in the majority of cases, with median values of 150 to 200 mg/dL. Occasionally, CSF protein values in excess of 1 to 2 g/dL are reported, usually in conjunction with spinal block (163). The identification of tuberculous organisms in CSF by specific stains is difficult because of the small population of organisms. In many series, fewer than 25% of specimens were smear-positive (159,160,162,167), although one review demonstrated positive smears in 52% of CSF specimens (161). The yield may be increased by staining the pellicle (if present) as well as layering the centrifuged sediment of large CSF volumes onto a single slide with repeated applications until the entire pellet can be stained at once. Obtaining repeated specimens may also increase the yield; an 86% rate of acid-fast smear positivity was demonstrated in one study when up to four separate specimens were examined for each patient (166), although this rate has not been consistently duplicated in the literature. Proof of infection requires isolation of the organism from CSF, although false-negative CSF cultures are common, with mycobacteria isolated from less than 50% of patients with a clinical diagnosis of tuberculous meningitis (159). Higher culture yields may be obtained by processing multiple specimens for each patient, although even with as many as four CSF specimens, almost 20% of patients with a clinical diagnosis of tuberculous meningitis have negative CSF cultures (166).

Based on the difficulty in making an etiologic diagnosis of tuberculous meningitis, several newer CSF diagnostic modalities have been developed (Table 6.4) (159,171). Some tests utilize biochemical assays to measure some feature of the organism or the host response to it (e.g., bromide partition test, adenosine deaminase assay). Other modalities are immunologic tests that detect mycobacterial antigen or antibody in the CSF (e.g., tuberculostearic acid antigen, enzyme-linked immunosorbent assay [ELISA], latex agglutination). However, there are problems with these immunodiagnostic tests as a result of the presence of cross-reacting antibodies against nonpathogenic mycobacteria, as well as with the presence of bacterial or fungal antigenic moieties. The technique of PCR for detecting fragments of mycobacterial DNA in CSF specimens appears to be an equally promising tool for the diagnosis of tuberculous meningitis (172–175). Before these tests can be considered useful in the diagnosis of tuberculous meningitis, however, large-scale confirmatory studies must be performed.

There are no pathognomonic radiologic changes for the diagnosis of tuberculous infection of the CNS. On CT scanning, hydrocephalus is frequently present at diagnosis or develops during the course of infection; following administration of intravenous contrast material, enhancement of the basal cisterns results, with widening and blurring of the basilar arterial structures. Periventricular lucencies may be evident, reflecting the presence of periventricular tuberculous exudate and tubercle formation adjacent to the ependyma and choroid. MR imaging with gadolinium enhancement has been shown to be more sensitive than CT in detecting the anatomic abnormalities of tuberculous meningitis (Fig. 6.3) (176). MR angiography has also been utilized to detect the characteristic vascular narrowing and the rare complication of aneurysm formation in patients with tuberculous meningitis (177). Both CT and MR imaging have also been useful in the localization of tuberculomas and tuberculous abscesses in the CNS (178).

Nontuberculous Mycobacteria

The nontuberculous or atypical mycobacteria may also be causes of CNS infection, although there are very few reported cases even in patients with disseminated disease (179). Isolated cases have occurred in both immunosuppressed and immunocompetent patients (162,180,181), in whom CNS infection was presumed to be a result of hematogenous dissemination of the organism. Most nontuberculous mycobacterial infections of the CNS have been caused by *M. avium* complex, although CNS infections have also been reported to be caused by *M. kansasii, M. fortuitum, M. gondonae, M. genavense,* and *M. terrae* complex (181). The diagnosis of CNS infection caused by these organisms requires stricter criteria than for infection caused by *M. tuberculosis*; repeated isolation of multiple colonies of nontuberculous mycobacteria must be demonstrated in the absence of other pathogens to implicate these agents as the cause of CNS disease (181).

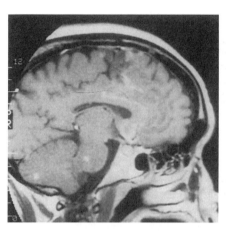

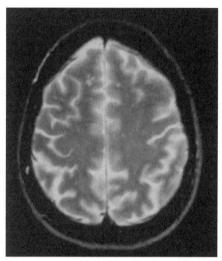

FIG. 6.3. T$_1$-weighted MR imaging study of the brain (sagittal view) in a patient with tuberculous meningitis, revealing extensive meningeal enhancement particularly in the interhemispheric fissure. Additional lesions are present in the pons and cerebellum.

FIG. 6.4. T$_2$-weighted MR imaging study of the brain (axial view) in a patient with Lyme disease, revealing punctate areas of increased signal intensity in the cerebral white matter.

SPIROCHETES

Treponema pallidum

Clinical CNS syndromes caused by *Treponema pallidum* can be divided into four distinct syndromes (182): syphilitic meningitis, meningovascular syphilis, parenchymatous neurosyphilis, and gummatous neurosyphilis. The incidence of syphilitic meningitis is greatest in the first 2 years following infection and is estimated to occur in only 0.3% to 2.4% of syphilis cases. In contrast, meningovascular syphilis is found in 10% to 12% of individuals with CNS involvement (182,183), occurring months to years following syphilis acquisition (peak incidence of approximately 7 years). Parenchymatous neurosyphilis (which includes the variants of general paresis and tabes dorsalis) is relatively rare today and usually becomes apparent 10 to 20 years after acquisition of infection. Gummata are late manifestations of tertiary syphilis and may occur anywhere, although gummatous neurosyphilis is rare. Recently, the overall incidence of neurosyphilis has increased, with many of the reported cases seen in patients with HIV-1 infection (184–186). In one report, 44% of all patients with neurosyphilis had AIDS and 1.5% of AIDS patients were found to have neurosyphilis at some point during the course of their disease (187). In a more recent review of neurosyphilis cases in San Francisco from 1985 to 1992, 75% of patients with neurosyphilis were either infected with HIV-1 or in a high-risk group for HIV-1 acquisition (188).

The clinical presentation of neurosyphilis is based on studies compiled before the availability of penicillin, and there is some debate as to whether the clinical presentations of symptomatic neurosyphilis have been modified in the antibiotic era and by associated HIV infection (182). Patients with syphilitic meningitis usually present with headache, nausea, and vomiting. In one series, these findings were present in 91% of patients, with meningismus and fever occurring in 59% and fewer than 50% of patients, respectively (189). Seizures occurred in 17% of patients, whereas cranial nerve palsies were found in 45% of cases (most commonly cranial nerves VII and VIII, followed by II, III, VI, and V). Less common findings include hemiplegia, aphasia, and mental status changes. In contrast, in meningovascular syphilis, most patients experience weeks to months of episodic prodromal symptoms and signs, including headache or vertiginous episodes, personality changes (e.g., apathy or inattention), behavioral changes (e.g., irritability or memory impairment), insomnia, or seizures (182,183,190). Focal deficits, reflecting episodes of ischemia to regions of the brain by involved blood vessels (usually in the distribution of the middle cerebral artery), may also occur and may progress to a stroke syndrome with attendant irreversible neurologic deficits in untreated patients. Coinfection with HIV-1 may modify the clinical spectrum of syphilis because patients with HIV-1 infection may be more likely to progress to neurosyphilis and to show accelerated disease courses (182–184,191). However, in one study of patients with syphilis at sexually transmitted disease clinics in Baltimore, no significant differences were observed in clinical stage or in disease progression between HIV-1-infected and noninfected patients (192).

No single routine laboratory test is definitive for the diagnosis of CNS involvement in patients with syphilis. CSF abnormalities are common in patients with syphilitic meningitis but are nonspecific (Table 6.5). Findings include a mononuclear pleocytosis (>10 cells/mm^3 in the majority of patients), elevated CSF protein concentrations (78% of patients), and mild decreases in CSF glucose concentrations (<50 mg/dL in 55% of patients) (189). Isolation of *T. pallidum* from CSF specimens is difficult, expensive, time-consuming, and not routinely performed (186). Given the difficulties in the diagnosis of neurosyphilis based on routine CSF studies, serologic testing (i.e., venereal disease research laboratory [VDRL] and fluorescent treponemal antibody [FTA] tests) of CSF has been utilized (186,189,193), although serologic testing of CSF in patients with syphilis is problematic. For example, CSF collected by lumbar puncture is subject to blood contamination in about 10% of patients, which may lead to contamination of CSF and, therefore, a false-positive serologic test result (182). For patients with a serum VDRL of 1:256 or less, sufficient blood contamination to be visible

TABLE 6.5. *Cerebrospinal fluid findings in syphilitic meningitis*

Parameter	Typical findings
White blood cell count	10–500/mm^3
Mononuclear cells	50% to 100%
Glucose	35–75 mg/dL
Protein	30–300 mg/dL
VDRL	Positive in 50% to 85%
FTA	Positive in 75% to 95%

to the naked eye is required to cause false-positive CSF VDRL results. Although the sensitivity of the CSF VDRL for the diagnosis of neurosyphilis is low, the specificity is high (193). Therefore a reactive CSF VDRL test in the absence of blood contamination is sufficient to diagnose neurosyphilis, but a nonreactive result does not exclude the diagnosis. The CSF FTA-ABS test has also been examined as a possible diagnostic test for neurosyphilis (182,193,194). A nonreactive test effectively rules out the likelihood of neurosyphilis. However, the specificity of the test is much less than that of the CSF VDRL because of the possibility of leakage of small amounts of antibody from the serum into CSF, and there are no compelling data that define the significance of a reactive CSF FTA-ABS as useful for the diagnosis of neurosyphilis (182). PCR has been used to detect *T. pallidum* DNA in CSF samples in patients with acute symptomatic neurosyphilis (195), although further large-scale studies are needed to determine the sensitivity and specificity of this technique. Based on the low sensitivity of the CSF VDRL and until further studies demonstrate the usefulness of rapid diagnostic techniques, the diagnosis of neurosyphilis is based on elevated CSF concentrations of white blood cells and/or protein in the appropriate clinical and serologic setting.

Borrelia burgdorferi

The nervous system is eventually involved clinically in at least 10% to 15% of patients with infection caused by *Borrelia burgdorferi,* the etiologic agent of Lyme disease (196–198). Meningitis is the most important neurologic abnormality of acute disseminated Lyme disease, usually following erythema migrans by 2 to 10 weeks, although only about 40% (range of 10% to 90%) of cases of Lyme meningitis are preceded by this characteristic rash (198,199).

In patients with Lyme meningitis, headache is the single most common symptom (30% to 90% of patients), with neck stiffness seen in only 10% to 20% of cases (196–199). Photophobia, nausea, and vomiting are intermediate in frequency between headache and neck stiffness. About two-thirds of patients have accompanying systemic symptoms, including malaise, fatigue, myalgias, fever, arthralgias, and involuntary weight loss. In untreated cases, the duration of symptoms ranges from 1 to 9 months; these patients typically experience recurrent attacks of meningeal symptoms lasting several weeks, alternating with similar periods of milder symptoms. About 50% of patients with Lyme meningitis have mild cerebral symptoms consisting most commonly of somnolence, emotional lability, depression, impaired memory and concentration, and behavioral symptoms (196–199). Transverse myelitis, spastic paraparesis or quadriparesis, disturbances of micturition, and Babinski's signs are also reported during this stage. Cranial neuropathies are also seen in 50% of patients. Facial nerve palsy is the most common (80% to 90%) of the cranial nerve palsies; the facial palsy is bilateral in 30% to 70% of cases, although the two sides are affected asynchronously in most patients. Other cranial nerves affected less commonly are cranial nerves II, III, the sensory portion of V, VI, and the acoustic portion of VIII.

The typical CSF changes in patients with Lyme meningitis are a pleocytosis (usually fewer than 500 cells/mm^3, but up to 3,500 cells/mm^3), with more than 90%

lymphocytes in 75% of cases (196); plasma cells may also be present. There is usually an elevated CSF protein (up to 620 mg/dL) and a normal CSF glucose, although the glucose can be low in patients with illness of long duration. The best currently available laboratory test for the diagnosis of Lyme disease is demonstration of specific serum antibody to *B. burgdorferi,* in which a positive test in a patient with a compatible neurologic abnormality is strong evidence for the diagnosis (196,199). However, these tests are not standardized, and there is marked variability between laboratories performing the test (200). It is currently recommended that when the pretest probability of Lyme disease is 0.20 to 0.80, sequential testing with ELISA and Western blot is the most accurate method for ruling in or out the diagnosis (201,202). Specific antibody against *B. burgdorferi* also appears in CSF and calculation of a specific antibody/IgG index for serum and CSF may indicate intrathecal antibody synthesis (196), although demonstration of the usefulness of CSF antibody must await prospective studies with adequate sample size (201). The technique of PCR on CSF samples has also been used successfully to identify *B. burgdorferi* DNA in patients with Lyme neuroborreliosis (203–205). A recent study utilizing PCR also detected spirochetal DNA in CSF samples from eight of 12 patients with acute (<2 weeks) disseminated Lyme borreliosis (206). However, PCR must still be considered experimental in the diagnosis of CNS Lyme disease.

Radiologic studies may also be useful in patients with CNS manifestations of Lyme disease. CT has shown both enhancing and nonenhancing low-density lesions, mass effect, and cerebral demyelination. MR imaging may reveal punctate hyperresonant areas, without mass effect, within the cerebral white matter (Fig. 6.4).

FUNGI

Cryptococcus neoformans

Cryptococcus neoformans is the most common fungal cause of clinically recognized meningitis, occurring most commonly in persons who are immunosuppressed (e.g., those with reticuloendothelial malignancies, sarcoidosis, organ transplantation, collagen vascular diseases, diabetes mellitus, chronic hepatic failure, chronic renal failure, and patients receiving corticosteroids) (207–209). Cases have also been documented in apparently healthy individuals. Currently, patients with HIV-1 infection are in the highest-risk group (210–215). Clinical studies suggest that 5% to 10% of AIDS patients develop cryptococcal meningitis (216).

The clinical presentation of cryptococcal meningitis is somewhat different in patients with and without AIDS (208,210–213,217). In non-AIDS patients, cryptococcal meningitis is typically a subacute process with days to weeks of symptoms. Headache is the most frequent complaint (87% of patients), and fever, meningismus, and personality changes may also occur. Confusion, irritability, and other personality changes reflecting meningoencephalitis are found in about 50% of cases. Ocular abnormalities occur in about 40% of patients and include papilledema (with or without loss of visual acuity) and cranial nerve palsies. Rare findings include seizures and focal

TABLE 6.6. *Cerebrospinal fluid findings in non-AIDS and AIDS patients with cryptococcal meningitis*

Parameter	% Patients with finding	
	Non-AIDS	AIDS
Opening pressure >200 mm H_2O	72	62–66
White blood cells >20/mm^3	70	13–31
Glucose <40 mg/dL	73	33
Protein >45 mg/dL	89	35–61
Positive India ink	60	72–88
Positive cryptococcal antigen	86	91–100
Positive culture	96	95

Data from Sabetta JR, Andriole VT. Cryptococcal infection of the central nervous system. *Med Clin North Am* 1985;69:333–345; Zugar A, Louie E, Holzman RS, et al. Cryptococcal disease in patients with the acquired immunodeficiency syndrome: diagnostic features and outcome of treatment. *Ann Intern Med* 1986;104:234–240; Chuck SL, Sande MA. Infections with *Cryptococcus neoformans* in the acquired immunodeficiency syndrome. *N Engl J Med* 1989;321:794–799; and Patterson TF, Andriole VT. Current concepts in cryptococcosis. *Eur J Clin Microbiol Infect Dis* 1989;8:457–465, with permission.

neurologic deficits. In AIDS patients, the presentation of cryptococcal meningitis can be very subtle, with minimal, if any, symptoms. AIDS patients may present with only headache and lethargy. Although fever is common (62% to 88% of cases), meningeal signs occur in only a minority (22% to 31%) of patients. Photophobia and cranial nerve palsies are often absent. On the African continent, AIDS patients with cryptococcal meningitis have higher rates of neurologic compromise (218,219), possibly because of the advanced stage of illness at the time of presentation.

The CSF findings in non-AIDS and AIDS patients with cryptococcal meningitis are shown in Table 6.6 (208,210–213,217). On CSF examination, most non-AIDS patients with cryptococcal meningitis have a pleocytosis with white cell counts ranging from 20 to 500 cells/mm^3; the proportion of neutrophils is usually less than 50%. In contrast, AIDS patients may have very low or even normal CSF leukocyte counts during active infection. As many as 65% of AIDS patients with cryptococcal meningitis exhibit fewer than 5 white blood cells/mm^3 in CSF. CSF protein concentrations are generally elevated, with concentrations above 1 g/dL suggesting subarachnoid block. CSF glucose concentrations may be reduced but may be normal in up to two-thirds of AIDS patients with cryptococcal meningitis. Therefore the CSF white blood cell count, glucose, and protein may all be normal in AIDS patients with cryptococcal meningitis. Normal CSF indices were found in 17% of HIV-1-infected patients with cryptococcal meningitis in one study from South Africa (218).

The yield of CSF culture in cryptococcal meningitis is excellent for both non-AIDS and AIDS patients, although cultures may require long periods before positive results are noted. Therefore several rapid tests are available for the diagnosis of cryptococcal meningitis (220). CSF India ink examination remains a rapid, effective test that is

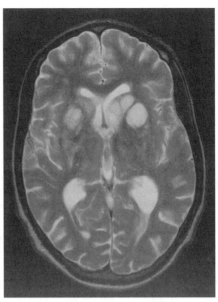

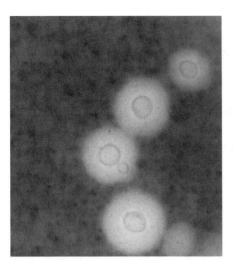

FIG. 6.5. India ink preparation of cerebrospinal fluid, demonstrating the prominent capsule of *Cryptococcus neoformans.*

FIG. 6.6. T_2-weighted MR imaging study of the brain (axial view) in a patient with AIDS and cryptococcal meningitis, revealing multiple nonenhancing cystic periventricular masses located within the lentiform nuclei bilaterally and in the left caudate nucleus, consistent with cryptococcal infection.

positive in 50% to 75% of cases of cryptococcal meningitis (Fig. 6.5); the yield may be as high as 88% in patients with AIDS. The latex agglutination test for cryptococcal polysaccharide antigen is both sensitive and specific for the diagnosis of cryptococcal meningitis when samples are first heated to eliminate rheumatoid factor (221,222). Titers of 1:8 or more by latex agglutination indicate a presumptive diagnosis of cryptococcal meningitis. Cryptococcal polysaccharide antigen can also be found in the serum as well as the CSF, usually in severely immunosuppressed patients such as those with AIDS. Serum cryptococcal antigen detection has been used as a screen for possible CNS infection in AIDS patients (220), although the value of serum antigen in screening patients suspected of having meningeal disease has not been definitively established. *C. neoformans* can also cause focal lesions within the CNS (i.e., cryptococcomas), which may be demonstrated by CT or MR imaging (Fig. 6.6).

Coccidioides immitis

The etiologic agent of coccidioidomycosis is *Coccidioides immitis,* an organism endemic to the semiarid regions of the Americas and desert areas of the southwestern United States (California, Arizona, New Mexico, Texas) (223–225). The initial pulmonary infection caused by *C. immitis* is usually asymptomatic or self-limited, with fewer than 1% of patients developing disseminated disease within the first 3 to 6 months after initial infection; one-third to one-half of patients with disseminated disease have meningeal involvement (226,227). Predisposition to the development of disseminated disease has been associated with infancy and old age, male gender, non-white race, pregnancy, corticosteroid therapy, antineoplastic chemotherapy, immune suppression for organ transplantation, and HIV-1 infection (225).

Meningeal coccidioidomycosis most often follows a subacute or chronic course, although it may present acutely, and is invariably fatal if not treated (226,227). Patients generally complain of headache, low-grade fever, weight loss, and mental status changes. Signs of meningeal irritation are usually absent, although this symptom has been reported in as many as one-third of cases. About 50% of patients develop disorientation, lethargy, confusion, or memory loss; nausea, vomiting, focal neurologic deficits, and seizures may also develop.

The diagnosis of disseminated *C. immitis* infection depends upon demonstration of elevated serum concentrations of complement-fixing antibodies; serum titers above 1:32 to 1:64 suggest dissemination (220). However, the titers may be low when other body sites are not involved. Routine CSF findings in coccidioidal meningitis include a pleocytosis (frequently lymphocytic), increased protein, and decreased glucose, although normal CSF findings do not exclude the diagnosis (226). Occasionally in coccidioidal meningitis, CSF examination may reveal prominent eosinophilia (227,228). CSF complement-fixing antibodies are present in at least 70% of patients with early coccidioidal meningitis and from virtually all patients as the infection progresses, paralleling the course of meningeal disease (226). However, patients who relapse after an initial response to antifungal therapy generally develop CSF pleocytosis or abnormal protein or glucose concentrations before detectable CSF antibody recurs. Patients with immunodeficiencies may also fail to develop complement-fixing antibodies in either serum or CSF. CSF cultures are positive in only 25% to 50% of patients with coccidioidal meningitis.

Histoplasma capsulatum

Histoplasma capsulatum is a dimorphic fungus endemic to fertile river valleys, principally the Mississippi and Ohio river basins (229), where humans are readily and presumably repeatedly infected by inhaling spores. Hematogenous dissemination tends to occur in immunocompromised individuals with impaired cell-mediated immunity (230–233), with CNS involvement occurring in 10% to 20% of cases (234). CNS disease may occur more frequently in patients infected with HIV-1.

The clinical presentation of *Histoplasma* meningitis is nonspecific (229,233). Symptoms usually include headache and fever. Only about one-half of patients have neurologic symptoms, and seizures or focal neurologic deficits occur in 10% to 30% of cases (234). Mental status abnormalities include reduced level of consciousness, confusion, personality changes, and memory impairment.

CSF findings in *Histoplasma* meningitis include a lymphocytic pleocytosis, elevated protein, and decreased glucose. Recovery of *H. capsulatum* from the CSF is accomplished in only 25% to 65% of documented cases (223,229,234). Therefore fungal cultures of blood, bone marrow, sputum, and urine should also be obtained in an attempt to diagnose disseminated disease. Antibody detection in CSF has been used for the diagnosis of *Histoplasma* meningitis (235). These tests (complement fixation and radioimmunoassay [RIA]) have excellent sensitivity for diagnosis but are less specific, with cross-reactivity seen in infections caused by other fungal pathogens (about 50% of cases). *Histoplasma* antigen detection in urine, CSF, and serum may be useful in the diagnosis of disseminated disease (236). However, one study utilizing an RIA for detection of *H. capsulatum* antigen in CSF from patients with meningitis revealed positive tests in only four of 12 patients (237).

Candida Species

Candida species are ubiquitous organisms that are normal commensals of humans and may cause tissue invasion and disseminate in persons with altered host defenses, including patients receiving corticosteroids, broad-spectrum antimicrobial therapy, or hyperalimentation; in premature infants; in patients with malignancy, neutropenia, chronic granulomatous disease, diabetes mellitus, or thermal injuries; and in patients with a central venous catheter in place (238–240). Widespread dissemination of *Candida* to multiple sites, including the CNS, may then ensue (241–243). Candidal meningitis is uncommon, occurring in fewer than 15% of patients with CNS candidiasis, although *Candida* is the most prevalent etiologic agent of fungal brain abscess; *Candida albicans* is the species most commonly found in CNS disease.

The clinical presentation of candidal meningitis is nonspecific (241–243). The onset of symptoms may be abrupt or insidious. The most common symptoms are fever, headache, and meningismus; some patients have depressed mental status, confusion, cranial neuropathies, and other focal neurologic signs.

In *Candida* meningitis, a CSF pleocytosis is commonly seen, with a mean of 600 cells/mm^3; lymphocytes or neutrophils may predominate. Yeast cells are detected in about 50% of cases on direct microscopy of CSF. Organisms can be readily grown from CSF in the majority of cases; a single positive culture from a patient with risk factors or symptoms is considered significant when CSF indices are compatible with meningitis and the fungus is isolated in pure culture (244). The value of antigen or antibody tests in the diagnosis of CNS candidiasis has not been established.

Aspergillus Species

Cases of intracranial infection caused by *Aspergillus* species have been reported worldwide, with most cases occurring in adults. The lungs are the usual site of primary infection, and intracranial seeding occurs following dissemination of the organism or by direct extension from an area anatomically adjacent to the brain (e.g., the paranasal sinuses) (245,246); of patients with disseminated disease, the brain is involved in 40% to 70% of cases. Most cases of invasive aspergillosis occur in neutropenic patients who have an underlying hematologic malignancy. Other risk groups include patients with hepatic disease, Cushing's syndrome, diabetes mellitus, HIV-1 infection, and chronic granulomatous disease, and those who are injection drug users, postcraniotomy patients, organ transplant recipients, and patients receiving chronic corticosteroid therapy (245–250). Some patients have no discernible risk factors (251).

The most common clinical presentation of CNS aspergillosis is brain abscess, in which patients most commonly manifest signs of a stroke referable to the involved area of brain (245). Headache, encephalopathy, and seizures may also occur. Fever is not a consistent feature, and signs of meningeal irritation are rare.

The diagnosis of *Aspergillus* brain abscesses is often difficult (245). CSF results are usually abnormal, but the findings are nonspecific. CT and MR imaging are quite sensitive in defining the lesions, but seldom show changes specific for fungal brain abscess, although some exceptions do exist. The finding of a cerebral infarct in a patient with risk factors for invasive aspergillosis should suggest that diagnosis. The areas of infarction typically develop into either single or multiple abscesses involving the cerebrum (usually frontal or temporal lobes) or cerebellum (Fig. 6.7). Definitive etiologic diagnosis requires biopsy of the lesion and examination by appropriate fungal stains (i.e., methenamine-silver) and cultures. *Aspergillus* species appear as septate hyphae with acute-angle, dichotomous branching in tissue sections.

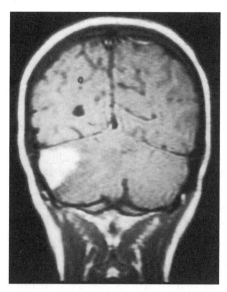

FIG. 6.7. T_1-weighted MR imaging study of the brain (coronal view) in a patient with chronic granulomatous disease, revealing an enhancing mass in the right cerebellum. Biopsy of the lesion revealed invasive aspergillosis.

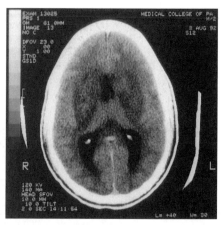

FIG. 6.8. CT scan of the head (axial view) in an injection drug user with focal cerebral mucormycosis, revealing bilateral infarction of the basal ganglia.

Mucoraceae

The Mucoraceae are ubiquitous fruit and bread molds that include the genera *Rhizopus, Absidia,* and *Mucor.* The genus *Rhizopus* is responsible for most cases of cerebral mucormycosis (252). Mucormycosis (zygomycosis, phycomycosis) is one of the most acute, fulminant fungal infections known. Conditions that predispose to mucormycosis include diabetes mellitus typically in association with acidosis (70% of cases), acidemia from profound systemic illnesses (e.g., sepsis, severe dehydration, severe diarrhea, chronic renal failure), hematologic neoplasms, renal transplantation, injection drug use, and deferoxamine use (245,252–254). Fewer than 5% of cases are found in normal hosts. CNS disease may occur from direct extension of the rhinocerebral form of mucormycosis or by hematogenous dissemination from other sites of primary infection.

Patients with rhinocerebral mucormycosis present initially with complaints referable to the eyes or sinuses, including headache (often unilateral), facial pain, diplopia, lacrimation, and nasal stuffiness or discharge (245,255). Initial signs include development of a nasal ulcer, facial swelling, nasal discharge, proptosis, and external ophthalmoplegia (as the infection begins to spread posteriorly to involve the orbit). Cranial nerve abnormalities (including cranial nerves II to VII, IX, and X) are common, and blindness may occur as a result of vascular compromise. Thrombosis is a striking feature of this disease because the organism has a proclivity for blood vessel invasion. Focal neurologic deficits such as hemiparesis, seizures, or monocular blindness suggest far-advanced disease. With further progression, invasion and occlusion of the cavernous sinus and internal carotid artery can occur (256).

In patients with rhinocerebral mucormycosis, CT and MR imaging may show sinus opacification, erosion of bone, cavernous sinus involvement, and obliteration of deep fascial planes (257,258). In injection drug users with cerebral mucormycosis, the basal ganglia are the most frequent site of CNS disease (Fig. 6.8) (253). Biopsy and stains of cerebral lesions in mucormycosis usually demonstrate irregular hyphae, right-angle branching, and lack of septae. Examination of scrapings or biopsies of necrotic nasal turbinates may also reveal the typical nonseptate hyphae of mucormycosis.

Pseudallescheria boydii

Pseudallescheria boydii is a common mold that may cause CNS disease in both normal and immunocompromised hosts (e.g., those with neutropenia or cellular immunodeficiency) (245). This organism is being increasingly referred to as *Scedosporium apiospermum,* the asexual form of *P. boydii. P. boydii* may enter the CNS by direct trauma, by hematogenous dissemination from a pulmonary route, via an intravenous catheter, or by direct extension from infected sinuses (259–262). Brain abscess is the usual CNS manifestation, although meningitis and ventriculitis have also been reported. There is an association between near drowning and subsequent illness caused by *P. boydii,* due to the pathogen's presence in contaminated water and manure.

CNS infection caused by *P. boydii* tends to become manifest 15 to 30 days after an episode of near drowning (260,261). Clinical presentations include seizures, altered consciousness, headache, meningeal irritation, focal neurologic deficits, abnormal behavior, and aphasia. Metastatic skin lesions may herald the fungemia as the organism spreads to the CNS.

In clinical specimens, *P. boydii* appears as septate hyphae, although the hyphae are narrower and, as a rule, do not show the characteristic dichotomous branching encountered in invasive aspergillosis. *P. boydii* can also be identified by staining the biopsy tissue with fluorescent antibodies, a sensitive method that does not cross-react with hyphae of other common pathogenic fungi.

PROTOZOA AND HELMINTHS

Amebae

Despite the hundreds of species of free-living amebae that are known, the most important are in the genera *Naegleria* and *Acanthamoeba* (263,264). *Naegleria fowleri* is the main protozoan causing primary amebic meningoencephalitis in humans. This organism has been recovered from lakes, puddles, pools, ponds, rivers, sewage sludge, tapwater, air-conditioner drains, and soil. Sporadic cases of primary amebic meningoencephalitis occur when people swim or play in water containing the amebae or when swimming pools or water supplies have become contaminated, often through failure of chlorination. The incidence of infection caused by *N. fowleri* is unknown, although one study found only seven documented cases of primary amebic meningoencephalitis in more than 1 billion swimming episodes in Florida lakes (265). Several cases have also been reported in HIV-1-infected patients; all patients had advanced disease at the time of amebic infection (266–269).

Primary amebic meningoencephalitis has two clinical presentations (263,264). In the acute form, following an incubation period of 3 to 8 days, there is the sudden onset of high fever, photophobia, and headache. This presentation is usually indistinguishable from acute bacterial meningitis, although focal signs and seizures are more common in amebic meningoencephalitis. Early symptoms of abnormal smell or taste may be reported because of early involvement of the olfactory area. Confusion, irritability, and restlessness progress rapidly to delirium, stupor, and finally coma. Death in untreated patients generally occurs within 2 to 3 days from the onset of symptoms. In contrast, the subacute or chronic form of primary amebic meningoencephalitis presents more insidiously, with low-grade fever, headache, and focal neurologic signs (e.g., hemiparesis, aphasia, cranial nerve palsies, visual field disturbances, diplopia, ataxia, and seizures) (263,264); the olfactory bulbs are usually spared. Deterioration occurs over a period of 2 to 4 weeks until death. However, longer durations of illness, ranging from 5 to 18 months, have also been reported.

The CSF findings in patients with the acute form of primary amebic meningoencephalitis typically reveal a neutrophilic pleocytosis, low glucose, elevated protein, and red blood cells (263,264); the Gram stain is always negative. However, examination of fresh, warm specimens of CSF can reveal the ameboid movements of the motile trophozoites (270). In patients with the subacute or chronic form of amebic meningoencephalitis, the CSF inflammatory response is less florid, with a leukocytosis that is predominantly mononuclear. The CSF protein concentration is elevated, and the glucose is often normal or slightly reduced. Because amebae are not found in CSF of patients with this form of the disease, the diagnosis usually requires examination of a biopsy specimen revealing the characteristic cysts. Serum immunofluorescence, amebic immobilization titers, and complement-fixing antibodies support the diagnosis, although demonstration of rising titers are necessary to establish the diagnosis since some normal persons have circulating antibodies (263).

Toxoplasma gondii

Toxoplasma gondii can infect the CNS in a variety of syndromes but is usually associated with development of intracerebral mass lesions or encephalitis in immunocompromised hosts. Most cases of CNS toxoplasmosis previously occurred from reactivation of disease in patients with reticuloendothelial malignancies (e.g., lymphoma, leukemia) (271–273), secondary either to the malignancy itself or to associated immunosuppressive or cytotoxic drug therapy. CNS disease has also occurred in patients receiving immunosuppressive therapy after organ transplantation and for treatment of collagen vascular disorders (271,273–275). Disease in organ transplant recipients may also occur after transfer of infected cysts in the allograft, most commonly in heart transplant recipients (276–278). The number of cases of CNS toxoplasmosis has increased dramatically since 1981, specifically in association with HIV-1 infection (279–283), although use of trimethoprim-sulfamethoxazole prophylaxis (284) and highly active antiretroviral therapy (285) has led to a decrease in the incidence of toxoplasmic encephalitis in this patient group.

The clinical manifestations of CNS toxoplasmosis in the immunocompromised patient may be variable, ranging from an insidious onset evolving over several weeks to an acute process associated with a confusional state (271). Furthermore, the initial CNS symptoms and signs may be focal, nonfocal, or both, and vary according to the pathogenesis of infection. Transplant recipients often have nonfocal disease that is diffuse and disseminated (273–277). Early signs and symptoms include weakness, lethargy, confusion, decreased responsiveness, generalized seizures, and headache, with localizing neurologic findings tending to occur late in the course of infection. In patients with underlying malignancies (e.g., Hodgkin's disease), the presentation of toxoplasmic encephalitis is evenly distributed between focal and nonfocal manifestations of encephalitis (271–273). AIDS patients with CNS toxoplasmosis often present with nonspecific symptoms such as neuropsychiatric complaints, headache, disorientation, confusion, and lethargy (279–283). The course is typically subacute, progressing over 2 to 8 weeks. Patients then develop evidence of focal CNS mass lesions with the clinical presentation dependent upon the intracranial location of the lesions. Findings include homonymous hemianopsia, diplopia, cranial nerve palsies, hemiparesis, hemiplegia, hemisensory loss, aphasia, focal seizures, personality changes, movement disorders, and cerebellar dysfunction. *T. gondii* also has a predilection to localize in the basal ganglia and brainstem, producing extrapyramidal symptoms resembling Parkinson's disease. In addition, AIDS patients may develop a more generalized encephalitis with increasing confusion, dementia, and stupor. Seizures are common with this syndrome and may be the presenting clinical manifestation of CNS toxoplasmosis.

In the immunosuppressed host, the value of serologic testing for the diagnosis of CNS toxoplasmosis depends on the pathogenesis of infection. In heart transplant recipients, toxoplasmic encephalitis most often follows acute acquisition of the organism from the transplanted allograft, such that seronegative recipients prior to transplant who receive an organ from a seropositive donor seroconvert and generally develop severe symptomatic disease (276–278,286). However, in many immunocompromised patients (e.g., those with AIDS or bone marrow transplant recipients), toxoplasmic encephalitis occurs as a result of recrudescence of a latent infection (279–283), in which the presence of anti-*Toxoplasma* antibody can be demonstrated almost uniformly prior to the development of the encephalitis. In AIDS patients, more than 97% of patients with toxoplasmic encephalitis have serum antibody titers against *T. gondii* ranging from 1:8 to greater than 1:1, 024 (271). The predictive value of a positive serology in patients with characteristic abnormalities on radiographic studies (see later) may be as high as 80% in the United States (281–287). In contrast, in a retrospective review of 115 patients with AIDS and CNS toxoplasmosis at San Francisco General Hospital between 1981 and 1990, four of 18 patients with pathologically confirmed disease had undetectable anti-*Toxoplasma* IgG antibody by an indirect immunofluorescence assay (283). The predictive value of a positive serology may be much lower in populations in whom other CNS processes are more prevalent (288). In populations where the overall seroprevalence for *T. gondii* is very high, there is a lower predictive value of a positive serology in distinguishing toxoplasmic encephalitis from other infectious and noninfectious etiologies that cause similar neuroradiologic abnormalities.

CT and MR imaging are both extremely useful in the diagnosis of CNS toxoplasmosis (271,281,289). The characteristic CT appearance (seen in 90% of patients) is that of rounded isodense or hypodense lesions with ring enhancement after the administration of contrast material, although homogeneous enhancement or no enhancement can also be seen. There are multiple lesions in approximately 75% of cases, often involving the corticomedullary junction and the basal ganglia, although any part of the CNS may be involved. Unfortunately, CT usually underestimates the number of lesions documented pathologically at autopsy (280). MR imaging has a greater sensitivity than CT (Fig. 6.9) and should be performed in AIDS patients with neurologic symptoms and antibody to *T. gondii* in which CT reveals no abnormality. MR imaging may also be useful in cases of diffuse toxoplasmic encephalitis (Fig. 6.10).

Definitive diagnosis of toxoplasmic encephalitis requires the demonstration of the organism in clinical specimens. Pseudocysts and tachyzoites, which are easily identifiable by histopathologic stains, are best identified at the periphery of the lesion or within normal brain tissue. A sensitive test for rapid diagnosis is the immunofluorescence technique, using monoclonal antitoxoplasmic antibodies on brain tissue touch

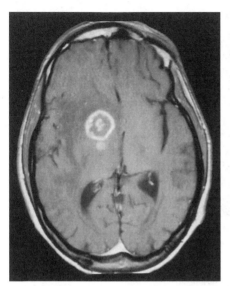 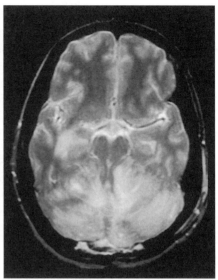

FIG. 6.9. T$_1$-weighted MR imaging study of the brain (axial view) in a patient with toxoplasmic encephalitis revealing ring enhancement of a large 2-cm lesion in the right lentiform nucleus. A small second lesion is also seen. There is associated cerebral edema and midline shift to the left.

FIG. 6.10. T$_2$-weighted MR imaging study of the brain (axial view) in an HIV-infected patient with diffuse toxoplasmic encephalitis, revealing massive cerebellitis with prominent signal change in the medial and posterior cerebellum bilaterally, and evidence of diffuse focal bilateral cortical lesions.

preparations (290). However, in HIV-1-infected patients with the presumptive diagnosis of toxoplasmic encephalitis, the diagnostic approach is somewhat different. When contrast CT or MR imaging reveals the presence of multiple ring-enhancing lesions and the patient has positive anti-*Toxoplasma* IgG serologic tests, empiric therapy for toxoplasmic encephalitis should be initiated. Clinical and radiographic improvement should be observed within 10 to 14 days in patients with toxoplasmic encephalitis (291). For patients with positive anti-*Toxoplasma* IgG serologic tests and a single lesion identified by MR imaging, consideration should be given to thallium-201 single photon emission computed tomography (^{201}Tl-SPECT) scanning (292,293) or to positron emission tomography scanning employing ^{18}F-fluorodeoxyglucose (^{18}FDG-PET) (294). These scans are highly specific for the diagnosis of primary CNS lymphoma and would warrant stereotactic brain biopsy to make a definitive diagnosis. In AIDS patients with mass lesions and negative anti-*Toxoplasma* IgG serologic tests, the diagnosis of toxoplasmic encephalitis is possible, but unlikely, and brain biopsy should be performed. However, some experts have recommended a therapeutic trial for toxoplasmic encephalitis, with brain biopsy performed in patients who fail to respond (295). Patients with single lesions on MR imaging and negative serologic tests should undergo a stereotactic brain biopsy for definitive diagnosis.

Angiostrongylus cantonensis

Infection of humans by the larvae of the nematode *Angiostrongylus cantonensis* can lead to development of an eosinophilic meningitis (296,297). *A. cantonensis* is widespread and human infections are fairly common, reported from many parts of the world (Thailand; India; Malaysia; Vietnam; Indonesia; Papua New Guinea; and the Pacific Islands, including Hawaii) (296–298). The parasites may spread to many countries as rats move freely from port to port on ships (296,299). The larvae invade the CNS either directly from the bloodstream or after migrating through other organs before reaching the spinal cord and brain, and then mature into adult worms.

Symptoms of meningitis begin 6 to 30 days after ingestion of raw mollusks or other sources of the parasite (297,300). Presenting symptoms include severe headache (90%), stiff neck (56%), paresthesias (54%), and vomiting (56%). Moderate fever is present in about half of the cases.

The combination of a history of ingestion of suspected food, moderate to high peripheral eosinophilia, and CSF eosinophilia (range of 16% to 72%) leads to the

---

TABLE 6.7. *Etiologies of eosinophilic meningitis*

Major parasitic etiologies
  Angiostrongylus cantonensis
  Gnathostoma spinigerum
  Baylisascaris procyonis
  Taenia solium
  Paragonimus westermani
  Schistosoma sp.
  Trichinella spiralis
  Toxocara cati
  Toxocara canis
Other infectious etiologies
  Lymphocytic choriomeningitis virus
  Mycobacterium tuberculosis
  Treponema pallidum
  Mycoplasma pneumoniae
  Rickettsia rickettsii
  Coccidioides immitis
  Other fungal meningitides
Noninfectious and diseases of unknown etiology
  Idiopathic eosinophilic meningitis
  Granulomatous meningitis
  Lymphoma
  Leukemia
  Multiple sclerosis
  Subarachnoid hemorrhage
  Obstructive hydrocephalus with shunt
  Antimicrobial agents
  Nonsteroidal antiinflammatory agents

Data from Weller PF. Eosinophilic meningitis. *AM J Med* 1993;95:250–253; and Greenlee JE, Carroll KC. Cerebrospinal fluid in CNS infections. In: Scheld WM, Whitley RJ, Durack DT, eds. *Infections of the central nervous system,* 2nd ed. Philadelphia: Lippincott-Raven Publishers, 1997:899–922, with permission.

suspicion of angiostrongyloidiasis (263). However, a number of other conditions, infectious and noninfectious, should be considered in the differential diagnosis of eosinophilic meningitis (Table 6.7) (301,302). Larvae of *A. cantonensis* are occasionally found in CSF.

REFERENCES

1. Connolly KJ, Hammer SM. The acute aseptic meningitis syndrome. *Infect Dis Clin North Am* 1990;4:599–622.
2. Tunkel AR, Scheld WM. Central nervous system infections. In: Reese RE, Betts RF, eds. *A practical approach to infectious diseases,* 4th ed. Boston: Little, Brown, 1996:133–183.
3. Moris G, Garcia-Monco JC. The challenge of drug-induced aseptic meningitis. *Arch Intern Med* 1999;159:1185–1194.
4. Scheld WM, Whitley RJ, Durack DT, eds. *Infections of the central nervous system,* 2nd ed. Philadelphia: Lippincott-Raven, 1997.
5. Scheld HA. Viral meningitis and the aseptic meningitis syndrome. In: Scheld WM, Whitley RJ, Durack DT, eds. *Infections of the central nervous system,* 2nd ed. Philadelphia: Lippincott-Raven, 1997:23–46.
6. Strikas RA, Anderson LJ, Parker RA. Temporal and geographic patterns of isolates of nonpolio enterovirus in the United States, 1970–1983. *J Infect Dis* 1986;153:346–351.
7. Ho M, Chen ER, Hsu KH, et al. An epidemic of enterovirus 71 infection in Taiwan. *N Engl J Med* 1999;341:929–935.
8. Huang CC, Liu CC, Chang UC, et al. Neurologic complications in children with enterovirus 71 infection. *N Engl J Med* 1999;341:936–942.
9. Dolin R. Enterovirus 71: emerging infections and emerging questions. *N Engl J Med* 1999;341: 984–985.
10. Rotbart HA, Brennan PJ, Fife KH, et al. Enterovirus meningitis in adults. *Clin Infect Dis* 1998;27: 896–898.
11. Kaplan MH, Klein SW, McPhee J, et al. Group B coxsackievirus infections in infants younger than three months of age: a serious childhood illness. *Rev Infect Dis* 1983;5:1019–1032.
12. Wilfert CM, Lehrman SN. Enteroviruses and meningitis. *Pediatr Infect Dis* 1983;2:333–341.
13. Jaffe M, Srugo I, Tirosh E, et al. The ameliorating effect of lumbar puncture in viral meningitis. *Am J Dis Child* 1989;143:682–685.
14. McKinney RE Jr, Katz SL, Wilfert CM. Chronic enteroviral meningoencephalitis in agammaglobulinemic patients. *Rev Infect Dis* 1987;9:334–356.
15. Dagan R, Henista JA, Menegus MA. Association of clinical presentation, laboratory findings, and virus serotypes with the presence of meningitis in hospitalized infants with enterovirus infection. *J Pediatr* 1988;113:975–978.
16. Negrini B, Kelleher KJ, Wald ER. Cerebrospinal fluid findings in aseptic versus bacterial meningitis. *Pediatrics* 2000;105:316–319.
17. Chonmaitree T, Baldwin CD, Lucia HL. Role of the virology laboratory in diagnosis and management of patients with central nervous system disease. *Clin Microbiol Rev* 1989;2:1–14.
18. Rotbart HA. Diagnosis of enteroviral meningitis with the polymerase chain reaction. *J Pediatr* 1990;117:85–89.
19. Sawyer MH, Holland D, Aintablian N. Diagnosis of enteroviral central nervous system infection by polymerase chain reaction during a large community outbreak. *Pediatr Infect Dis J* 1994;13:177–182.
20. Ahmed A, Brito F, Goto C, et al. Clinical utility of polymerase chain reaction for diagnosis of enteroviral meningitis in infancy. *J Pediatr* 1997;131:393–397.
21. Gorgievski-Hrisoho M, Schumacher JD, Vilimonovic N, et al. Detection of PCR of enteroviruses in cerebrospinal fluid during a summer outbreak of aseptic meningitis in Switzerland. *J Clin Microbiol* 1998;36:2408–2412.
22. Van Vliet KE, Glimaker M, Lebon P, et al. Multicenter evaluation of the amplicor enterovirus PCR test with cerebrospinal fluid from patients with aseptic meningitis. *J Clin Microbiol* 1998;36:2652–2657.
23. Gnann JW Jr. Meningitis and encephalitis caused by mumps virus. In: Scheld WM, Whitley RJ, Durack DT, eds. *Infections of the central nervous system,* 2nd ed. Philadelphia: Lippincott-Raven, 1997:169–180.

24. Miller E, Goldacre M, Pugh S, et al. Risk of aseptic meningitis after measles, mumps, and rubella vaccine in UK children. *Lancet* 1993;341:979–982.
25. Levitt LP, Rich TA, Kinde SW, et al. Central nervous system mumps. *Neurology* 1970;20:829–834.
26. Deibel R, Woodall JP, Decher WJ, et al. Lymphocytic choriomeningitis virus in man: serologic evidence of association with pet hamsters. *JAMA* 1975;232:501–504.
27. Vanzee BE, Douglas RG Jr, Betts RF, et al. Lymphocytic choriomeningitis in university hospital personnel: clinical features. *Am J Med* 1975;58:803–809.
28. Hirsch MS, Moellering RC Jr, Pope HG, et al. Lymphocytic-choriomeningitis-virus infection traced to a pet hamster. *N Engl J Med* 1974;291:610–612.
29. Dykewicz CA, Dato VM, Fisher-Hoch SP, et al. Lymphocytic choriomeningitis outbreak associated with nude mice in a research institute. *JAMA* 1992;267:1349–1353.
30. Ratzan KR. Viral meningitis. *Med Clin North Am* 1985;69:399–413.
31. Corey L, Spear PG. Infections with herpes simplex viruses (second of two parts). *N Engl J Med* 1986; 314:749–757.
32. Olsen LC, Beuscher EL, Artenstein MS, et al. Herpesvirus infections of the human central nervous system. *N Engl J Med* 1967;277:1271–1277.
33. Craig CP, Nahmias AJ. Different patterns of neurologic involvement with herpes simplex virus types 1 and 2: isolation of herpes simplex virus type 2 from the buffy coat of two adults with meningitis. *J Infect Dis* 1973;127:365–372.
34. Corey L, Adams HG, Brown ZA, et al. Genital herpes simplex virus infection: clinical manifestations, course, and complications. *Ann Intern Med* 1983;98:958–972.
35. Bergsträm T, Vahlne A, Alestig K, et al. Primary and recurrent herpes simplex virus type 2–induced meningitis. *J Infect Dis* 1990;162:322–330.
36. Steel JG, Dix RD, Baringer JR. Isolation of herpes simplex virus type 1 in recurrent (Mollaret) meningitis. *Ann Neurol* 1982;11:17–21.
37. Yamamoto LJ, Tedder DG, Ashley R, et al. Herpes simplex virus type 1 DNA in cerebrospinal fluid of a patient with Mollaret's meningitis. *N Engl J Med* 1991;325:1082–1085.
38. Tedder DG, Ashley R, Tyler KL, et al. Herpes simplex virus infection as a cause of benign recurrent lymphocytic meningitis. *Ann Intern Med* 1994;121:334–338.
39. Picard FJ, Dekaban GA, Silva J, et al. Mollaret's meningitis associated with herpes simplex type 2 infection. *Neurology* 1993;43:1722–1727.
40. Boston Interhospital Virus Study Group and the NIAID-Sponsored Cooperative Antiviral Clinical Study. Failure of high dose 5-iodo-2'-deoxyuridine in the therapy of herpes simplex virus encephalitis: evidence of unacceptable toxicity. *N Engl J Med* 1975;292:599–603.
41. Whitley RJ. Herpes simplex virus. In: Scheld WM, Whitley RJ, Durack DT, eds. *Infections of the central nervous system,* 2nd ed. Philadelphia: Lippincott-Raven, 1997:73–89.
42. Whitley RJ, Tilles J, Linneman C, et al. Herpes simplex encephalitis: clinical assessment. *JAMA* 1982;247:317–320.
43. Whitley RJ, Cobbs CG, Alford CA Jr, et al. Diseases that mimic herpes simplex encephalitis: diagnosis, presentation, and outcome. *JAMA* 1989;262:234–239.
44. Johnson M, Valyi-Nagy T. Expanding the clinicopathologic spectrum of herpes simplex encephalitis. *Hum Pathol* 1998;29:207–210.
45. Ch'ien LT, Boehm RM, Robinson H, et al. Characteristic early electroencephalographic changes in herpes simplex encephalitis. *Arch Neurol* 1977;34:361–364.
46. Smith JB, Westmoreland BF, Reagan TJ, et al. A distinctive clinical EEG profile in herpes simplex encephalitis. *Mayo Clin Proc* 1975;50:469–474.
47. Enzmann DR, Ransom B, Norman D, et al. Computed tomography of herpes simplex encephalitis. *Radiology* 1978;129:419–425.
48. Zimmerman RD, Russell EJ, Leeds N, et al. CT in the early diagnosis of herpes simplex encephalitis. *Am J Roentgenol* 1980;134:61–66.
49. Schlesinger Y, Buller RS, Brunstrom JE, et al. Expanded spectrum of herpes simplex encephalitis in childhood. *J Pediatr* 1995;126:234–241.
50. Johnson RT. Acute encephalitis. *Clin Infect Dis* 1996;23:219–226.
51. Boos J, Esiri MM. Biopsy histopathology in herpes simplex encephalitis and in encephalitis of undefined etiology. *Yale J Biol Med* 1984;57:751–755.
52. Garcia JH, Colon LE, Whitley RJ, et al. Diagnosis of viral encephalitis by brain biopsy. *Semin Diagn Pathol* 1984;1:71–80.
53. Nahmias AJ, Whitley RJ, Visintine AN, et al. Herpes simplex virus encephalitis: laboratory evaluations and their diagnostic significance. *J Infect Dis* 1982;145:829–836.

54. Griffith JF, Ch'ien LT. Herpes simplex virus encephalitis: diagnostic and treatment considerations. *Med Clin North Am* 1983;647:991–1008.
55. Whitley RJ. Viral encephalitis. *N Engl J Med* 1990;323:242–250.
56. Lakeman FD, Koga J, Whitley RJ. Detection of antigen to herpes simplex virus in cerebrospinal fluid from patients with herpes simplex encephalitis. *J Infect Dis* 155:1172–1178.
57. Rowley A, Lakeman F, Whitley RJ, et al. Diagnosis of herpes simplex encephalitis by DNA amplification of cerebrospinal fluid cells. *Lancet* 1990;335:440–441.
58. Lakeman FD, Whitley RJ, NIAID Collaborative Antiviral Study Group. Diagnosis of herpes simplex encephalitis: application of polymerase chain reaction to cerebrospinal fluid from brain biopsied patients and correlation with disease. *J Infect Dis* 1995;171:857–863.
59. Gnann JW Jr, Whitley RJ. Neurologic manifestations of varicella and herpes zoster. In: Scheld WM, Whitley RJ, Durack DT, eds. *Infections of the central nervous system,* 2nd ed. Philadelphia: Lippincott-Raven, 1997:91–105.
60. Barnes DW, Whitley RJ. CNS diseases associated with varicella zoster virus and herpes simplex virus infection: pathogenesis and current therapy. *Neurol Clin* 1986;4:265–283.
61. Mazur MH, Dolin R. Herpes zoster at the NIH: a 20-year experience. *Am J Med* 1978;65:738–744.
62. Jemsek J, Greenberg SB, Taber L, et al. Herpes zoster–associated encephalitis: clinicopathologic report of 12 cases and review of the literature. *Medicine (Baltimore)* 1983;62:81–97.
63. Echevarria JM, Martinez-Martin P, Tellaz A, et al. Aseptic meningitis due to varicella-zoster virus: serum antibody levels and local synthesis of specific IgG, IgM, and IgA. *J Infect Dis* 1987;155:959–967.
64. Mayo DR, Booss J. Varicella zoster–associated neurologic disease without skin disease. *Arch Neurol* 1989;46:313–315.
65. Karp SJ. Meningitis and cutaneous disseminated zoster complicating herpes zoster infection. *J Neurol Neurosurg Psychiatry* 1983;46:582–590.
66. Tenser RB. Herpes simplex and herpes zoster: nervous system involvement. *Neurol Clin* 1984;2:215–240.
67. Patresi R, Freemon FR, Lowry JL. Herpes zoster ophthalmicus with contralateral hemiplegia. *Arch Neurol* 1977;34:640–641.
68. Walker RJ, Gammal TE, Allen MB. Cranial arteritis associated with herpes zoster. *Radiology* 1973;107:109–110.
69. Ophir O, Seigman-Igra Y, Vardinon N, et al. Herpes zoster encephalitis: isolation of virus from cerebrospinal fluid. *Isr J Med Sci* 1984;20:1189–1192.
70. Andiman WA, White-Greenwald M, Tinghitella T. Zoster encephalitis: isolation of virus and measurement of varicella-zoster specific antibodies in cerebrospinal fluid. *Am J Med* 1982;73:769–772.
71. Steele RW, Keeney RE, Bradsher RW, et al. Treatment of varicella-zoster meningoencephalitis with acyclovir: demonstration of virus in cerebrospinal fluid by electron microscopy. *Am J Clin Pathol* 1983;80:57–60.
72. Bieger RC, Van Scoy RE, Smith TF. Antibodies to varicella zoster in cerebrospinal fluid. *Arch Neurol* 1977;34:489–491.
73. Mathiesen T, Linde A, Olding-Stenvisk E, et al. Antiviral IgM and IgG subclasses in varicella-zoster–associated neurological syndromes. *J Neurol Neurosurg Psychiatry* 1989;52:578–582.
74. Kuroiwa Y, Furukawa T. Hemispheric infarction after herpes zoster ophthalmicus: computed tomography and angiography. *Neurology* 1981;31:1030–1032.
75. Echevarria JM, Cases I, Tenoirio A, et al. Detection of varicella-zoster virus–specific DNA sequences in cerebrospinal fluid from patients with acute aseptic meningitis and no cutaneous lesions. *J Med Virol* 1994;43:331–335.
76. Shoji H, Honda Y, Murai I, et al. Detection of varicella-zoster virus DNA by polymerase chain reaction in cerebrospinal fluid of patients with herpes zoster meningitis. *J Neurol* 1992;239:69–70.
77. Glenn J. Cytomegalovirus infections following renal transplantation. *Rev Infect Dis* 1981;3:1151–1178.
78. Winston DJ, Gale RP, Meyer DV, et al. Infectious complications of human bone marrow transplantation. *Medicine (Baltimore)* 1979;58:1–31.
79. Jacobson MA, Mills J. Serious cytomegalovirus disease in the acquired immunodeficiency syndrome (AIDS): clinical findings, diagnosis, and treatment. *Ann Intern Med* 1988;108:585–594.
80. Schneck SA. Neuropathological features of human organ transplantation. I. Possible cytomegalovirus infection. *J Neuropathol Exp Neurol* 1965;24:415–429.
81. Schober R, Herman MM. Neuropathology of cardiac transplantation. *Lancet* 1973;1:962–967.

82. Moskowitz LB, Gregorios JB, Hensley GT, et al. Cytomegalovirus induced demyelination associated with acquired immune deficiency syndrome. *Arch Pathol Lab Med* 1984;108:873–877.

83. Post MJD, Hensley GT, Moskowitz LB, et al. Cytomegalic inclusion virus encephalitis in patients with AIDS: CT, clinical and pathologic correlation. *Am J Neuroradiol* 1986;7:275–280.

84. Holland NR, Power C, Mathews VP, et al. Cytomegalovirus encephalitis in acquired immunodeficiency syndrome (AIDS). *Neurology* 1994;44:507–514.

85. Grassi MP, Clerici F, Perin C, et al. Microglial nodular encephalitis and ventriculoencephalitis due to cytomegalovirus infection in patients with AIDS: two distinct clinical patterns. *Clin Infect Dis* 1998;27:504–508.

86. Kalayjian RC, Cohen ML, Bonomo RA, et al. Cytomegalovirus ventriculoencephalitis in AIDS: a syndrome with distinct clinical and pathologic features. *Medicine (Baltimore)* 1993;72: 67–77.

87. Causey JQ. Spontaneous cytomegalovirus mononucleosis-like syndrome and aseptic meningitis. *South Med J* 1976;69:1384–1387.

88. Masdeu JC, Small CB, Weiss L, et al. Multifocal cytomegalovirus encephalitis in AIDS. *Ann Neurol* 1988;23:97–99.

89. Levy RM, Bredesen DE. Central nervous system dysfunction in acquired immunodeficiency syndrome. *J Acquir Immune Defic Syndr* 1988;1:41–64.

90. Clifford DB, Buller RS, Mohammed S, et al. Use of polymerase chain reaction to demonstrate cytomegalovirus DNA in CSF of patients with human immunodeficiency virus infection. *Neurology* 1993;43:75–79.

91. Cinque P, Vago L, Brytting M, et al. Cytomegalovirus infection of the central nervous system in patients with AIDS: diagnosis by DNA amplification from cerebrospinal fluid. *J Infect Dis* 1992;166:1408–1411.

92. Wolf DG, Spector SA. Diagnosis of human cytomegalovirus central nervous system disease in AIDS patients by DNA amplification from cerebrospinal fluid. *J Infect Dis* 1992;166:1412–1415.

93. Wildemann B, Haas J, Lynen N, et al. Diagnosis of cytomegalovirus encephalitis in patients with AIDS by quantitation of cytomegalovirus genomes in cells of cerebrospinal fluid. *Neurology* 1998;50: 693–697.

94. Silverstein A, Steinberg G, Nathanson M. Nervous system involvement in infectious mononucleosis. *Arch Neurol* 1972;26:353–358.

95. Ross JP, Cohen JI. Epstein-Barr virus. In: Scheld WM, Whitley RJ, Durack DT, eds. *Infections of the central nervous system,* 2nd ed. Philadelphia: Lippincott-Raven; 1997:117–127.

96. Huang LM, Lee CY, Lee PI, et al. Meningitis caused by human herpesvirus-6. *Arch Dis Child* 1991;66:1443–1444.

97. McCullers JA, Lakeman FD, Whitley RJ. Human herpesvirus 6 is associated with focal encephalitis. *Clin Infect Dis* 1995;21:571–576.

98. Kondo KH, Nagafuji A, Hata C, et al. Association of human herpesvirus 6 infection of the central nervous system with recurrence of febrile convulsions. *J Infect Dis* 1993;167:1197–2000.

99. Wang FZ, Linde A, Hagglund H, et al. Human herpesvirus 6 DNA in cerebrospinal fluid specimens from allogeneic bone marrow transplant patients: does it have clinical significance? *Clin Infect Dis* 1999;28:562–568.

100. Caserta MT, Hall CB, Schnabel K, et al. Neuroinvasion and persistence of human herpesvirus 6 in children. *J Infect Dis* 1994;170:1586–1589.

101. Braun DK, Dominguez G, Pellett PE. Human herpesvirus 6. *Clin Microbiol Rev* 1997;10:521–567.

102. Whitley RJ. B virus. In: Scheld WM, Whitley RJ, Durack DT, eds. *Infections of the central nervous system,* 2nd ed. Philadelphia: Lippincott-Raven, 1997:139–145.

103. Berger JR, Simpson DM. Neurologic complications of AIDS. In: Scheld WM, Whitley RJ, Durack DT, eds. *Infections of the central nervous system,* 2nd ed. Philadelphia: Lippincott-Raven, 1997: 255–271.

104. Janssen RS. Epidemiology and neuroepidemiology of human immunodeficiency virus infection. In: Berger JR, Levy RM, eds. AIDS and the nervous system, 2nd ed. Philadelphia: Lippincott-Raven, 1997:13–37.

105. Price RW. Neurologic complications of HIV infection. *Lancet* 1996;348:445–452.

106. McArthur JC. Neurologic manifestations of AIDS. *Medicine (Baltimore)* 1987;66:407–437.

107. Gabuzda DH, Hirsch MS. Neurologic manifestations of infection with human immunodeficiency virus: clinical features and pathogenesis. *Ann Intern Med* 1987;107:383–391.

108. Lantos PL, McLaughlin JE, Scholtz CL, et al. Neuropathology of the brain in HIV infection. *Lancet* 1989;1:309–311.

109. Malouf R, Jacquette G, Dobkin J, et al. Neurologic disease in human immunodeficiency virus-infected drug abusers. *Arch Neurol* 1990;47:1002–1007.
110. Carne CA, Tedder RS, Smith A, et al. Acute encephalopathy coincident with seroconversion for anti-HTLV-III. *Lancet* 1985;2:1206–1208.
111. Hollander H, Stringari S. Human immunodeficiency virus-associated meningitis: clinical course and correlations. *Am J Med* 1987;83:813–816.
112. Navia BA, Jordan BD, Price RW. The AIDS dementia complex. I. Clinical features. *Ann Neurol* 1986;19:517–524.
113. Navia BA, Price RW. The acquired immunodeficiency syndrome dementia complex as the presenting or sole manifestation of human immunodeficiency virus infection. *Arch Neurol* 1987;44:65–69.
114. Bacellar H, Munoz A, Miller E, et al. Temporal trends in the incidence of HIV-1-related neurologic diseases: multicenter AIDS Cohort Study, 1985–1992. *Neurology* 1994;44:1892–1900.
115. Belman AL, Ultmann MH, Horoupian D, et al. Neurologic complications in infants and children with acquired immune deficiency syndrome. *Ann Neurol* 1985;18:560–566.
116. Epstein LG, Sharer LR, Joshi VV, et al. Progressive encephalopathy in children with acquired immune deficiency syndrome. *Ann Neurol* 1985;17:488–496.
117. Epstein LG, Sharer LR, Goudsmit J. Neurological and neuropathological features of human immunodeficiency virus infection in children. *Ann Neurol* 1988;23:S19–S23.
118. Koralnik IJ, Beaumanoir A, Hausler R, et al. A controlled study of early neurologic abnormalities in men with asymptomatic human immunodeficiency virus infection. *N Engl J Med* 1990;323: 864–870.
119. Hollander H. Cerebrospinal fluid normalities and abnormalities in individuals infected with human immunodeficiency virus. *J Infect Dis* 1988;158:855–858.
120. Appelman ME, Marshall DW, Brey RL, et al. Cerebrospinal fluid abnormalities in patients without AIDS who are seropositive for human immunodeficiency virus. *J Infect Dis* 1988;158:193–199.
121. Chalmers AC, Aprill BS, Shephard H. Cerebrospinal fluid and human immunodeficiency virus: findings in healthy, asymptomatic, seropositive men. *Arch Intern Med* 1990;150:1538–1540.
122. Resnick L, Berger JR, Shapshak P, et al. Early penetration of the blood-brain-barrier by HIV. *Neurology* 1988;38:9–14.
123. Hollander H, Levy JA. Neurologic abnormalities and recovery of human immunodeficiency virus from cerebrospinal fluid. *Ann Intern Med* 1987;106:692–695.
124. Resnick L, diMarzo-Veronese F, Schüpbach J, et al. Intra-blood-brain-barrier synthesis of HTLV-III-specific IgG in patients with neurologic symptoms associated with AIDS or AIDS-related complex. *N Engl J Med* 1985;313:1498–1504.
125. Portegies P, Epstein LG, Hung ST, et al. Human immunodeficiency virus type 1 antigen in cerebrospinal fluid: correlation with clinical neurologic status. *Arch Neurol* 1989;46:261–264.
126. Brew BJ, Bhalla RB, Fleisher M, et al. Cerebrospinal fluid β_2—microglobulin in patients infected with human immunodeficiency virus. *Neurology* 1989;39:830–834.
127. Heyes MP, Rubinow D, Lane C, et al. Cerebrospinal fluid quinolinic acid concentrations are increased in acquired immune deficiency syndrome. *Ann Neurol* 1989;26:275–277.
128. Ellis RJ, Hsia K, Spector SA, et al. Cerebrospinal fluid human immunodeficiency virus type 1 RNA levels are elevated in neurocognitively impaired individuals with acquired immunodeficiency syndrome. *Ann Neurol* 1997;42:679–688.
129. McArthur JC, McClernon DR, Cronin MF, et al. Relationship between human immunodeficiency virus–associated dementia and viral load in cerebrospinal fluid and brain. *Ann Neurol* 1997;42: 689–698.
130. Price RW, Staprans S. Measuring the "viral load" in cerebrospinal fluid in human immunodeficiency virus infection: window into brain infection? *Ann Neurol* 1997;42:675–678.
131. Bossi P, Dupin N, Coutellier A, et al. The level of human immunodeficiency virus (HIV) type 1 RNA in cerebrospinal fluid as a marker of HIV encephalitis. *Clin Infect Dis* 1998;26:1072–1073.
132. Greenlee JE. Progressive multifocal leukoencephalopathy. In: Remington JS, Swartz MN, eds. *Current clinical topics in infectious diseases.* Boston: Blackwell Scientific, 1989:140–156.
133. Greenlee JE. Progressive multifocal leukoencephalopathy: progress made and lessons relearned. *N Engl J Med* 1998;338:1378–1380.
134. Seong D, Bruner JM, Lee KH, et al. Progressive multifocal leukoencephalopathy after autologous bone marrow transplantation in a patient with chronic myelogenous leukemia. *Clin Infect Dis* 1996;23:402–403.
135. Chikezie PU, Greenberg AL. Idiopathic CD4$^+$ T lymphocytopenia presenting as progressive multifocal leukoencephalopathy: case report. *Clin Infect Dis* 1997;24:526–527.

136. Bezrodnik L, Samara R, Krasovec S, et al. Progressive multifocal leukoencephalopathy in a patient with hypogammaglobulinemia. *Clin Infect Dis* 1998;27:181–184.
137. Berger JR, Kaszovitz B, Post MJD, et al. Progressive multifocal leukoencephalopathy associated with human immunodeficiency virus infection: a review of the literature with a report of sixteen cases. *Ann Intern Med* 1987;107:78–87.
138. Chaisson RE, Griffin DE. Progressive multifocal leukoencephalopathy in AIDS. *JAMA* 1990;264: 79–82.
139. Berger JR, Concha M. Progressive multifocal leukoencephalopathy: the evolution of a disease once considered rare. *J Neurovirol* 1995;1:5–18.
140. Parr J, Horoupian DS, Winkelman AC. Cerebellar form of progressive multifocal leukoencephalopathy. *Can J Neurol Sci* 1979;6:123–128.
141. Baqi M, Kucharczyk W, Walmsley SL. Regression of progressive multifocal leukoencephalopathy with highly active antiretroviral therapy. *AIDS* 1997;11:1526–1527.
142. Elliot B, Aromin I, Gold R, et al. Two to five year remission of AIDS-associated progressive multifocal leukoencephalopathy with combined antiretroviral therapy. *Lancet* 1997;349:850.
143. Albrecht H, Hoffmann C, Degen O, et al. Highly active antiretroviral therapy significantly improves the prognosis of patients with HIV-associated progressive multifocal leukoencephalopathy. *AIDS* 1998;12:1149–1154.
144. Cinque P, Casari S, Bertelli D. Progressive multifocal leukoencephalopathy, HIV, and highly active antiretroviral therapy. *N Engl J Med* 1998;339:848–849.
145. Koeppen S. Progressive multifocal leukoencephalopathy: neurological findings and evaluation of magnetic resonance imaging and computed tomography. *Neurosurg Rev* 1987;10:127–132.
146. Guilleux MH, Seiner RE, Young I. MR imaging in progressive multifocal leukoencephalopathy. *Am J Neuroradiol* 1986;7:1033–1035.
147. Mark AS, Atlas SW. Progressive multifocal leukoencephalopathy in patients with AIDS: appearance on MR images. *Radiology* 1989;173:517–520.
148. Schlitt M, Morawetz RB, Bonnin J, et al. Progressive multifocal leukoencephalopathy: three patients diagnosed by brain biopsy, with prolonged survival in two. *Neurosurgery* 1986;18:407–414.
149. Aksamit AJ, Sever JL, Major EO. Progressive multifocal leukoencephalopathy: JC virus detection by in situ hybridization compared with immunohistochemistry. *Neurology* 1986;36:499–504.
150. Aksamit A, Major EO, Ghatak NR, et al. Diagnosis of progressive multifocal leukoencephalopathy by brain biopsy with biotin labeled DNA:DNA *in situ* hybridization. *J Neuropathol Exp Neurol* 1987;46:556–566.
151. Weber T, Turner RW, Frye S, et al. Specific diagnosis of progressive multifocal leukoencephalopathy by polymerase chain reaction. *J Infect Dis* 1994;169:1138–1141.
152. Hammarin AL, Bogdanovic G, Svedhem V, et al. Analysis of PCR as a tool for detection of JC virus DNA in cerebrospinal fluid for diagnosis of progressive multifocal leukoencephalopathy. *J Clin Microbiol* 1996;34:2929–2932.
153. Bogdanovic G, Priftakis P, Hammarin AL, et al. Detection of JC virus in cerebrospinal fluid (CSF) samples from patients with progressive multifocal leukoencephalopathy but not in CSF samples from patients with herpes simplex encephalitis, enteroviral meningitis, or multiple sclerosis. *J Clin Microbiol* 1998;36:1137–1138.
154. Leonard JM, Des Prez RM. Tuberculous meningitis. *Infect Dis Clin North Am* 1990;4:769–787.
155. Singh N, Paterson DL. *Mycobacterium tuberculosis* infection in solid-organ transplant recipients: impact and implications for management. *Clin Infect Dis* 1998;27:1266–1277.
156. Markowitz N, Hansen NI, Hopewell PC, et al. Incidence of tuberculosis in the United States among HIV-infected persons. *Ann Intern Med* 1997;126:123–132.
157. Barnes PF, Bloch AB, Davidson PT, et al. Tuberculosis in patients with human immunodeficiency virus infection. *N Engl J Med* 1991;324:1644–1650.
158. Gracey DR. Tuberculosis in the world today. *Mayo Clin Proc* 1988;63:1251–1255.
159. Zugar A, Lowy FD. Tuberculosis of the central nervous system. In: Scheld WM, Whitley RJ, Durack DT, eds. *Infections of the central nervous system,* 2nd ed. Philadelphia: Lippincott-Raven, 1997: 417–443.
160. Ogawa SK, Smith MA, Brennessel DJ, et al. Tuberculous meningitis in an urban medical center. *Medicine (Baltimore)* 1987;63:317–326.
161. Kent SJ, Crowe SM, Yung A, et al. Tuberculous meningitis: a 30-year review. *Clin Infect Dis* 1993;17:987–994.

162. Klein NC, Damsker B, Hirschman SZ. Mycobacterial meningitis: retrospective analysis from 1970–1983. *Am J Med* 1985;79:29–34.
163. Alvarez S, McCabe WR. Extrapulmonary tuberculosis revisited: a review of experience at Boston City and other hospitals. *Medicine (Baltimore)* 1984;63:25–54.
164. Idriss ZH, Sinno AA, Kronfol NM. Tuberculous meningitis in childhood. *Am J Dis Child* 1976;130:364–367.
165. Haas EJ, Madhavan T, Quinn EL, et al. Tuberculous meningitis in an urban general hospital. *Arch Intern Med* 1977;137:1518–1521.
166. Kennedy DH, Fallon RJ. Tuberculous meningitis. *JAMA* 1979;241:264–268.
167. Verdon R, Chevret S, Laissy JP, et al. Tuberculous meningitis in adults: review of 48 cases. *Clin Infect Dis* 1996;22:982–988.
168. Leiguarda R, Berthier M, Starkstein S, et al. Ischemic infarction in 25 children with tuberculous meningitis. *Stroke* 1988;19:200–204.
169. Berenguer J, Moreno S, Laguna F, et al. Tuberculous meningitis in patients infected with human immunodeficiency virus. *N Engl J Med* 1992;326:668–672.
170. Dube MP, Holtom PD, Larsen RA. Tuberculous meningitis in patients with and without human immunodeficiency virus infection. *Am J Med* 1992;93:520–524.
171. Daniel TM. New approaches to the rapid diagnosis of tuberculous meningitis. *J Infect Dis* 1987;155:599–602.
172. Kaneko K, Onodera O, Miyatake T, et al. Rapid diagnosis of tuberculous meningitis by polymerase chain reaction (PCR). *Neurology* 1990;40:1617–1618.
173. Liu PY, Shi Z, Lau Y, et al. Rapid diagnosis of tuberculous meningitis by a nested amplification protocol. *Neurology* 1994;44:1161–1164.
174. Folgueira L, Delgado R, Palenque E, et al. Polymerase chain reaction for rapid diagnosis of tuberculous meningitis in AIDS patients. *Neurology* 1994;44:1336–1338.
175. Bonington A, Strang JIG, Klapper PE, et al. Use of Roche AMPLICOR *Mycobacterium tuberculosis* PCR in early diagnosis of tuberculous meningitis. *J Clin Microbiol* 1998;36:1251–1254.
176. Offenbacher H, Fazekas F, Schmidt R, et al. MRI in tuberculous meningoencephalitis: report of four cases and review of the neuroimaging literature. *J Neurol* 1991;238:340–344.
177. Gupta RK, Gupta S, Singh D, et al. MR imaging and angiography in tuberculous meningitis. *Neuroradiology* 1994;36:87–92.
178. Whiteman MLH. Neuroimaging of central nervous system tuberculosis in HIV-infected patients. *Neuroimaging Clin North Am* 1997;7:199–214.
179. Horsburgh CR, Mason UG, Farhi DC, et al. Disseminated infection with *Mycobacterium avium-intracellulare:* a report of 13 cases and a review of the literature. *Medicine (Baltimore)* 1985;64:36–48.
180. Wolinsky E. Nontuberculous mycobacteria and associated diseases. *Am Rev Respir Dis* 1979;119:107–159.
181. Cegielski JP, Wallace RJ Jr. Infections due to nontuberculous mycobacteria. In: Scheld WM, Whitley RJ, Durack DT, eds. *Infections of the central nervous system,* 2nd ed. Philadelphia: Lippincott-Raven, 1997:445–461.
182. Hook EW III. Central nervous system syphilis. In: Scheld WM, Whitley RJ, Durack DT, eds. *Infections of the central nervous system,* 2nd ed. Philadelphia: Lippincott-Raven, 1997:669–684.
183. Simon RP. Neurosyphilis. *Arch Neurol* 1985;42:606–613.
184. Hook EW III. Syphilis and HIV infection. *J Infect Dis* 1989;160:530–534.
185. Musher DM, Hamill RJ, Baughn RE. Effect of human immunodeficiency virus (HIV) infection on the course of syphilis and on the response to treatment. *Ann Intern Med* 1990;113:872–881.
186. Hook EW III, Marra CM. Acquired syphilis in adults. *N Engl J Med* 1992;326:1060–1069.
187. Katz DA, Berger JR. Neurosyphilis in acquired immunodeficiency syndrome. *Arch Neurol* 1989;46:895–898.
188. Flood JM, Weinstock HS, Guroy ME, et al. Neurosyphilis during the AIDS epidemic, San Francisco, 1985–1992. *J Infect Dis* 1998;177:931–940.
189. Merritt HH, Moore M. Acute syphilitic meningitis. *Medicine (Baltimore)* 1935;14:119–183.
190. Holmes MD, Zawadzki B, Simon RP. Clinical features of meningovascular syphilis. *Neurology* 1984;34:553–555.
191. Johns DR, Tierney M, Felsenstein D. Alteration in the natural history of neurosyphilis by concurrent infection with the human immunodeficiency virus. *N Engl J Med* 1987;316:1569–1572.

192. Hutchinson CM, Rompalo AM, Reichart CA, et al. Characteristics of patients with syphilis attending Baltimore STD clinics: multiple, high-risk subgroups and interactions with human immunodeficiency virus infection. *Arch Intern Med* 1991;151:511–516.

193. Hart G. Syphilis tests in diagnostic and therapeutic decision making. *Ann Intern Med* 1986;104: 368–376.

194. Davis LE, Schmitt JW. Clinical significance of cerebrospinal fluid tests for neurosyphilis. *Ann Neurol* 1989;25:50–55.

195. Noordhoek GT, Wolters EC, de Jonge MEJ, et al. Detection by polymerase chain reaction of *Treponema pallidum* DNA in cerebrospinal fluid from neurosyphilis patients before and after antibiotic treatment. *J Clin Microbiol* 1991;29:1976–1984.

196. Reik L Jr. Lyme disease. In: Scheld WM, Whitley RJ, Durack DT, eds. *Infections of the central nervous system,* 2nd ed. Philadelphia: Lippincott-Raven, 1997:685–718.

197. Reik L, Steere AC, Bartenhagen NH, et al. Neurologic abnormalities of Lyme disease. *Medicine (Baltimore)* 1979;58:281–294.

198. Pachner AR, Steere AC. The triad of neurologic manifestations of Lyme disease: meningitis, cranial neuritis and radiculoneuritis. *Neurology* 1985;35:47–53.

199. Reik L, Burgdorfer W, Donaldson JO. Neurologic abnormalities in Lyme disease without erythema chronicum migrans. *Am J Med* 1986;81:73–78.

200. Steere AC. Lyme disease. *N Engl J Med* 1989;321:586–596.

201. Corpuz M, Hilton E, Lardis MP, et al. Problems in the use of serologic tests for the diagnosis of Lyme disease. *Arch Intern Med* 1991;151:1837–1840.

202. American College of Physicians. Guidelines for laboratory evaluation in the diagnosis of Lyme disease. *Ann Intern Med* 1997;127:1106–1108.

203. Tugwell P, Dennis DT, Weinstein A, et al. Laboratory evaluation in the diagnosis of Lyme disease. *Ann Intern Med* 1997;127:1109–1123.

204. Keller TL, Halperin JJ, Whitman M. PCR detection of *Borrelia burgdorferi* DNA in cerebrospinal fluid of Lyme neuroborreliosis patients. *Neurology* 1992;42:32–42.

205. Lebech AM, Hansen K. Detection of *Borrelia burgdorferi* DNA in urine samples and cerebrospinal fluid samples from patients with early and late Lyme neuroborreliosis by polymerase chain reaction. *J Clin Microbiol* 1992;30:1646–1653.

206. Luft BJ, Steinman CR, Neimark HC, et al. Invasion of the central nervous system by *Borrelia burgdorferi* in acute disseminated infection. *JAMA* 1992;267:1364–1367.

207. Diamond RD, Bennett JE. Prognostic factors in cryptococcal meningitis: a study of 111 patients. *Ann Intern Med* 1974;80:176–181.

208. Sabetta JR, Andriole VT. Cryptococcal infection of the central nervous system. *Med Clin North Am* 1985;69:333–345.

209. Perfect JR, Durack DT, Gallis HA. Cryptococcemia. *Medicine (Baltimore)* 1983;62:98–109

210. Kovacs JA, Kovacs AA, Polis M, et al. Cryptococcosis in the acquired immunodeficiency syndrome. *Ann Intern Med* 1985;103:533–538.

211. Zugar A, Louie E, Holzman RS, et al. Cryptococcal disease in patients with the acquired immunodeficiency syndrome: diagnostic features and outcome of treatment. *Ann Intern Med* 1986;104: 234–240.

212. Eng RHK, Bishburg E, Smith SM, et al. Cryptococcal infections in patients with acquired immune deficiency syndrome. *Am J Med* 1986;81:19–23.

213. Chuck SL, Sande MA. Infections with *Cryptococcus neoformans* in the acquired immunodeficiency syndrome. *N Engl J Med* 1989;321:794–799.

214. Clark RA, Greer D, Atkinson W, et al. Spectrum of *Cryptococcus neoformans* infection in 68 patients with human immunodeficiency virus. *Rev Infect Dis* 1990;12:768–777.

215. Mitchell TG, Perfect JR. Cryptococcosis in the era of AIDS 100 years after the discovery of *Cryptococcus neoformans. Clin Microbiol Rev* 1995;8:515–548.

216. Powderly WG. Cryptococcal meningitis and AIDS. *Clin Infect Dis* 1993;17:837–842.

217. Patterson TF, Andriole VT. Current concepts in cryptococcosis. *Eur J Clin Microbiol Infect Dis* 1989;8:457–465.

218. Moosa MYS, Coovadia YM. Cryptococcal meningitis in Durban, South Africa: a comparison of clinical features, laboratory findings, and outcome for human immunodeficiency virus (HIV)-positive and HIV-negative patients. *Clin Infect Dis* 1997;24:131–134.

219. Heyderman RS, Gangaidzo IT, Hakim JG, et al. Cryptococcal meningitis in human immunodeficiency virus–infected patients in Harare, Zimbabwe. *Clin Infect Dis* 1998;26:284–289.

220. Perfect JR. Diagnosis and treatment of fungal meningitis. In: Scheld WM, Whitley RJ, Durack DT, eds. *Infections of the central nervous system*, 2nd ed. Philadelphia: Lippincott-Raven, 1997:721–739.
221. Goodman JS, Kaufman L, Loening MG. Diagnosis of cryptococcal meningitis: detection of cryptococcal antigen. *N Engl J Med* 1971;285:434–436.
222. Snow RM, Dismukes WE. Cryptococcal meningitis: diagnostic value of cryptococcal antigen in cerebrospinal fluid. *Arch Intern Med* 1975;135:1155–1157.
223. Treseler CB, Sugar AM. Fungal meningitis. *Infect Dis Clin North Am* 1990;4:789–808.
224. Kirkland TN, Fierer J. Coccidioidomycosis: a reemerging infectious disease. *Emerg Infect Dis* 1996;2:192–199.
225. Galgiani JN. Coccidioidomycosis: a regional disease of national importance. Rethinking approaches to control. *Ann Intern Med* 1999;130:293–300.
226. Bouza E, Dreyer JS, Hewitt WL, et al. Coccidioidal meningitis: an analysis of thirty-one cases and review of the literature. *Medicine (Baltimore)* 1981;60:139–172.
227. Ampel NM, Wieden MA, Galgiani JN. Coccidioidomycosis: clinical update. *Rev Infect Dis* 1989;11:897–911.
228. Schermoly MJ, Hinthorn DR. Eosinophilia in coccidioidomycosis. *Arch Intern Med* 1988;148: 895–896.
229. Wheat LJ. Histoplasmosis. *Infect Dis Clin North Am* 1988;2:841–859.
230. Kauffman CA, Israel KS, Smith JW, et al. Histoplasmosis in immunosuppressed patients. *Am J Med* 1978;64:923–932.
231. Wheat LJ, Slama TG, Norton JA, et al. Risk factors for disseminated or fatal histoplasmosis. *Ann Intern Med* 1982;96:159–163.
232. Johnson PC, Khardori N, Najjar AF, et al. Progressive disseminated histoplasmosis in patients with acquired immunodeficiency syndrome. *Am J Med* 1988;85:152–158.
233. Wheat LJ, Connolly-Stringfield PA, Baker RL, et al. Disseminated histoplasmosis in the acquired immune deficiency syndrome: clinical findings, diagnosis and treatment, and review of the literature. *Medicine (Baltimore)* 1990;69:361–374.
234. Wheat J. Histoplasmosis. Experience during outbreaks in Indianapolis and review of the literature. *Medicine (Baltimore)* 1997;76:339–354.
235. Wheat LJ, French M, Batteiger B, et al. Cerebrospinal fluid *Histoplasma* antibodies in central nervous system histoplasmosis. *Arch Intern Med* 1985;145:1237–1240.
236. Wheat LJ, Kohler RB, Tewari RP. Diagnosis of disseminated histoplasmosis by detection of *Histoplasma capsulatum* antigen in serum and urine specimens. *N Engl J Med* 1986;314:83–88.
237. Wheat LJ, Kohler RB, Tewari RP, et al. Significance of *Histoplasma* antigen in the cerebrospinal fluid of patients with meningitis. *Arch Intern Med* 1989;149:302–304.
238. Meunier-Carpentier I, Kiehn TE, Armstrong D. Fungemia in the immunocompromised host: changing patterns, antigenemia, high mortality. *Am J Med* 1981;71:363–370.
239. Wey SB, Mori M, Pfaller MA, et al. Risk factors for hospital-acquired candidemia: a matched case-control study. *Arch Intern Med* 1989;149:2349–2353.
240. Lee BE, Cheung PY, Robinson JL, et al. Comparative study of mortality and morbidity in premature infants (birth weight, <1,250 g) with candidemia or candidal meningitis. *Clin Infect Dis* 1998;27:559–565.
241. Bayer AS, Edwards JE Jr, Seidel JS, et al. *Candida* meningitis: report of seven cases and review of the English literature. *Medicine (Baltimore)* 1976;55:477–486.
242. Lipton SA, Hickey WF, Morris JH, et al. Candidal infection in the central nervous system. *Am J Med* 1984;76:101–108.
243. Walsh TJ, Hier DB, Caplan LP. Fungal infections of the central nervous system: comparative analysis of risk factors and clinical signs in 57 patients. *Neurology* 1985;35:1654–1657.
244. Geers TA, Gordon SM. Clinical significance of *Candida* species isolated from cerebrospinal fluid following neurosurgery. *Clin Infect Dis* 1999;28:1139–1147.
245. Sepkowitz K, Armstrong D. Space-occupying fungal lesions of the central nervous system. In: Scheld WM, Whitley RJ, Durack DT, eds. *Infections of the central nervous system,* 2nd ed. Philadelphia: Lippincott-Raven, 1997:741–762.
246. Denning DW. Invasive aspergillosis. *Clin Infect Dis* 1998;26:781–805.
247. Salaki JS, Louria DB, Chmel H. Fungal and yeast infections of the central nervous system: a clinical review. *Medicine (Baltimore)* 1984;63:108–132.
248. Beal MF, O'Carroll P, Kleinman GM, et al. Aspergillosis of the nervous system. *Neurology* 1982;32:473–479.

249. Denning DW, Follansbee SE, Scolaro M, et al. Pulmonary aspergillosis in the acquired immuno-deficiency syndrome. *N Engl J Med* 1991;324:654–662.
250. Minamoto GY, Barlam TF, Vander Els NJ. Invasive aspergillosis in patients with AIDS. *Clin Infect Dis* 1992;14:66–74.
251. Walsh TJ, Hier DB, Caplan LR. Aspergillosis of the central nervous system: clinicopathological analysis of 17 patients. *Ann Neurol* 1985;18:574–582.
252. Sugar AM. Mucormycosis. *Clin Infect Dis* 1992;14:S126–S129.
253. Stave GM, Heimberger T, Kerkering TM. Zygomycosis of the basal ganglia in intravenous drug users. *Am J Med* 1989;86:115–117.
254. Daly AL, Velazquez LA, Bradley SF, et al. Mucormycosis: association with deferoxamine therapy. *Am J Med* 1989;87:468–471.
255. Rangel-Guerra R, Martinez HR, Saenz C. Mucormycosis: report of 11 cases. *Arch Neurol* 1985; 42:578–581.
256. Anaissie EJ, Shikhani AH. Rhinocerebral mucormycosis with internal carotid occlusion: report of two cases and review of the literature. *Laryngoscope* 1985;95:1107–1113.
257. Anderson D, Matick H, Naheedy MH, et al. Rhinocerebral mucormycosis with CT scan findings. *Comput Radiol* 1984;8:113–117.
258. Press GA, Weindling SM, Hesselink JR, et al. Rhinocerebral mucormycosis: MR manifestations. *J Comput Assist Tomogr* 1988;12:744–749.
259. Travis LB, Roberts GD, Wilson WR. Clinical significance of *Pseudallescheria boydii*: a review of ten years' experience. *Mayo Clin Proc* 1985;60:531–537.
260. Berenguer J, Diaz-Mediavilla J, Urra D, et al. Central nervous system infection caused by *Pseudallescheria boydii*. *Rev Infect Dis* 1989;11:890–896.
261. Dworzack DL, Clark RB, Borkowski WJ, et al. *Pseudallescheria boydii* brain abscess: association with near-drowning and efficacy of high-dose, prolonged miconazole therapy in patients with multiple abscesses. *Medicine (Baltimore)* 1989;68:218–224.
262. Kershaw P, Freeman R, Templeton D, et al. *Pseudallescheria boydii* infection of the central nervous system. *Arch Neurol* 1990;47:468–472.
263. Niu MT, Duma RJ. Meningitis due to protozoa and helminths. *Infect Dis Clin North Am* 1990;4:809–841.
264. Durack DT. Amebic infections. In: Scheld WM, Whitley RJ, Durack DT, eds. *Infections of the central nervous system,* 2nd ed. Philadelphia: Lippincott-Raven, 1997:831–844.
265. Wellings FM, Amuso PT, Chang SL, et al. Isolation and identification of pathogenic *Naegleria* from Florida lakes. *Appl Environ Microbiol* 1977;34:661–667.
266. Gardner HAR, Martinez AJ, Visvesvara GS, et al. Granulomatous amebic encephalitis in an AIDS patient. *Neurology* 1991;41:1993–1995.
267. Di Gregorio C, Rivasi R, Mongiardo N, et al. *Acanthamoeba* meningoencephalitis in a patient with acquired immunodeficiency syndrome. *Arch Pathol Lab Med* 1992;116:1363–1365.
268. Gordon SM, Steinberg JP, DuPuis MH, et al. Culture isolation of *Acanthamoeba* species and leptomyxid amebas from patients with amebic meningoencephalitis, including two patients with AIDS. *Clin Infect Dis* 1992;15:1024–1030.
269. Hawley HB, Czachor JS, Malhotra V, et al. *Acanthamoeba* encephalitis in patients with AIDS. *The AIDS Reader* 1997;7:137–142.
270. Martinez AJ, Visvesvara GS. Laboratory diagnosis of pathogenic free-living amoebas: *Naegleria, Acanthamoeba,* and *Leptomyxid. Clin Lab Med* 1991;11:861–872.
271. Dukes CS, Luft BJ, Durack DT. Toxoplasmosis of the central nervous system. In: Scheld WM, Whitley RJ, Durack DT, eds. *Infections of the central nervous system,* 2nd ed. Philadelphia: Lippincott-Raven, 1997:785–806.
272. Carey RM, Kimball AC, Armstrong D, et al. Toxoplasmosis: clinical experiences in a cancer hospital. *Am J Med* 1973;54:30–38.
273. Ruskin J, Remington JS. Toxoplasmosis in the compromised host. *Ann Intern Med* 1976;84:193–199.
274. Reynolds ES, Walls KW, Pfeiffer RI. Generalized toxoplasmosis following renal transplantation. *Arch Intern Med* 1966;118:401–405.
275. Deleze M, Mintz G, Carmen Majia MD. *Toxoplasma gondii* encephalitis in systemic lupus erythe-matosus, a neglected cause of treatable nervous system infection. *J Rheumatol* 1985;12:994–996.
276. Hakim M, Esmore D, Wallwork J, et al. Toxoplasmosis in cardiac transplantation. *Br Med J* 1986;292:1108.

277. Luft BJ, Naot Y, Araujo FG, et al. Primary and reactivated *Toxoplasma* infection in patients with cardiac transplants. *Am Coll Physicians* 1983;99:27–31.
278. Nagington J, Martin AL. Toxoplasmosis and heart transplantation. *Lancet* 1983;2:679.
279. Luft BJ, Brooks RG, Conley FK, et al. Toxoplasmic encephalitis in patients with acquired immune deficiency syndrome. *JAMA* 1984;252:913–917.
280. Navia BA, Petito CK, Gold JWM, et al. Cerebral toxoplasmosis complicating the acquired immune deficiency syndrome: clinical and neuropathological findings in 27 patients. *Ann Neurol* 1986;19:224–238.
281. Luft BJ, Remington JS. Toxoplasmic encephalitis in AIDS. *Clin Infect Dis* 1992;15:211–222.
282. Renold C, Sugar A, Chave JP, et al. *Toxoplasma* encephalitis in patients with acquired immunodeficiency syndrome. *Medicine (Baltimore)* 1992;71:224–239.
283. Porter SB, Sande MA. Toxoplasmosis of the central nervous system in the acquired immunodeficiency syndrome. *N Engl J Med* 1992;327:1643–1648.
284. Carr A, Tindall B, Brew BJ, et al. Low dose trimethoprim sulfamethoxazole prophylaxis for toxoplasmic encephalitis in patients with AIDS. *Ann Intern Med* 1992;117:106–111.
285. Furrer H, Egger M, Opravil M, et al. Discontinuation of primary prophylaxis against *Pneumocystis carinii* pneumonia in HIV-1-infected adults treated with combination antiretroviral therapy. *N Engl J Med* 1999;340:1301–306.
286. Rose AG, Uys CJ, Novitsky D, et al. Toxoplasmosis of donor and recipient hearts after heterotopic cardiac transplantation. *Arch Pathol Lab Med* 1990;107:368–373.
287. Cohn JA, McMeeking A, Cohen W, et al. Evaluation of the policy of empiric treatment of suspected *Toxoplasma* encephalitis in patients with the acquired immunodeficiency syndrome. *Am J Med* 1989;86:521–527.
288. Bishburg E, Eng RHK, Slim J, et al. Brain lesions in patients with acquired immunodeficiency syndrome. *Arch Intern Med* 1989;149:941–943.
289. Post MJD, Sheldon JJ, Hensley GT, et al. Central nervous system disease in acquired immunodeficiency syndrome: prospective correlation using CT, MR imaging and pathologic studies. *Radiology* 1986;158:141–148.
290. Sun T, Greenspan J, Tenenbaum M, et al. Diagnosis of cerebral toxoplasmosis using fluorescein-labeled antitoxoplasma monoclonal antibodies. *Am J Surg Pathol* 1986;10:312–316.
291. Luft BJ, Hafner R, Korzun AH, et al. Toxoplasmic encephalitis in patients with the acquired immunodeficiency syndrome. *N Engl J Med* 1993;329:995–1000.
292. Ruiz A, Ganz WI, Post MJD, et al. Use of thallium-201 brain SPECT to differentiate cerebral lymphoma from *Toxoplasma* encephalitis in AIDS patients. *Am J Neuroradiol* 1994;15:1885–1894.
293. Berry I, Gaillard JF, Guo Z, et al. Cerebral lesions in AIDS. What can be expected from scintigraphy? Cerebral tomographic scintigraphy using thallium-201: a contribution to the differential diagnosis of lymphomas and infectious lesions. *J Neuroradiol* 1995;22:218–228.
294. Pierce MA, Johnson MD, Maciunas RJ, et al. Evaluating contrast-enhancing brain lesions in patients with AIDS by using positron emission tomography. *Ann Intern Med* 1995;123:594–598.
295. Quality Standards Subcommittee of the American Academy of Neurology. Evaluation and management of intracranial mass lesions in AIDS. *Neurology* 1998;50:21–26.
296. Koo J, Pien F, Kliks MM. *Angiostrongylus (Parastrongylus)* eosinophilic meningitis. *Rev Infect Dis* 1998;10:1155–1162.
297. Cameron ML, Durack DT. Helminthic infections of the central nervous system. In: Scheld WM, Whitley RJ, Durack DT, eds. *Infections of the central nervous system,* 2nd ed. Philadelphia: Lippincott-Raven, 1997:845–878.
298. Kliks MM, Palumbo NE. Eosinophilic meningitis beyond the Pacific basin: the global dispersal of a peridomestic zoonosis caused by *Angiostrongylus cantonensis,* the nematode lungworm of rats. *Soc Sci Med* 1992;34:199–212.
299. Campbell BG, Little MD. The finding of *Angiostrongylus cantonensis* in rats in New Orleans. *Am J Trop Med Hyg* 1988;38:568–573.
300. Kuberski T, Wallace GD. Clinical manifestations of eosinophilic meningitis due to *Angiostrongylus cantonensis. Neurology* 1979;29:1566–1570.
301. Weller PF. Eosinophilic meningitis. *Am J Med* 1993;95:250–253.
302. Greenlee JE, Carroll KC. Cerebrospinal fluid in CNS infections. In: Scheld WM, Whitley RJ, Durack DT, eds. *Infections of the central nervous system,* 2nd ed. Philadelphia: Lippincott-Raven, 1997:899–922.

7

Initial Management

The initial management approach to the patient with acute bacterial meningitis depends upon early recognition of the meningitis syndrome, rapid diagnostic evaluation, and emergent antimicrobial therapy. In the following sections, I will review the principles of antimicrobial therapy in bacterial meningitis, make recommendations for emergent use of specific antimicrobial agents, and discuss the situations for use of adjunctive dexamethasone therapy.

PRINCIPLES OF ANTIMICROBIAL THERAPY

Many factors influence the choice of an antimicrobial agent in the therapy of bacterial meningitis. Through utilization of animal models of infection, the principles of use of antimicrobial agents in bacterial meningitis have been elucidated (1–3). Although susceptibility testing may give information regarding the *in vitro* activity of an antimicrobial agent against a specific meningeal pathogen, the *in vivo* effectiveness of a particular drug may be very different. The most common animal model of meningitis utilized for therapeutic studies is the rabbit model (4,5). In this model, animals are anesthetized, and a helmet formed with dental acrylic is attached to the skull by screws. The helmet secures the animal in a stereotactic frame that holds a geared electrode introducer with a spinal needle, facilitating puncture of the cisterna magna. This intracisternal route of microorganism inoculation is quite reliable for producing experimental meningitis, although a number of disadvantages are apparent (Table 7.1). In addition, other predisposing conditions (e.g., head trauma, immunosuppression, splenectomy) that may be present in patients with bacterial meningitis are not taken into consideration in experimental animal models and may have significant roles in the pathogenesis of bacterial meningitis (2). Despite these disadvantages, the experimental rabbit model is easy to use and relatively inexpensive. Furthermore, the presence of sufficient cerebrospinal fluid (CSF) volume in the rabbit allows frequent sampling of CSF for measurement of leukocyte counts and chemical parameters, determination of quantitative antimicrobial and bacterial concentrations during the treatment period, quantitation of the relative penetration of drug into CSF and the effects of meningitis on this entry parameter, and determination of the relative bactericidal efficacy (defined

TABLE 7.1. *Advantages and disadvantages of the experimental rabbit model for studying the efficacy of specific antimicrobial agents in bacterial meningitis*

Advantages	Disadvantages
Reliable method (i.e., intracisternal route) for producing meningitis	Natural route of infection to cerebrospinal fluid (CSF) is bypassed so pathogenesis is artificial
Easy handling of animals	Early bacteremia and death may supervene prior to CSF inflammation
Relative lack of expense	Extravasation into surrounding tissues may ensue
Presence of sufficient CSF volume for frequent sampling	Direct trauma to the medulla oblongata may result in cardiopulmonary arrest
Ability to determine CSF penetration of drugs, effects of meningitis on this parameter, and bactericidal activity in purulent CSF	Use of analgesics and anesthetics during experiments may alter the pathophysiology of meningitis by inducing hypotension and/or hypoventilation

as the rate of bacterial eradication) within purulent CSF. Bacterial eradication from CSF determines the efficacy of the antimicrobial agent, and several factors determine whether this is achieved.

Cerebrospinal Fluid Penetration and Elimination

The first factor relates to penetration of the antimicrobial agent into CSF (1,3,5), which depends, to a great extent, on the status of the blood-brain barrier (BBB). For example, β-lactam antibiotics such as penicillin penetrate into CSF poorly (about 0.5% to 2.0% of peak serum concentrations) when the BBB is normal. In the presence of meningeal inflammation, CSF penetration of many antimicrobial agents is enhanced as a result of increased drug permeability across the BBB, perhaps as a result of separation of intercellular tight junctions and increased numbers of pinocytotic vesicles in cerebral microvascular endothelial cells as observed in the experimental rat model (6). Antimicrobial entry decreases as inflammation subsides, indicating that maximal parenteral doses of antimicrobial agents should be continued throughout the course of therapy to maintain adequate CSF concentrations. In addition, any process that decreases meningeal inflammation (e.g., administration of dexamethasone) can diminish BBB penetration of an antimicrobial agent (7). For example, CSF concentrations of vancomycin were reduced by 42% to 77% by the administration of dexamethasone (8, 9). CSF concentrations of ampicillin and gentamicin were also reduced by 57% and 30%, respectively, in the experimental rabbit model (10).

Antimicrobial entry into and removal from CSF are also affected as follows (1,3,5,7):

1. Entry into CSF is enhanced if the antimicrobial agent has a low molecular weight and simple chemical structure. Drugs with a high molecular weight (e.g., vancomycin, polymyxin B) penetrate poorly even in the presence of meningeal inflammation.

2. Drugs with a high degree of ionization have poor CSF penetration. For example,

weak acids such as the β-lactams are highly ionized at physiologic pH in plasma, making them hydrophobic and limiting their penetration through an intact BBB. Because the pH of plasma is higher than that of purulent CSF in bacterial meningitis, β-lactams (e.g., the penicillins) tend to pass more readily from the CSF into the plasma than to pass in the reverse direction.

3. Drugs with a high lipid solubility (e.g., the fluoroquinolones, chloramphenicol, rifampin, the sulfonamides, metronidazole) have enhanced CSF penetration. For example, the methoxymethyl ester of hetacillin, which is highly lipid soluble and rapidly hydrolyzed in solution to ampicillin, has a much greater CSF penetration than ampicillin (5.5% versus 0.7% in the experimental rabbit model). CSF penetration of these lipophilic agents is also affected very little by concomitant steroid administration.

4. Antibacterial entry into CSF is decreased with drugs that have a high degree of protein binding (e.g., ceftriaxone). Protein-bound drugs have difficulty penetrating the BBB because of the hydrophobic nature of proteins and resultant increase in molecular weight. It is the amount of free (i.e., non-protein-bound) drug in serum, rather than the total amount, that is important for CSF penetration under normal conditions. Following disruption of the BBB during bacterial meningitis, there is an influx of proteins from serum to CSF that is associated with increased penetration of antimicrobial agents into CSF.

5. An active transport system in cerebral capillaries transports penicillin and ceftriaxone from blood to CSF, although the pump has a low capacity and transports only very small amounts of these drugs into CSF.

6. An active transport system in the choroid plexus removes penicillins and cephalosporins from CSF to blood. This transport system is saturable and can be competitively inhibited by probenecid, leading to increased CSF concentrations of β-lactam agents. Active transport systems play only a small role in the elimination of the aminoglycosides and the fluoroquinolones from CSF; these agents exit the CSF predominantly by passive diffusion.

The penetration of antimicrobial agents into CSF has been studied in a number of experimental animal models and in patients (Table 7.2) (1, 3, 5, 7, 11, 12). In experimental animal model studies, continuous intravenous infusion of an antimicrobial agent is performed to attain serum concentrations approximating those found in humans. The percent penetration of the antimicrobial agent is then calculated as follows:

$$\frac{\text{CSF antimicrobial concentration}}{\text{Serum antimicrobial concentration}} \times 100$$

In some studies, this calculation is based on peak concentrations attained in the serum and CSF, although peak concentrations do not always coincide if drawn simultaneously, and the concentration time curves in serum and CSF do not run parallel. For example, the percent penetration of meropenem (as determined by the preceding formula) was 7.8% when measured within 2 hours of drug administration but

TABLE 7.2. *Percent penetration of selected antimicrobial agents into cerebrospinal fluid (CSF) of rabbits and humans with meningitis*

Antimicrobial agent	Percent penetration (range)	
	Rabbits	Humans
Penicillins		
Penicillin G	2.6–4.9	7.8
Ampicillin	12.1–18.4	4–65
Nafcillin	1.8–2.9	5–27
Ticarcillin	6.1–14.6	40
Mezlocillin	13.5–23.1	3
Piperacillin	15.7	22.7–32.0
Cephalosporins		
Cephalothin	0.7	—
Cefazolin	3.1	0–4
Cefuroxime	8.7	11.6–88.0
Cefotaxime	2.1–8.4	4–55
Ceftriaxone	2.7–12.0	1.5–16.0
Ceftazidime	7.6–11.1	14–45
Cefepime	16–22	10–11.8
Monobactams		
Aztreonam	22.9	5–17
Carbapenems		
Imipenem	3–13	10.6–41.0
Meropenem	6.4	10.7–21.0
Aminoglycosides		
Gentamicin	18.9–28.7	<1.0–2.5
Tobramycin	24.4–26.6	<1.0–0.9
Amikacin	19.0–35.5	20–34
Fluoroquinolones		
Ciprofloxacin	15.0–27.5	6–37
Ofloxacin	20	28–87
Pefloxacin	46.0–51.3	52–58
Trovafloxacin	19–27	22
Gatifloxacin	46–56	—
Moxifloxacin	34–81	—
Gemifloxacin	28–33	—
Rufloxacin	—	72–84
Other Antimicrobial Agents		
Vancomycin	8.4–11.7	<1–53
Chloramphenicol	23.8–34.3	30–66
Metronidazole	—	42–90
Doxycycline	—	13–26
Rifampin	17.2–19.1	4–25
Trimethoprim	35.6–39.0	30–53
Sulfamethoxazole	17.0–27.1	19–72

Data from Tunkel AR, Scheld WM. Applications of therapy in animal models to bacterial infection in human disease. *Infect Dis Clin North Am* 1989;3:441–459; Chowdhury MH, Tunkel AR. Antibacterial agents in infections of the central nervous system. *Infect Dis Clin North Am* 2000;14:391–408; Schmidt T, Täuber MG. Pharmacodynamics of antibiotics in the therapy of meningitis: infection model observations. *J Antimicrob Chemother* 1993;31:61–70; Andes DR, Craig WA. Pharmacokinetics and pharmacodynamics of antibiotics in meningitis. *Infect Dis Clin North Am* 1999;13:595–618; Thea D, Barza M. Use of antibacterial agents in infections of the central nervous system. *Infect Dis Clin North Am* 1989;3:553–570; and Lutsar I, McCracken GH Jr, Friedland IR. Antibiotic pharmacodynamics in cerebrospinal fluid. *Clin Infect Dis* 1998;27:1117–1129, with permission.

was 23.9% when determined after 2 hours (13). In other studies, the area under the concentration curve (AUC) is calculated, which requires multiple sampling of serum and CSF at multiple time points. In one study of children with bacterial meningitis, the penetration of ampicillin was 13.4% when expressed as a ratio of peak concentrations in CSF and blood but was 25.1% when calculated as a ratio of AUC values (14). Although use of AUC is more accurate for the calculation of percent penetration, it is not feasible for the determination of CSF penetration of drugs in humans. In addition, studies in humans should only be considered to give a rough indication of percent penetration because of differences in underlying diseases, dosage of drug administered, frequency of drug administration, and timing of sample acquisition. Although measurement of peak serum and CSF concentrations may circumvent these differences in human studies, it is not clear that peak concentrations were measured in most clinical studies.

Bactericidal Activity in Cerebrospinal Fluid

The second factor is the bactericidal activity of the antimicrobial agent within purulent CSF. This may be influenced as follows (1, 3, 5):

1. As a result of the accumulation of lactate in CSF during bacterial meningitis, the pH of CSF is decreased, thereby inhibiting the bactericidal activity of the aminoglycosides. This likely contributed to the poor response observed with the aminoglycosides in the therapy of meningitis in experimental animal models (15) and in patients. In addition, the newer macrolide clarithromycin had absolutely no bactericidal activity in the CSF of animals with pneumococcal meningitis, despite the fact that clarithromycin had *in vitro* activity against the test strain and that CSF clarithromycin concentrations exceeded the minimal bacterial concentration (MBC) several hundred fold (16). It was suggested that the MBC of clarithromycin was substantially increased in the acidified medium of CSF.

2. Elevated CSF protein concentrations may decrease the efficacy of antimicrobial agents that are highly protein bound because free drug is needed for the antibacterial effect.

3. The growth rates of bacteria in CSF are slower than maximal growth rates *in vitro*. A slower generation time may reduce the bactericidal effects of β-lactam agents *in vivo*.

4. Drugs that penetrate into the CSF may be metabolized *in vivo* to inactive or active metabolites. For example, cephalothin is converted *in vivo* to desacetylcephalothin, which is less active *in vitro* than the parent compound (17). In contrast, cefotaxime is metabolized *in vivo* to desacetylcefotaxime, which is nearly as active *in vitro* as the parent compound, as demonstrated in the experimental rabbit model of *Escherichia coli* meningitis (18).

5. Other drugs may influence antimicrobial activity within purulent CSF. In experimental animal models of meningitis, antagonism has been demonstrated when a bactericidal agent is coadministered with a bacteriostatic agent. In an experimental

canine model of meningitis, the combination of penicillin and chloramphenicol was antagonistic, especially when administration of chloramphenicol preceded that of penicillin. In an experimental rabbit model of *Proteus mirabilis* meningitis, chloramphenicol also antagonized the action of gentamicin (15), an experience that was confirmed in a review of patients with meningitis caused by members of the Enterobacteriaceae family, in which case fatality rates were highest when chloramphenicol was included in the therapeutic regimen (19). However, in other instances the combination of antimicrobial agents may be synergistic, as in the combination of penicillin or ampicillin with gentamicin in *Listeria monocytogenes* meningitis, ampicillin plus mecillinam against *E. coli*, and ampicillin plus gentamicin against *Streptococcus agalactiae* (1, 3).

6. Bactericidal activity may be modified by the so-called inoculum effect, in which the minimal inhibitory concentration (MIC) of an antimicrobial agent against the test strain increases dramatically as the inoculum of the test strain is increased from 10^5 to 10^7 colony-forming units (CFU)/mL under standardized *in vitro* conditions. Therefore the enormous CSF concentrations of bacteria attained during meningitis ($\geq 10^8$ CFU/mL) may contribute to antimicrobial failure and may have contributed to the observed failure of cefamandole in *Haemophilus influenzae* meningitis (20).

Rapid bactericidal activity in CSF is required for optimal therapy, because bacterial meningitis represents an infection in an area of impaired host defense, allowing bacteria to attain enormous population densities in purulent CSF. Multiple studies in experimental animal models have shown that rapid bacterial killing is observed *in vivo* only when CSF concentrations of β-lactams or aminoglycosides exceed the MBC by about 10- to 30-fold (5, 7, 12). The reasons for this reduced activity of these antimicrobial agents in CSF compared with that observed *in vitro* are not completely clear, but the environment of the CSF may be a contributing factor, since time/kill curves performed in CSF *ex vivo* with penicillin G against *Streptococcus pneumoniae* revealed that three to 10 times higher concentrations of penicillin G were needed to reach the same maximal bactericidal activity as that in broth (21). The effect of this CSF bactericidal activity on the cure rate in an experimental rabbit model of pneumococcal meningitis was examined using two different strains of *S. pneumoniae* (22). The *in vitro* susceptibility of each strain to ampicillin was identical, and the ampicillin dosage used (250 mg intramuscularly every 8 hours) produced mean CSF concentrations approximately five times greater than the MBC of both isolates. In contrast, the strains had different *in vitro* susceptibilities to chloramphenicol (16 μg/mL and 2 μg/mL). The administered dosages of chloramphenicol achieved CSF concentrations that produced a bactericidal effect against one strain and a bacteriostatic effect against the other. Cure was achieved only with regimens that achieved bactericidal activity in CSF.

The importance of this rapid bacterial killing has also been examined in patients with bacterial meningitis. One study that compared the outcome in infants and children with bacterial meningitis who had negative or positive CSF cultures 18 to 36 hours after initiation of antimicrobial therapy revealed an increased rate of neurologic

TABLE 7.3. *Influence of delayed sterilization of cerebrospinal fluid (CSF) on outcome of infants and children with bacterial meningitis*

	CSF cultures at 18–36 h	
	Positive	Negative
Neurologic abnormalities at discharge	45%	19%
Neurologic abnormalities at 6-week follow-up		
Ataxia	18%	3%
Hemiparesis	18%	2%
Developmental delay	29%	7%
Moderate to severe hearing impairment	35%	15%

$P < 0.05$ comparing those with negative to positive cultures in all categories.

Data from Lebel MH, McCracken GH Jr. Delayed cerebrospinal fluid sterilization and adverse outcome of bacterial meningitis in infants and children. *Pediatrics* 1989;83:161–167, with permission.

complications (i.e., ataxia, hemiparesis, developmental delay, moderate to severe hearing impairment) in the group in whom the causative microorganism could still be recovered after this time interval (Table 7.3) (23), indicating that rapid bactericidal activity may be critical in improving outcome in patients with bacterial meningitis.

Pharmacodynamics in Cerebrospinal Fluid

A final factor that may contribute to response to antimicrobial therapy in bacterial meningitis is pharmacodynamics, which is concerned with the time course of antimicrobial activity at the site of infection (7, 12). An understanding of the pharmacodynamic properties of a single antimicrobial agent (which may be different in CSF because of poor CSF penetration and low CSF concentrations of antibody and complement) may be useful to determine a dosing regimen for optimal effectiveness. In general, two major patterns of antimicrobial activity have been described. The first pattern is time-dependent, in which the bactericidal activity of an antimicrobial agent is dependent upon the time that its concentration exceeds the MIC; this is the pattern observed with the β-lactam agents (7, 12). As stated earlier, CSF concentrations of β-lactams need to exceed the MBC by 10- to 30-fold to obtain the maximum bactericidal effect in experimental models of meningitis (21, 24–26). However, peak CSF antimicrobial concentrations and the time that the antimicrobial concentrations exceed the MBC (T > MBC) are interrelated; it is likely in these studies that T > MBC increased in parallel with peak CSF concentrations. This would explain why the bactericidal effect did not improve with larger antimicrobial doses and suggests that the activity of β-lactam agents in CSF is time dependent rather than concentration dependent. This concept was supported in an experimental rabbit model of pneumococcal meningitis in which the administration of ampicillin in more frequent smaller doses increased the CSF bacterial killing rate (26). Although earlier studies failed to demonstrate the superiority of continuous over bolus administration of various β-lactam antimicrobial agents (27–29), these studies should be interpreted with caution because CSF concentrations achieved with either mode of administration exceeded the MBC of the infecting microorganism for the entire study period, further supporting the notion that the activity of β-lactams is time dependent. This was recently studied in an experimental animal model of cephalosporin-resistant pneumococcal meningitis, in which ceftriaxone was administered at four different dosage regimens (30). The duration of time that the CSF concentrations of ceftriaxone exceeded the MBC was the only parameter that independently correlated with the bacterial kill rate. The maximal bacterial kill rate was achieved only when CSF ceftriaxone concentrations exceeded the MBC for 95% to 100% of the dosing interval. Based on these results, it has been suggested that time-dependent bactericidal activity is likely to be characteristic of all β-lactam agents (12).

The second pattern of antimicrobial activity is concentration-dependent killing, which is characterized by bacterial killing over a wide range of antimicrobial concentrations and a prolonged recovery period (i.e., a postantibiotic effect) after drug concentrations fall below the MIC; this pattern is seen with the aminoglycosides and fluoroquinolones (7, 12). A direct correlation between gentamicin concentrations and bacterial killing rates in CSF was demonstrated in an experimental model of *E. coli* meningitis (31). Single-dose gentamicin therapy was as effective as divided dosing regimens despite different times that CSF gentamicin concentrations exceeded the MBC. The applicability of these findings to meningitis in humans, however, needs to be established. The pharmacodynamic characteristics of the fluoroquinolones are very similar to the aminoglycosides. Increasing CSF concentrations of various fluoroquinolones have resulted in higher rates of bacterial killing in several animal models of bacterial meningitis (32, 33). However, features of both time dependency and concentration dependency have been demonstrated with the fluoroquinolones in animal models of meningitis. In two studies utilizing experimental models of pneumococcal meningitis, the CSF concentrations of trovafloxacin and gatifloxacin needed to exceed the MBC for the entire dosing interval to achieve maximal bactericidal activity (34, 35); divided dosing regimens of gatifloxacin appeared superior to single-dose regimens (35). These findings are likely the result of the short sub-MIC effects of fluoroquinolones against pneumococci in CSF. Further studies of these pharmacodynamic properties are needed to examine the time-dependent and concentration-dependent bacterial killing of antimicrobial agents in CSF during bacterial meningitis.

INITIAL ANTIMICROBIAL THERAPY

Empiric and Targeted Antimicrobial Therapy

The initial approach to management of a patient with presumed bacterial meningitis begins with a careful history and physical examination to determine whether the clinical presentation is consistent with the diagnosis (see Chapter 4). Once the diagnosis is considered, the clinician must quickly determine whether bacterial meningitis is indeed present. As shown in the management algorithm (Fig. 7.1) (36, 37), for patients

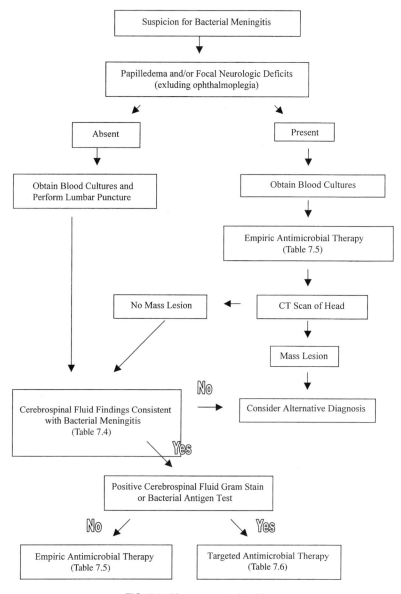

FIG. 7.1. Management algorithm.

in whom there is no clinical suspicion of an intracranial mass lesion (i.e., absence of papilledema and/or focal neurologic deficits), blood cultures are obtained and a lumbar puncture performed. If the CSF findings are consistent with the diagnosis of bacterial meningitis (Table 7.4), empiric antimicrobial therapy (based on various predisposing factors or conditions) is begun if the CSF Gram stain and bacterial

TABLE 7.4. *Typical cerebrospinal fluid (CSF) findings in children and adults with bacterial meningitis*

Cerebrospinal fluid parameter	Typical findings
Opening pressure	200–500 mm H_2O
Appearance	Turbid and/or discolored
White blood cell count	1,000–5,000/mm^3 (range <100/mm^3 to >10,000/mm^3)
Percentage of neutrophils	≥80%
Protein	100–500 mg/dL
Glucose	<40 mg/dL
CSF: serum glucose	≤0.4

antigen tests are negative (Table 7.5), and targeted antimicrobial therapy is initiated if a likely microorganism is identified by Gram stain or bacterial antigen test (Table 7.6). Recommended dosages of antimicrobial agents commonly used in bacterial meningitis in neonates, infants and children, and adults are shown in Table 7.7. The choice of specific antimicrobial agents for empiric or targeted therapy is based on current knowledge of antimicrobial susceptibility patterns. For initial therapy, the assumption is that antimicrobial resistance is likely and the specific agents utilized must treat these resistant microorganisms until *in vitro* susceptibility tests are performed. A detailed discussion of the rationale for use of specific antimicrobial agents for each meningeal pathogen is found in Chapter 8.

In patients who present with a focal neurologic examination or who have papilledema or other features of increased intracranial pressure but in whom bacterial meningitis is suspected, a computed tomographic (CT) scan of the head should be performed prior to lumbar puncture because of the potential risk of cerebral herniation in the presence of an intracranial mass lesion (36–38). However, the time involved in waiting for a CT scan significantly delays definitive diagnosis, with the potential for increased morbidity and mortality in patients with bacterial meningitis in whom antimicrobial therapy is delayed. Therefore after obtaining blood cultures, emergent empiric antimicrobial therapy should be initiated (Table 7.5) before sending the patient to the CT scanner. The effects of administration of antimicrobial agents prior to performance of the lumbar puncture on establishing the diagnosis of bacterial meningitis has been examined in a number of studies (39). Although CSF cultures may become sterile after initiation of antimicrobial therapy, pretreatment blood cultures and the CSF parameters, Gram stain, and/or bacterial antigen tests will likely provide evidence for or against a diagnosis of bacterial meningitis. In one series of children with *H. influenzae* type b meningitis, comparison was made between the CSF profile on admission and after 48 hours of adequate antimicrobial therapy (i.e., culture-negative CSF on repeat examination) (40). After 48 hours, 100% of patients had persistent CSF pleocytosis (14% had more than 50% neutrophils) and 89% had a persistently elevated CSF protein, although 71% had resolution of hypoglycorrhachia and 98% of patients with a positive CSF Gram stain on initial CSF examination converted to no microorganisms visualized on repeat Gram staining of

TABLE 7.5. *Recommended empiric antimicrobial therapy of purulent meningitis*[a]

Predisposing factor	Common bacterial pathogens	Antimicrobial therapy
Age		
<1 mo	*Streptococcus agalactiae, Escherichia coli, Listeria monocytogenes, Klebsiella* species	Ampicillin plus cefotaxime; or ampicillin plus an aminoglycoside
1–23 mo	*Streptococcus pneumoniae, Neisseria meningitidis, Streptococcus agalactiae, Haemophilus influenzae, Escherichia coli*	Third-generation cephalosporin[b]; or ampicillin plus chloramphenicol
2–50 yr	*Neisseria meningitidis, Streptococcus pneumoniae*	Third-generation cephalosporin[b]
>50 yr	*Streptococcus pneumoniae, Neisseria meningitidis, Listeria monocytogenes,* aerobic gram-negative bacilli	Ampicilin plus a third-generation cephalosporin[b]
Nosocomial acquisition	Aerobic gram-negative bacilli (including *Pseudomonas aeruginosa*), staphylococci (*Staphylococcus aureus* and coagulase-negative staphylococci)	Vancomycin plus either ceftazidime or cefepime
Head trauma		
Basilar skull fracture	*Streptococcus pneumoniae, Haemophilus influenzae,* group A β-hemolytic streptococci	Third-generation cephalosporin[b]
Penetrating trauma	*Staphylococcus aureus, Staphylococcus epidermidis,* aerobic gram-negative bacilli (including *Pseudomonas aeruginosa*)	Vancomycin plus either ceftazidime or cefepime
Postneurosurgery	Aerobic gram-negative bacilli (including *Pseudomonas aeruginosa*), *Staphylococcus aureus, Staphylococcus epidermidis*	Vancomycin plus either ceftazidime or cefepime
Cerebrospinal fluid shunt	*Staphylococcus epidermidis, Staphylococcus aureus,* aerobic gram-negative bacilli (including *Pseudomonas aeruginosa*), *Propionibacterium acnes*	Vancomycin plus either ceftazidime or cefepime
Immunocompromised state[c]		
Cellular immunodeficiency	*Listeria monocytogenes, Nocardia* species	Ampicillin plus a third-generation cephalosporin[b] (±trimethoprim-sulfamethoxazole)
Humoral immunodeficiency	*Streptococcus pneumoniae, Haemophilus influenzae, Neisseria meningitidis, Staphylococcus aureus,* other streptococci	Vancomycin plus a third-generation cephalosporin[b]

TABLE 7.5. *Continued*

Predisposing factor	Common bacterial pathogens	Antimicrobial therapy
Neutropenia	Aerobic gram-negative bacilli (including *Pseudomonas aeruginosa*), *Staphylococcus aureus*	Vancomycin plus either ceftazidime or cefepime

[a] Vancomycin should be added to empiric therapeutic regimens when highly penicillin- or cephalosporin-resistant strains of *Streptococcus pneumoniae* are suspected.
[b] Cefotaxime or ceftriaxone.
[c] Age must also be considered when choosing empiric antimicrobial regimens in immunocompromised patients.

CSF. Other studies, however, have documented no significant changes in CSF total white blood cells counts, or CSF glucose or protein concentrations within 48 hours of initiation of adequate antimicrobial therapy (41, 42).

Other patients presenting with the suspicion of acute bacterial meningitis may have received antimicrobial therapy (usually orally administered) prior to performance of the lumbar puncture, so-called partially treated bacterial meningitis. The association between administration of oral antimicrobial therapy and CSF findings was investigated in 281 children with *H. influenzae* type b meningitis from two prospective studies (43); 94 children were pretreated, with 59% of pretreated children receiving ampicillin or amoxicillin. Although pretreated children had significant decreases in

TABLE 7.6. *Recommended antimicrobial therapy for acute bacterial meningitis based on presumptive pathogen identified by positive gram stain or bacterial antigen test[a]*

Microorganism	Standard antimicrobiol therapy	Alternate antimicrobial therapies
Streptococcus pneumoniae	Vancomycin plus a third-generation cephalosporin[b]	Meropenem
Neisseria meningitidis	Penicillin G or ampicillin[c]	Third-generation cephalosporin[b]; chloramphenicol; fluoroquinolone
Listeria monocytogenes	Ampicillin or penicillin G[d]	Trimethoprim-sulfamethoxazole
Streptococcus agalactiae	Ampicillin or penicillin G[d]	Third-generation cephalosporin[b]; vancomycin
Haemophilus influenzae type b	Third-generation cephalosporin[b]	Chloramphenicol; fluoroquinolone; meropenem
Escherichia coli	Third-generation cephalosporin[b]	Aztreonam, fluoroquinolone, trimethoprim-sulfamethoxazole, meropenem

[a] Choice of a targeted antimicrobial regimen should be based on the assumption that a resistant microorganism is possible. See text for details.
[b] Cefotaxime or ceftriaxone.
[c] Some authorities would prefer a third-generation cephalosporin if a resistant organism is suspected; the superiority of a third-generation cephalosporin over penicillin for these microorganisms has not been proven.
[d] Addition of an aminoglycoside should be considered.

TABLE 7.7. *Recommended dosages of antimicrobial agents for bacterial meningitis in patients with normal renal and hepatic function[a]*

Antimicrobial agent	Total daily dosing (dosing interval in h)			
	Neonates (0–7 d old)[b]	Neonates (8–28 d old)[b]	Infants and children	Adults
Amikacin[c]	15–20 mg/kg (12)	20–30 mg/kg (8)	20–30 mg/kg (8)	15 mg/kg (8)
Ampicillin	100–150 mg/kg (8–12)	150–200 mg/kg (6–8)	200–300 mg/kg (6)	12 g (4)
Aztreonam	—	—	—	6–8 g (6–8)
Cefepime			50 mg/kg (8)	6 g (8)
Cefotaxime	100 mg/kg (12)	150–200 mg/kg (6–8)	200 mg/kg (6–8)	8–12 g (4–6)
Ceftazidime	60 mg/kg (12)	90 mg/kg (8)	125–150 mg/kg (8)	6 g (8)
Ceftriaxone	—	—	80–100 mg/kg (12–24)	4 g (12–24)
Chloramphenicol	25 mg/kg (24)	50 mg/kg (12–24)	75–100 mg/kg (6)	4–6 g (6)[d]
Ciprofloxacin	—	—	—	800–1200 mg (8–12)
Gentamicin[c]	5 mg/kg (12)	7.5 mg/kg (8)	7.5 mg/kg (8)	3–5 mg/kg (8)
Meropenem	—	—	120 mg/kg (8)	6 g (8)
Nafcillin	100–150 mg/kg (8–12)	150–200 mg/kg (6–8)	200 mg/kg (6)	9–12 g (4)
Penicillin G	0.1–0.15 mU/kg (8–12)	0.15–0.2 mU/kg (6–8)	0.25 mU/kg (4–6)	24 mU (4)
Rifampin[e]	—	—	10–20 mg/kg (12–24)	600 mg (24)
Tobramycin[c]	5 mg/kg (12)	7.5 mg/kg (8)	7.5 mg/kg (8)	3–5 mg/kg (8)
Trimethoprim-sulfamethoxazole[f]	—	—	10–20 mg/kg (6–12)	10–20 mg/kg (6–12)
Vancomycin[c,g]	20 mg/kg (12)	30–40 mg/kg (8)	50–60 mg/kg (6)	2–3 g (8–12)

[a] Unless indicated, therapy is administered intravenously.
[b] Smaller doses and longer intervals may be advisable for very-low-birth-weight neonates (<2,000 g).
[c] Need to monitor peak and trough serum concentrations.
[d] Higher dose recommended for pneumococcal meningitis.
[e] Oral administration; maximum daily dose of 600 mg.
[f] Dosage based on trimethoprim component.
[g] May need to monitor cerebrospinal fluid concentrations in severely ill patients.

the percentages of CSF neutrophils, protein concentration, and positive Gram stain or culture when compared with untreated children, oral antibiotics given prior to admission did not alter the CSF findings in most patients, such that a diagnosis of *H. influenzae* type b meningitis could be established. In a retrospective review of 178 patients (39 of whom had received prior antimicrobial therapy) with CSF culture—proven bacterial meningitis (44), the combination of blood culture, CSF Gram strain, and/or latex agglutination test identified the causative bacterium in 92% of patients. These data indicate that in patients with bacterial meningitis in whom antimicrobial therapy is administered prior to lumbar puncture, pretreatment blood cultures and CSF analysis can help in the subsequent identification of the causative microorganism.

Timing of Antimicrobial Administration

There are no prospective clinical data on the relationship of the timing of administration of antimicrobial agents to clinical outcome in patients with bacterial meningitis (45). All existing studies examined only the duration of symptoms, not the duration of meningitis, prior to antimicrobial administration, making it difficult to make definitive conclusions as to the optimal timing of drug administration to prevent an adverse clinical outcome. Most physicians would intuitively agree that the longer the duration of symptoms in bacterial meningitis, the more likely is the possibility of experiencing an adverse outcome, although there are no definitive data to support this belief. This concept is supported by results of studies that poor outcome is associated with greater amounts of antigen or a larger number of microorganisms in CSF obtained before initiation of antimicrobial therapy (46, 47), and that delayed sterilization of CSF after 24 hours of antimicrobial therapy is a risk for subsequent neurologic sequelae (23, 48). However, ethical considerations preclude the design of human studies in which the effect of a delay in the administration of antimicrobial therapy upon the outcome of bacterial meningitis could be studied.

To address the question of whether a delay in diagnosis and therapy affects outcome in bacterial meningitis, several large reviews examined the available published literature on this topic. In one review of 22 studies involving 4,707 patients, the duration of symptoms before initiation of antimicrobial therapy was compared with subsequent sequelae (49). The studies were heterogeneous with regard to patient demographics, study numbers, causative microorganisms, and length of follow-up. In addition, the reporting of relevant data was often incomplete and not all studies contained elemental study design components. It was suggested that any connection between a delay in treatment and outcome depends upon one of the following presenting clinical patterns: (a) if the presentation was that of a nonspecific illness with general symptoms, a short delay of less than 3 to 5 days did not appear to alter the risk of sequelae or death; (b) in the case of fulminant meningitis, a delay in the initiation of antimicrobial therapy seemed unconnected to outcome; and (c) for patients with a history of clinically overt meningitis, an inappropriate delay incrementally increased the risk of permanent injury. However, in a subsequent literature review of 27 studies analyzing a total of 5,585 patients (including many patients in the studies of the previous analysis) up to August 1995 (50), only 20% of all studies specifically defined any "symptoms" in their analyses, and could not specify whether "symptoms" denoted a premeningitic phase or heralded the onset of bacterial seeding of the CNS. It was suggested that because there are no pathognomonic clinical features of bacterial meningitis, opinions based on reviews of an individual patient's clinical course and symptomatic progression were interpretive at best and could not dictate with certainty when bacteremic seeding of the CNS occurred.

These issues were also examined in several recent retrospective studies from the United Kingdom after implementation of specific recommendations for therapy of meningococcal infections. In the United Kingdom in the 1980s, notifications of cases of meningococcal meningitis to the Office of Population of Censuses and Surveys increased, leading the chief medical officer in 1988 to write to all general practitioners to advise them to consider giving parenteral benzylpenicillin before transferring the patient to the hospital if the diagnosis of a meningococcal infection was suspected. Based on these recommendations, results from two retrospective studies documented a reduction in the case fatality rate from meningococcal disease in patients who received parenteral penicillin before hospital admission (51, 52). In one study, none of the 13 patients given parenteral penicillin by the referring doctor before admission died, compared with eight deaths (24%) in 33 patients admitted without such treatment (52). In another retrospective review of 305 patients admitted to the hospital in the United Kingdom with a diagnosis of bacterial meningitis, 53 (17.4%) received an antibiotic prior to admission; there was only one death (1.9%) in the 53 who received an antibiotic versus 30 deaths (12%) in the 252 who had not (53). These results led the British Infection Society Working Party to recommend parenteral administration of appropriate antimicrobial therapy without delay to all adult patients in whom the diagnosis of bacterial meningitis is suspected while arranging urgent transfer to the hospital (54).

In another recent retrospective cohort study of 269 patients with community-acquired bacterial meningitis in the United States, the baseline clinical features of hypotension, altered mental status, and seizures were independently associated with adverse clinical outcome and were used to create a prognostic model that predicted clinical outcome (55). Patients were stratified into the three prognostic stages of low risk, intermediate risk, and high risk for adverse outcome based on these clinical features. The results demonstrated that a delay in initiation of antimicrobial therapy after patient arrival in the emergency room was associated with adverse clinical outcome when the patient's condition advanced from a low- or intermediate-risk stage to a high-risk stage of prognostic severity, supporting the assumption that treatment of bacterial meningitis before it advances to a high level of clinical severity improves clinical outcome.

What can be gleaned from the preceding studies to make decisions on the timing of administration of antimicrobial therapy to patients with suspected or proven bacterial meningitis? The key factor would appear to be the need to administer antimicrobial therapy before the patient's condition advances to a high level of clinical severity, during which the patient is less likely to respond to appropriate antimicrobial therapy. This information, however, cannot be based on the duration of symptoms prior to clinical presentation. Clinical experience shows that the outcome of bacterial meningitis is multifactorial and does not always correlate with duration of symptoms, since some patients who are diagnosed and treated within a few hours of developing symptoms experience significant sequelae, whereas others who are symptomatic for days before presentation have a seemingly normal outcome (50). Therefore it is impossible to determine when a high level of clinical severity will be reached in any individual patient. The logical and intuitive approach makes sense; that is, to administer antimicrobial therapy as emergently as possible after the diagnosis of bacterial meningitis is suspected or proven. This should include drug administration prior to admission if the patient initially presents outside of the hospital. There are inadequate data to determine specific guidelines for a defined time period from initial encounter to antimicrobial administration. The assumption that any delay in administration of antimicrobial therapy might be associated with an adverse clinical outcome has been the basis for malpractice claims against physicians who have been accused of failure to promptly diagnose and treat bacterial meningitis (45). In a meningitis case, there is the need to determine whether the physician has breached the standard of care, which is the level of care rendered by a majority of competent physicians practicing in a given set of circumstances, in making the diagnosis and initiating appropriate therapy (56). In three published reports describing a population of more than 300 children (57–59), the mean time from initial presentation to antimicrobial administration generally ranged from 2 to 3 hours; the time that encompassed 95% of such cases was about 6 hours in one study (59). In another analysis of 122 children and adults evaluated in the emergency department and admitted with a diagnosis of bacterial meningitis, the mean time from emergency department registration until antimicrobial administration was 2.7 hours (60). These standards are reasonable to utilize in making recommendations for the optimal timing of antimicrobial administration in patients with suspected or proven acute bacterial meningitis.

ADJUNCTIVE DEXAMETHASONE THERAPY

In certain patients who present with acute bacterial meningitis, consideration should be given to administration of adjunctive dexamethasone therapy, given either concomitant with or just before the first dose of an antimicrobial agent, to reduce the risks of audiologic or neurologic sequelae in some patient groups. Recommendations for use of adjunctive dexamethasone are based on data obtained from experimental animal models of meningitis and clinical trials.

Experimental Studies

The rationale for the use of adjunctive dexamethasone is derived from experimental animal models of infection, which have shown that the subarachnoid space inflammatory response during bacterial meningitis is a major factor contributing to morbidity and mortality (Chapter 3). For example, generation of pneumococcal cell wall components in an experimental animal model of pneumococcal meningitis after treatment with bacteriolytic antibiotics may contribute to the inflammatory response in the subarachnoid space; the inflammatory response was reduced by agents (e.g., methylprednisolone, oxindanac) that inhibit the cyclooxygenase pathway of arachidonic acid metabolism (61). In addition, the administration of either dexamethasone or oxindanac lessened the massive influx of serum albumin and other proteins of high and low molecular weight into the CSF during the early stages of experimental pneumococcal meningitis (62).

Several corticosteroid agents have been examined in experimental animal models of meningitis. Early studies revealed that methylprednisolone administration led to a significant reduction in the mass of leukocytes within the meninges of rabbits with pneumococcal meningitis (63). Another study demonstrated that CSF outflow resistance was reduced by methylprednisolone therapy and to a greater extent than in untreated or penicillin-treated rabbits with pneumococcal meningitis (64). In further studies that examined the effects of corticosteroids (methylprednisolone or dexamethasone) on brain water content, CSF pressure, and CSF lactate in rabbits with pneumococcal meningitis, it was found that both agents completely reversed the development of brain edema, but only dexamethasone led to a reduction in CSF pressure and lactate (65). However, neither agent was superior to therapy with ampicillin alone in reducing cerebral edema or intracranial pressure, and no comparison was made between ampicillin alone and the combination of ampicillin plus corticosteroids, a comparison that would have been relevant to the potential clinical usefulness of adjunctive corticosteroid therapy in bacterial meningitis. A subsequent study did examine treatment with ceftriaxone compared with ceftriaxone plus dexamethasone in an experimental rabbit model of *H. influenzae* meningitis (66). Although combination therapy consistently reduced the brain water content, CSF pressure, and CSF lactate to a greater degree than ceftriaxone alone, the differences were not statistically significant. The authors suggested, however, that adjunctive dexamethasone might be more beneficial if administered early, or even before antibiotic-induced bacterial lysis and release of microbial products. In a subsequent analysis using the experimental rabbit model of *H. influenzae* type b meningitis (67), ceftriaxone administration led to a significant increase in CSF endotoxin concentrations 2 hours after administration, which was followed by a rise in CSF TNF concentrations. Simultaneous administration of dexamethasone and ceftriaxone did not affect release of endotoxin into CSF but markedly attenuated CSF concentrations of TNF measured 8 hours later. Adjunctive dexamethasone therapy also resulted in a significant decrease in CSF leukocytosis and a trend toward earlier improvement in CSF concentrations of glucose, lactate, and protein. These parameters improved without any apparent decrease in the rate of bacterial killing within the CSF *in vivo*. Adjunctive dexamethasone has also been shown to prevent hearing loss in experimental animal models of pneumococcal meningitis (68, 69), especially if instituted early in the course of infection.

Clinical Studies

On the basis of these experimental observations, numerous clinical trials were undertaken to determine the effects of adjunctive corticosteroids (most commonly, dexamethasone) on outcome in patients with bacterial meningitis (Table 7.8) (70–86). A recently published meta-analysis of clinical studies published from 1988 to 1996 confirmed the benefit of adjunctive dexamethasone (0.15 mg/kg every 6 hours for 2 to 4 days) for *H. influenzae* type b meningitis and, if commenced with or before parenteral antimicrobial therapy, suggested benefit for pneumococcal meningitis in childhood (87). Evidence of clinical benefit was strongest for hearing outcomes. In patients with meningitis caused by *H. influenzae* type b, dexamethasone reduced hearing impairment overall (combined odds ratio 0.31; 95% confidence interval 0.14 to 0.69), whereas in patients with pneumococcal meningitis, dexamethasone only suggested protection for severe hearing loss if given early (combined odds ratio 0.09; 95% confidence interval 0.0 to 0.71). Dexamethasone therapy does not appear to be compromised by significant adverse effects if the duration of treatment is limited to 2 days, which is likely to be as effective as 4 days of therapy (88).

When using dexamethasone, the timing of administration is crucial. Administration before or concomitant with antimicrobial therapy is optimal for attenuating the subarachnoid space inflammatory response. In addition, patients should be carefully monitored for the possibility of gastrointestinal hemorrhage. Despite the conclusions of the preceding metaanalysis, the routine use of adjunctive dexamethasone cannot be recommended in adults or in patients with meningitis caused by microorganisms other than *H. influenzae* type b, pending results of ongoing studies. Although some authors recommend their use in all cases of meningitis with a likely bacterial etiology (i.e., demonstrable bacteria on CSF Gram stain, which may predict the patients at greatest risk of bacteriolysis-induced exacerbation of inflammation) (89), there are no clinical data to support this recommendation. Adults with severely impaired mental status (stupor or coma), documented cerebral edema (e.g., by CT scan), and/or markedly elevated intracranial pressure (e.g., high opening pressure on lumbar puncture, palsy of cranial nerve VI) may benefit from adjunctive dexamethasone (90), although again data are lacking.

Pneumococcal Meningitis

The use of adjunctive dexamethasone is of particular concern in patients with pneumococcal meningitis caused by highly penicillin- and cephalosporin-resistant strains, in which patients may require antimicrobial therapy with vancomycin. In this instance, a diminished CSF inflammatory response following dexamethasone administration might significantly reduce vancomycin penetration into CSF and delay CSF sterilization, as shown in an experimental rabbit model of penicillin- and cephalosporin-resistant pneumococcal meningitis (8). This was confirmed in another rabbit model of pneumococcal meningitis in which significantly lower CSF vancomycin concentrations and differences in bacterial killing were found in the dexamethasone-treated

TABLE 7.8. *Outcome in patients receiving adjunctive corticosteroid therapy for bacterial meninitis*

Study (ref.)	Design	Antimicrobial regimen	Corticosteroid regimen	Results	Concerns
deLemos et al. (70)	Randomized, placebo-controlled; 117 patients >1 month of age; 20% of cases caused by H. influenzae, 31% of cases by S. pneumoniae, and 6% of cases by N. meningitidis	Chloramphenicol for H. influenzae, sulfa-diazine or penicillin for N. meningitidis, and penicillin for S. pneumoniae	Methylprednisolone 40 mg every 6 h for 3 d	No differences in time for CSF sterilization; no significant differences between treated and placebo groups either at discharge or 1–4 yr later; at time of final evaluation, 9 of 48 patients in the steroid group and 2 of 57 placebo patients had frank neurologic abnormalities	No data on time of admin-istration of steroid dose in relation to first dose of antibiotic; 46% of placebo- and 35% of steroid-treated patients received antibiotics prior to diagnosis
Belsey et al. (71)	Randomized, placebo-controlled; 102 infants and children; 57% of cases caused by H. influenzae, 27% by N. meningitidis, and 8% by S. pneumoniae	Penicillin + sulfadiazine for pneumococcal and meningococcal meningitis; and chlor-amphenicol + sulfadiazine for H. influenzae	Dexamethasone 1.2 mg/m² every 6 h for 4 d	Neurologic complications occurred in 8 patients treated with dexamethasone and 18 patients treated with placebo (P < 0.05); significantly more patients in the dexa-methasone group had a return to normal CSF glucose after 18–24 h of therapy, developed fewer subdural effusions, and were afebrile sooner	The placebo group was more severely ill at presentation and was more likely to have delayed initiation of antimicrobial therapy; no data on time of administration of dexemethasone in relation to first dose of antibiotic

182

Study	Study design	Antibiotic	Dexamethasone regimen	Results	Comments
Lebel et al. (72)	Randomized, placebo-controlled; 200 infants and children 2 mo to 16 yr of age; 77% of cases caused by H. influenzae type b	Cefuroxime or ceftriaxone	Dexamethasone 0.15 mg/kg every 6 h for 4 d	More rapid normalization of CSF parameters (glucose, protein, lactate) and temperature; lower incidence of moderate to severe bilateral sensorineural hearing loss (15.5% vs 3.3%; $P < 0.01$)	Audiologic sequelae only significantly reduced in patients receiving cefuroxime; 4 patients receiving dexamethasone developed gastrointestinal hemorrhage
Lebel et al. (73)	Randomized, placebo-controlled; 60 infants and children 3 mo to 16 yr of age; 75% of cases caused by H. influenzae type b	Cefuroxime	Dexamethasone 0.15 mg/kg every 6 h for 4 d	No significant differences in audiologic or neurologic sequelae	Small study size
Girgis et al. (74)	Randomized, not placebo-controlled; 429 children and adults 3 mo to 60 yr of age; 62% of cases caused by N. meningitidis; 25% by S. pneumoniae; 13% by H. influenzae type b	Ampicillin plus chloramphenicol	Dexamethasone 8 mg to children younger than 12 yr of age and 12 mg to adults every 12 h for 3 d	Lower mortality rate in patients with pneumococcal meningitis (13.5% vs 40.7%; $P < 0.01$); lower incidence of sensorineural hearing loss in patients with pneumococcal meningitis (0 vs 12.5%; $P < 0.05$)	No differences in normalization of CSF parameters; no documentation of possible adverse effects; high percentage (>60%) of patients presented in a comatose state, most patients (370 of 429) received inadequate therapy for 3–5 d before hospitalization; antibiotics administered intramuscularly; no differences in outcome in patients with meningitis caused by N. meningitidis or H. influenzae type b

continued

183

TABLE 7.8. *Continued.*

Study (ref.)	Design	Antimicrobial regimen	Corticosteroid regimen	Results	Concerns
Odio et al. (75)	Randomized, placebo-controlled; 101 infants and children 6 wk to 13 yr of age; 78% of cases caused by *H. influenzae* type b	Cefotaxime	Dexamethasone 0.15 mg/kg every 6 h for 4 d; dexamethasone given 15–20 min before first dose of antibiotic	Significantly better clinical condition and mean prognostic score at 24 h ($P \le 0.001$); by 12 h all indices of CSF inflammation improved with dexamethasone associated with a decrease in TNF-α and PAF; decreased incidence of one or more neurologic sequelae in patients followed a mean of 15 mo (10% vs 31%; $P = 0.008$; trend in reduction of audiologic sequelae in patients followed a mean of 15 mo (6% vs 16%; $P = 0.18$)	
Kennedy et al. (76)	Retrospective; 97 infants and children 2 mo to 15 yr of age; 100% of cases caused by *S. pneumoniae*	Cefotaxime, ceftriaxone, cefuroxime, ampicillin, or penicillin	Dexamethasone 0.15 mg/kg every 6 h for 4 d	Significant reduction in total long-term neurologic outcome (11% vs 33%; $P = 0.033$); trend to reduction in neurologic (6% vs 16%; $P = 0.18$) and audiologic outcome (9% vs 21%; $P = 0.14$)	Retrospective review; no data on differences with regard to specific antibiotic used

184

Study	Design and population	Antibiotic	Dexamethasone regimen	Outcome	Comments
Schaad et al. (77)	Randomized, placebo-controlled; 115 infants and children 3 mo to 16 yr of age; 58% of cases caused by *H. influenzae* type b, 24% by *N. meningitidis*	Ceftriaxone	Dexamethasone 0.4 mg/kg every 12 h for 2 d; dexamethasone given 10 min before first dose of antibiotic	Reduction in one or more neurologic or audiologic sequelae 15 mo after discharge (5% vs 16%; $P = 0.066$), relative risk of sequelae of 3.27 in patients receiving placebo	Dexamethasone given within 24 h of antibiotic (median of 11 h); only 8 of 50 patients received dexamethasone within 4 h; study stopped prematurely because standard of care became early administration of dexamethasone
King et al. (78)	Randomized, placebo-controlled; 101 children 1 mo to 18 yr of age; 55% of cases caused by *H. influenzae* type b, 18% by *N. meningitidis*, 13% by *S. pneumoniae*	Ceftriaxone	Dexamethasone 0.15 mg/kg every 6 h for 4 d	No significant reduction in audiologic sequelae (10.4% vs 11.1% in placebo recipients); no significant reduction in neurologic sequelae (10.9% vs 8.6% in placebo recipients)	
Wald et al. (79)	Randomized, placebo-controlled; 143 infants and children 8 wk to 12 yr of age; 53% of cases caused by *H. influenzae* type b, 23% by *S. pneumoniae*, 16% by *N. meningitidis*	Ceftriaxone	Dexamethasone 0.15 mg/kg every 6 h for 4 d	No significant differences in neurologic sequelae or developmental outcome; no significant differences in unilateral (10.3% vs 13.5% in placebo recipients) or bilateral (4.4% vs 9.4% in placebo recipients; $P = 0.33$) deafness; of 22 children who were deaf at entry, there were no significant differences in resolution of hearing impairment	Dexamethasone given within 4 h of first dose of antibiotic; lack of follow-up for 13% of study population and incomplete follow-up for an additional 18%

continued

185

TABLE 7.8. Continued.

Study (ref.)	Design	Antimicrobial regimen	Corticosteroid regimen	Results	Concerns
Kanra et al. (80)	Randomized, placebo-controlled; 56 children 2 to 16 yr of age; 100% of cases caused by *S. pneumoniae*	Ampicillin-sulbactam	Dexamethasone 0.15 mg/kg every 6 h for 4 d; dexamethasone given at least 15 minutes before the first dose of antibiotic	No significant differences in moderate or severe unilateral or bilateral sensorineural hearing loss or neurologic sequelae at 6 wk (7.4% vs 23% in the placebo group; $P = 0.11$) or 1 yr (7.4% vs 26.9% in the placebo group; $P = 0.062$); significant reduction in hearing impairment at 3 mo (3.7% vs 23%; $P = 0.044$)	Did not use standard antibiotic therapy for bacterial meningitis; no data on antimicrobial resistance of pneumococcal isolates; Glasgow coma score significantly lower in the dexamethasone group ($P = 0.004$)
Kilpi et al. (81)	Randomized, not placebo-controlled; 122 infants and children 3 mo to 15 yr of age; 53% of cases caused by *H. influenzae* type b, 33% by *N. meningitidis*, 10% by *S. pneumoniae*	Ceftriaxone	Dexamethasone 0.5 mg/kg every 8 h for 3 d; dexamethasone administered concomitantly with the first dose of antibiotic	Dexamethasone recipients showed only a tendency to less severe hearing impairment	Some patients in each group also received therapy with oral glycerol; small sample size

186

Reference	Study design/population	Antibiotic therapy	Corticosteroid regimen	Results	Comments
Macaluso et al. (82)	Retrospective; 179 children 1 mo to 16 yr of age; 37% of cases caused by *H. influenzae* type b, 22% by *N. meningitidis*, 9% by *S. pneumoniae*	Benzyl penicillin plus chloramphenicol	Dexamethasone 0.15 mg/kg every 6 h for 4 d	Rate of discharge without sequelae was higher in the dexamethasone group (70% vs. 56%; *P* = 0.07); in children aged 6–59 mo those treated with dexamethasone had a significantly lower case fatality rate (11% vs 25%; *P* = 0.05) and a better rate of discharge without sequelae (73% vs 52%; *P* = 0.02)	Retrospective; benefits observed only for children aged 6–59 mo; no causative organism identified in 27% of cases; no follow-up to assess the incidence of permanent neurologic sequelae
Qazi et al. (83)	Randomized, placebo-controlled; 89 children 2 mo to 12 yr of age; 20% of cases caused by *H. influenzae* type b, 9% by *N. meningitidis*, 7% by *S. pneumoniae*	Ampicillin plus chloramphenicol	Dexamethasone 0.15 mg/kg every 6 h for 4 d; dexamethasone given 10–15 min before the first dose of antibiotic	Higher mortality rate in patients treated with adjunctive dexamethasone (25% vs 12%); in the survivors who received dexamethasone, the frequency of neurologic sequelae was 26.5% (vs 24% in the placebo recipients) and the frequency of hearing impairment was 42.3% (vs 30% in the placebo recipients)	No causative organism identified in 55% of cases; differences in mortality were not statistically significant due to small sample size; no correlation of severity of illness with outcome; not all patients may have received appropriate intensive care

continued

TABLE 7.8. *Continued.*

Study (ref.)	Design	Antimicrobial regimen	Corticosteroid regimen	Results	Concerns
Arditi et al. (84)	Retrospective; children 3 d to 16.5 yr of age; 100% of cases caused by *S. pneumoniae*	Variable	Dexamethasone 0.15 mg/kg every 6 h for 2–4 d given within 60 min of first antibiotic dose	In the dexamethasone group there was a higher incidence of any moderate or severe hearing loss (46% vs 23%; $P = 0.016$) or of any neurologic deficits (55% vs 33%; $P = 0.02$); no significant differences in deafness ($P = 0.06$) or neurologic sequelae ($P = 0.10$) when data controlled for severity of disease	Retrospective; children in the dexamethasone group more frequently required intubation and mechanical ventilation, and had a lower initial CSF glucose concentration; no data on use of specific antimicrobial agents in each group; no long-term follow-up of patients with hearing loss or neurologic deficits
Daoud et al. (85)	Randomized, but not placebo-controlled; 52 full-term neonates	Cefotaxime plus ampicillin	Dexamethasone 0.15 mg/kg every 6 h for 4 d; dexamethasone given 10–15 min before the first dose of antibiotic	Mortality was 22% in the treated group versus 28% in the control group ($P = 0.87$); at follow-up examination up to age of 2 years, 30% of dexamethasone recipients and 39% of the control group had neurologic sequelae	Small study size

| Thomas et al. (86) | Randomized, placebo-controlled; 60 patients 18–79 yr of age; 52% of cases caused by S. pneumoniae and 30% caused by N. meningitidis | Amoxicillin | Dexamethasone 10 mg every 6 h for 3 d given within 3 h of initiation of an antibiotic | No significant differences in the rate of cured patients without any neurologic sequelae (74.2% in the dexamethasone group vs 51.7% in the placebo group; $P = 0.07$) | Study stopped prematurely because of a new recommendation to use vancomycin plus a third-generation cephalosporin in meningitis; amoxicillin may have been inadequate therapy for meningitis caused by resistant pneumococci; dexamethasone given within 3 h of first antibiotic dose; patients in the dexamethasone group were significantly younger and less ill |

CSF, cerebrospinal fluid; PAF, platelet-activating factor; TNF, tumor necrosis factor.

rabbits (91). However, CSF vancomycin penetration was not reduced by dexamethasone in a study in children with acute meningitis (92). In an attempt to further address the utility of vancomycin in the therapy of meningitis caused by penicillin- and cephalosporin-resistant *S. pneumoniae*, the pharmacodynamics of vancomycin were determined with the coadministration of dexamethasone in the experimental rabbit model (93). The coadministration of dexamethasone significantly reduced the CSF penetration of vancomycin by 29% and significantly lowered the rate of bacterial clearing during the first 6 hours. However, in animals receiving higher doses of vancomycin (40 mg/kg versus 20 mg/kg), therapeutic peak concentrations were obtained even with steroid use, suggesting that the effects of steroids on vancomycin penetration into CSF may be circumvented by the use of larger vancomycin doses. CSF concentrations of ceftriaxone are not significantly altered in animals or patients treated with adjunctive dexamethasone (8, 94, 95). In contrast, in an experimental rabbit model of cephalosporin-resistant pneumococcal meningitis (96), concomitant use of dexamethasone with ceftriaxone resulted in higher CSF bacterial counts and a higher number of therapeutic failures (57% with the 50 mg/kg/day dose and 28% with the 100 mg/kg/day dose of ceftriaxone), demonstrating that concomitant use of dexamethasone in pneumococcal meningitis caused by ceftriaxone-resistant strains was associated with a higher failure rate even when higher doses of ceftriaxone were utilized.

Despite these conflicting reports, many experts have expressed concern regarding the use of adjunctive dexamethasone in treating pneumococcal meningitis caused by penicillin- and cephalosporin-resistant strains (36, 37, 97, 98). An ongoing study in the Netherlands is evaluating the efficacy of adjunctive dexamethasone for community-acquired meningitis in adults (99), and may help to answer these questions. For any patient receiving adjunctive dexamethasone who is not improving as expected or who has a pneumococcal isolate for which the cefotaxime or ceftriaxone MIC is ≥2.0 μg/mL, a repeat lumbar puncture 36 to 48 hours after initiation of antimicrobial therapy is recommended to document sterility of CSF (100).

REFERENCES

1. Tunkel AR, Scheld WM. Applications of therapy in animal models to bacterial infection in human disease. *Infect Dis Clin North Am* 1989;3:441–459.
2. Koedel U, Pfister HW. Models of experimental bacterial meningitis: role and limitations. *Infect Dis Clin North Am* 1999;13:549–577.
3. Chowdhury MH, Tunkel AR. Antibacterial agents in infections of the central nervous system. *Infect Dis Clin North Am* 2000;14:391–408.
4. Dacey RG, Sande MA. Effect of probenecid on cerebrospinal fluid concentrations of penicillin and cephalosporin derivatives. *Antimicrob Agents Chemother* 1974;6:437–441.
5. Schmidt T, Täuber MG. Pharmacodynamics of antibiotics in the therapy of meningitis: infection model observations. *J Antimicrob Chemother* 1993;31:61–70.
6. Quagliarello VJ, Long WJ, Scheld WM. Morphologic alterations of the blood-brain barrier with experimental meningitis in the rat. *J Clin Invest* 1986;77:1084–1095.
7. Andes DR, Craig WA. Pharmacokinetics and pharmacodynamics of antibiotics in meningitis. *Infect Dis Clin North Am* 1999;13:595–618.
8. Paris MM, Hickey SM, Uscher MI, et al. Effect of dexamethasone on therapy of experimental penicillin- and cephalosporin-resistant pneumococcal meningitis. *Antimicrob Agents Chemother* 1994;38:1320–1324.

9. Cabellos C, Martinez-Lacasa J, Martos A, et al. Influence of dexamethasone on efficacy of ceftriaxone and vancomycin therapy in experimental pneumococcal meningitis. *Antimicrob Agents Chemother* 1995;39:2158–2160.
10. Scheld WM, Brodeur JP. Effect of methylprednisolone on entry of ampicillin and gentamicin into cerebrospinal fluid in experimental pneumococcal and *Escherichia coli* meningitis. *Antimicrob Agents Chemother* 1983;23:108–112.
11. Thea D, Barza M. Use of antibacterial agents in infections of the central nervous system. *Infect Dis Clin North Am* 1989;3:553–570.
12. Lustar I, McCracken GH Jr, Friedland IR. Antibiotic pharmacodynamics in cerebrospinal fluid. *Clin Infect Dis* 1998;27:1117–1129.
13. Dagan R, Velghe L, Rodda JL, et al. Penetration of meropenem into cerebrospinal fluid of patients with inflamed meninges. *J Antimicrob Chemother* 1994;34:175–179.
14. Wilson HD, Haltalin KC. Ampicillin in *Haemophilus influenzae* meningitis. *Am J Dis Child* 1975;129:208–215.
15. Strausbaugh LJ, Sande MA. Factors influencing the therapy of experimental *Proteus mirabilis* meningitis in rabbits. *J Infect Dis* 1978;137:251–260.
16. Schmidt T, Froula J, Täuber MG. Clarithromycin lacks bactericidal activity in cerebrospinal fluid in experimental pneumococcal meningitis. *J Antimicrob Chemother* 1993;32:627–632.
17. Nolan CM, Ulmer CW Jr. A study of cephalothin and desacetylcephalothin in cerebrospinal fluid in therapy for experimental pneumococcal meningitis. *J Infect Dis* 1980;141:326–330.
18. Nolan CM, Ulmer CW Jr. Penetration of cefotaxime and moxalactam into cerebrospinal fluid of rabbits with experimentally induced *Escherichia coli* meningitis. *Rev Infect Dis* 1982;4:S396–S400.
19. Cherubin CE, Marr JS, Sierra MF, et al. *Listeria* and gram-negative bacillary meningitis in New York City, 1972–1979. Frequent causes of meningitis in adults. *Am J Med* 1981;71:199–209.
20. Steinberg E, Overturf GD, Wilkins J, et al. Failure of cefamandole in treatment of meningitis due to *Haemophilus influenzae* type b. *J Infect Dis* 1978;137:S180–S186.
21. Täuber MG, Doroshow CA, Hackbarth CA, et al. Antibacterial activity of β-lactam antibiotics in experimental meningitis due to *Streptococcus pneumoniae*. *J Infect Dis* 1984;149:568–574.
22. Scheld WM, Sande MA. Bactericidal versus bacteriostatic antibiotic therapy of experimental pneumococcal meningitis in rabbits. *J Clin Invest* 1983;71:411–419.
23. Lebel MH, McCracken GH Jr. Delayed cerebrospinal fluid sterilization and adverse outcome of bacterial meningitis in infants and children. *Pediatrics* 1989;83:161–167.
24. Decazes JM, Ernst JD, Sande MA. Correlation of *in vitro* time—kill curves and kinetics of bacterial killing in cerebrospinal fluid during ceftriaxone therapy in experimental *Escherichia coli* meningitis. *Antimicrob Agents Chemother* 1983;24:463–467.
25. Scheld WM, Täuber MG, Zak O, et al. The influence of dosing schedules and cerebrospinal fluid bactericidal activity on the therapy of bacterial meningitis. *J Antimicrob Chemother* 1985;15:303–312.
26. Täuber MG, Kunz S, Zak O, et al. Influence of antibiotic dose, dosing interval, and duration of therapy on outcome in experimental pneumococcal meningitis in rabbits. *Antimicrob Agents Chemother* 1989;33:418–423.
27. McCracken GH, Nelson JD, Grimm L. Pharmacokinetics and bacteriological efficacy of cefoperazone, cefuroxime, ceftriaxone, and moxalactam in experimental *Streptococcus pneumoniae* and *Haemophilus influenzae* meningitis. *Antimicrob Agents Chemother* 1982;21:262–267.
28. McCracken GH, Sakata Y. Antimicrobial therapy of experimental meningitis caused by *Streptococcus pneumoniae* strains with different susceptibilities to penicillin. *Antimicrob Agents Chemother* 1985;27:141–145.
29. Sande MA, Korzeniowski OM, Allegro GM, et al. Intermittent or continuous therapy of experimental meningitis due to *Streptococcus pneumoniae* in rabbits: preliminary observations on the postantibiotic effect *in vivo*. *Rev Infect Dis* 1981;3:98–109.
30. Lustar I, Ahmed A, Friedland IR, et al. Pharmacodynamics and bactericidal activity of ceftriaxone therapy in experimental cephalosporin-resistant pneumococcal meningitis. *Antimicrob Agents Chemother* 1997;41:2414–447.
31. Ahmed A, Paris MM, Trujilo M, et al. Once-daily gentamicin therapy for experimental *Escherichia coli* meningitis. *Antimicrob Agents Chemother* 1997;41:49–53.
32. Hackbarth CJ, Chambers HF, Stella F, et al. Ciprofloxacin in experimental *Pseudomonas aeruginosa* meningitis. *J Antimicrob Chemother* 1986;18:65–69.
33. Nau R, Schmidt T, Kaye K, et al. Quinolone antibiotics in therapy of experimental pneumococcal meningitis in rabbits. *Antimicrob Agents Chemother* 1995;39:593–597.

34. Kim YS, Liu Q, Chow L, et al. Trovafloxacin treatment of rabbits with experimental meningitis caused by high-level penicillin resistant *Streptococcus pneumoniae*. *Antimicrob Agents Chemother* 1997;41:1186–1189.
35. Lustar I, Friedland IR, Wubbel L, et al. Pharmacodynamics of gatifloxacin in cerebrospinal fluid in experimental cephalosporin-resistant pneumococcal meningitis. *Antimicrob Agents Chemother* 1998;42:2650–2655.
36. Tunkel AR, Scheld WM. Acute bacterial meningitis. *Lancet* 1995;346:1675–1680.
37. Tunkel AR, Scheld WM. Acute meningitis. In: Mandell GL, Bennett JE, Dolin R, eds. *Principles and practice of infectious diseases,* 5th ed. Philadelphia: Churchill-Livingstone, 2000:959–997.
38. Mellor DH. The place of computed tomography and lumbar puncture in suspected bacterial meningitis. *Arch Dis Child* 1992;67:1417–1419.
39. Bonadio WA. The cerebrospinal fluid: physiologic aspects and alterations associated with bacterial meningitis. *Pediatr Infect Dis J* 1992;11:423–432.
40. Bonadio WA. Cerebrospinal fluid changes after 48 hours of effective therapy for *Haemophilus influenzae* type b meningitis. *Am J Clin Pathol* 1990;94:426–428.
41. Marks WA, Stutman HR, Marks MI, et al. Cefuroxime versus ampicillin plus chloramphenicol in childhood bacterial meningitis: a multicenter randomized controlled trial. *J Pediatr* 1986;109:123–130.
42. Jacobs RF, Wells TG, Steele RW, et al. A prospective randomized comparison of cefotaxime vs ampicillin and chloramphenicol for bacterial meningitis in children. *J Pediatr* 1985;107:129–133.
43. Kaplan SL, O'Brian Smith E, Willis C, et al. Association between preadmission oral antibiotic therapy and cerebrospinal fluid findings and sequelae caused by *Haemophilus influenzae* type b meningitis. *Pediatr Infect Dis J* 1986;5:626–632.
44. Coant PN, Kornberg AE, Duffy LC, et al. Blood culture results as determinants in the organism identification of bacterial meningitis. *Pediatr Emerg Care* 1992;8:200–205.
45. Feigin RD, Kaplan SL. Commentary. *Pediatr Infect Dis J* 1992;11:698–700.
46. Feigin RD, Stechenberg BW, Chang MJ, et al. Prospective evaluation of treatment of *Haemophilus influenzae* meningitis. *J Pediatr* 1976;88:542–548.
47. Feldman WE, Ginsburg CM, McCracken GH Jr. Relation of concentrations of *Haemophilus influenzae* type b in cerebrospinal fluid to late sequelae of patients with meningitis. *J Pediatr* 1982;100:209–212.
48. Schaad UB, Suter S, Gianella-Borradori A, et al. A comparison of ceftriaxone and cefuroxime for the treatment of bacterial meningitis in children. *N Engl J Med* 1990;322:141–147.
49. Radetsky M. Duration of symptoms and outcome in bacterial meningitis: an analysis of causation and the implications of a delay in diagnosis. *Pediatr Infect Dis J* 1992;11:694–698.
50. Bonadio WA. Medical-legal considerations related to symptom duration and patient outcome after bacterial meningitis. *Am J Emerg Med* 1997;15:420–423.
51. Cartwright K, Reilly S, White D, et al. Early treatment with parenteral penicillin in meningococcal disease. *Br Med J* 1992;305:143–147.
52. Strang JR, Pugh EJ. Meningococcal infections: reducing the case fatality rate by giving penicillin before admission to the hospital. *Br Med J* 1992;305:141–143.
53. The Research Committee of the British Society for the Study of Infection. Bacterial meningitis: causes for concern. *J Infect* 1995;30:89–94.
54. Begg N, Cartwright KAV, Cohen J, et al. Consensus statement on diagnosis, investigation, treatment and prevention of acute bacterial meningitis in immunocompetent adults. *J Infect* 1999;39:1–15.
55. Aronin SI, Peduzzi P, Quagliarello VJ. Community-acquired bacterial meningitis: risk stratification for adverse clinical outcome and effect of antibiotic timing. *Ann Intern Med* 1998;129:862–869.
56. Goodman JM. Commentary: legal aspects of bacterial meningitis. *Pediatr Infect Dis J* 1992;11:700–701.
57. Bryan CS, Reynolds KL, Crout L. Promptness of antibiotic therapy in acute bacterial meningitis. *Ann Emerg Med* 1986;15:544–557.
58. Talan DA, Guterman JJ, Overturf GD, et al. Analysis of emergency department management of suspected bacterial meningitis. *Ann Emerg Med* 1989;18:856–862.
59. Meadow WL, Lantos J, Tanz RR, et al. Ought "standard care" be the "standard of care"? A study of time to administration of antibiotics in children with meningitis. *Am J Dis Child* 1993;147:40–44.
60. Talan DA, Zibulewsky J. Relationship of clinical presentation to time to antibiotics for the emergency department management of suspected bacterial meningitis. *Ann Emerg Med* 1993;22:1733–1738.
61. Tuomanen E, Hengstler B, Rich R, et al. Nonsteroidal anti-inflammatory agents in the therapy for experimental pneumococcal meningitis. *J Infect Dis* 1987;155:985–990.

62. Kadurugamuwa JL, Hengstler B, Zak O. Cerebrospinal fluid protein profile in experimental pneumococcal meningitis and its alteration by ampicillin and anti-inflammatory agents. *J Infect Dis* 1989;159:26–34.
63. Nolan CM, McAllister CK, Walters E, et al. Experimental pneumococcal meningitis. IV. The effect of methylprednisolone on meningeal inflammation. *J Lab Clin Invest* 1978;91:979–988.
64. Scheld WM, Dacey RG, Winn HR, et al. Cerebrospinal fluid outflow resistance in rabbits with experimental meningitis: alterations with penicillin and methylprednisolone. *J Clin Invest* 1980;66:243–253.
65. Täuber MG, Khayam-Bashi H, Sande MA. Effects of ampicillin and corticosteroids on brain water content, cerebrospinal fluid pressure, and cerebrospinal fluid lactate levels in experimental pneumococcal meningitis. *J Infect Dis* 1985;151:528–534.
66. Syrogiannopoulos GA, Olsen KD, Reisch JS, et al. Dexamethasone in the treatment of experimental *Haemophilus influenzae* type b meningitis. *J Infect Dis* 1987;155:213–219.
67. Mustafa MM, Ramilo O, Mertsola J, et al. Modulation of inflammation and cachectin activity in relation to treatment of experimental *Haemophilus influenzae* type b meningitis. *J Infect Dis* 1989;160:818–825.
68. Bhatt SM, Cabellow C, Nadol JB Jr, et al. The impact of dexamethasone on hearing loss in experimental pneumococcal meningitis. *Pediatr Infect Dis J* 1995;14:93–96.
69. Rappaport JM, Bhatt SM, Burkard RF, et al. Prevention of hearing loss in experimental pneumococcal meningitis by administration of dexamethasone and ketorolac. *J Infect Dis* 1999;179:264–268.
70. DeLemos RA, Haggerty RJ. Corticosteroids as an adjunct to treatment in bacterial meningitis: a controlled clinical trial. *Pediatrics* 1969;44:30–34.
71. Belsey MA, Hoffpauir CW, Smith MHD. Dexamethasone in the treatment of acute bacterial meningitis: the effect of study design on the interpretation of results. *Pediatrics* 1969;44:503–513.
72. Lebel MH, Freij BJ, Syrogiannopoulos GA, et al. Dexamethasone therapy for bacterial meningitis: results of two double-blind, placebo-controlled trials. *N Engl J Med* 1988;319:964–971.
73. Lebel MH, Hoyt MJ, Waagner DC, et al. Magnetic resonance imaging and dexamethasone therapy for bacterial meningitis. *Am J Dis Child* 1989;143:301–306.
74. Girgis NI, Farid Z, Mikhail IA, et al. Dexamethasone treatment for bacterial meningitis in children and adults. *Pediatr Infect Dis J* 1989;8:848–851.
75. Odio CM, Faingezicht I, Paris M, et al. The beneficial effects of early dexamethasone administration in infants and children with bacterial meningitis. *N Engl J Med* 1991;324:1525–1531.
76. Kennedy WA, Hoyt MJ, McCracken GH Jr. The role of corticosteroid therapy in children with pneumococcal meningitis. *Am J Dis Child* 1991;145:1374–1378.
77. Schaad UB, Lips U, Gnehm HE, et al. Dexamethasone therapy for bacterial meningitis in children. *Lancet* 1993;342:1525–1531.
78. King SM, Law B, Langley JM, et al. Dexamethasone therapy for bacterial meningitis: better never than late? *Can J Infect Dis* 1994;5:1–7.
79. Wald ER, Kaplan SL, Mason EO Jr., et al. Dexamethasone therapy for children with bacterial meningitis. *Pediatrics* 1995;95:21–28.
80. Kanra GY, Ozen H, Secmeer G, et al. The beneficial effects of dexamethasone in children with pneumococcal meningitis. *Pediatr Infect Dis J* 1995;14:490–494.
81. Kilpi T, Peltola H, Jauhiainen T, et al. Oral glycerol and intravenous dexamethasone in preventing neurologic and audiologic sequelae of childhood bacterial meningitis. *Pediatr Infect Dis J* 1995;14:270–278.
82. Macaluso A, Pivetta S, Maggi RS, et al. Dexamethasone adjunctive therapy for bacterial meningitis in children: a retrospective study in Brazil. *Ann Trop Paediatr* 1996;16:193–198.
83. Qazi SA, Khan MA, Mughal N, et al. Dexamethasone and bacterial meningitis in Pakistan. *Arch Dis Child* 1996;75:482–488.
84. Arditi M, Mason EO Jr, Bradley JS, et al. Three-year multicenter surveillance of pneumococcal meningitis in children: clinical characteristics, and outcome related to penicillin susceptibility and dexamethasone use. *Pediatrics* 1998;102:1087–1097.
85. Daoud AS, Batieha A, Al-Sheyyab M, et al. Lack of effectiveness of dexamethasone in neonatal bacterial meningitis. *Eur J Pediatr* 1999;158:230–233.
86. Thomas R, Le Tulzo Y, Bouget J, et al. Trial of dexamethasone treatment for severe bacterial meningitis in adults. *Intensive Care Med* 1999;25:475–480.
87. McIntyre PB, Berkey CS, King SM, et al. Dexamethasone as adjunctive therapy in bacterial meningitis: a meta-analysis of randomized clinical trials since 1988. *JAMA* 1997;278:925–931.

88. Syrogiannopoulos GA, Lourida AN, Theodoridou MC, et al. Dexamethasone therapy for bacterial meningitis in children: 2- versus 4-day regimen. *J Infect Dis* 1994;169:853–858.
89. Quagliarello V, Scheld WM. Bacterial meningitis: pathogenesis, pathophysiology, and progress. *N Engl J Med* 1992;327:864–872.
90. Gary N, Powers N, Todd JK. Clinical identification and comparative prognosis of high-risk patients with *Haemophilus influenzae* meningitis. *Am J Dis Child* 1989;143:307–311.
91. Cabellos C, Martinez-Lacasa J, Martos A, et al. Influence of dexamethasone on efficacy of ceftriaxone and vancomycin therapy in experimental pneumococcal meningitis. *Antimicrob Agents Chemother* 1995;39:2158–2160.
92. Klugman KP, Friedland IR, Bradley JS. Bactericidal activity against cephalosporin-resistant *Streptococcus pneumoniae* in cerebrospinal fluid of children with acute bacterial meningitis. *Antimicrob Agents Chemother* 1995;39:1988–1992.
93. Ahmed A, Jafri H, Lustar I, et al. Pharmacodynamics of vancomycin for the treatment of experimental penicillin- and cephalosporin-resistant pneumococcal meningitis. *Antimicrob Agents Chemother* 1999;43:876–881.
94. Gaillard JL, Abadie V, Cheron G, et al. Concentrations of ceftriaxone in cerebrospinal fluid of children with meningitis receiving adjunctive dexamethasone therapy. *Antimicrob Agents Chemother* 1994;38:1209–1210.
95. Enting R, The Dutch Bacterial Meningitis Study Group. Dexamethasone for bacterial meningitis: we need the answer. *Lancet* 1997;349:1179–1180.
96. Cabellos C, Martinez-Lacasa J, Tubau F, et al. Evaluation of combined ceftriaxone and dexamethasone therapy in experimental cephalosporin-resistant pneumococcal meningitis. *J Antimicrob Chemother* 2000;45:315–320.
97. Prober CG. The role of steroids in the management of children with bacterial meningitis. *Pediatrics* 1995;95:29–31.
98. Schaad UB, Kaplan SL, McCracken GH Jr. Steroid therapy for bacterial meningitis. *Clin Infect Dis* 1995;20:685–690.
99. Coyle PK. Glucocorticoids in central nervous system bacterial infection. *Arch Neurol* 1999;56:796–801.
100. Kaplan SL, Mason EO Jr. Management of infections due to antibiotic-resistant *Streptococcus pneumoniae*. *Clin Microbiol Rev* 1998;11:628–644.

8

Therapy and Outcome

All patients with a suspected or confirmed diagnosis of acute bacterial meningitis should be hospitalized; admission to an intensive care unit is indicated by the presence of sepsis and/or neurologic compromise, manifested as clinical evidence of increased intracranial pressure, cranial nerve palsies, focal cerebral signs, and/or seizures. Following initiation of empiric or targeted antimicrobial therapy, the choice of continued antimicrobial therapy is based on the specific microorganism isolated and *in vitro* susceptibility testing. Other adjunctive measures in patients with a complicated course may also be required. These issues, and the expected response and outcome, are discussed later.

ANTIMICROBIAL THERAPY

Once the meningeal pathogen is isolated, *in vitro* susceptibility testing is critical to determine the optimal therapeutic regimen for continued treatment of bacterial meningitis. Reduced susceptibility of many meningeal pathogens to previously used antimicrobial agents has led to new therapeutic recommendations (Table 8.1), which continue to be in evolution. The epidemiology, mechanisms of resistance, and recommendations for antimicrobial therapy based on microorganism isolated are discussed later.

Streptococcus pneumoniae

The therapy of meningitis caused by the pneumococcus has been modified recently based on current *in vitro* pneumococcal susceptibility patterns (1,2). The National Committee for Clinical Laboratory Standards has set up definitions for minimal inhibitory concentration (MIC) breakpoints that define intermediate and high-level resistance to penicillin and other antimicrobial agents (Table 8.2) (3). In the past, pneumococci were uniformly susceptible to penicillin with MICs of ≤0.06 μg/mL. Numerous reports from throughout the world have now identified strains of pneumococci that are of intermediate (or relative) resistance to penicillin (MIC range of 0.1 to 1.0 μg/mL) as well as strains that are highly resistant to penicillin (MIC

TABLE 8.1. *Specific antimicrobial therapy of acute bacterial meningitis*

Microorganism	Standard therapy	Alternative therapies
Streptococcus pneumoniae		
Penicillin MIC <0.1 μg/mL	Penicillin G or ampicillin	Third-generation cephalosporin[a], chloramphenicol
Penicillin MIC 0.1–1.0 μg/mL	Third-generation cephalosporin[a]	Meropenem, cefepime
Penicillin MIC ≥2.0 μg/mL	Vancomycin plus a third-generation cephalosporin[a,b]	Meropenem; fluoroquinolone[c]
Cefotaxime or ceftriaxone MIC ≥1.0 μg/mL	Vancomycin plus a third-generation cephalosporin[a,b]	Meropenem; fluoroquinolone[c]
Neisseria meningitidis		
Penicillin MIC <0.1 μg/mL	Penicillin G or ampicillin	Third-generation cephalosporin[a]; chloramphenicol
Penicillin MIC 0.1–1.0 μg/mL	Third-generation cephalosporin[a,d]	Chloramphenicol; fluoroquinolone; meropenem
Streptococcus agalactiae	Ampicillin or penicillin G[e]	Third-generation cephalosporin[a]; vancomycin
Listeria monocytogenes	Ampicillin or penicillin G[e]	Trimethoprim-sulfamethoxazole; meropenem
Haemophilus influenzae		
β-lactamase negative	Ampicillin	Third-generation cephalosporin[a]; cefepime; chloramphenicol; aztreonam
β-lactamase positive	Third-generation cephalosporin[a]	Cefepime, chloramphenicol; aztreonam; fluoroquinolone[c]
Enterobacteriaceae	Third-generation cephalosporin[a]	Aztreonam; fluoroquinolone; trimethoprim-sulfamethoxazole; meropenem
Pseudomonas aeruginosa	Ceftazidime[e]	Aztreonam[e], fluoroquinolone[e], meropenem[e]
Staphylococcus aureus		
Methicillin-sensitive	Nafcillin or oxacillin	Vancomycin
Methicillin-resistant	Vancomycin	
Staphylococcus epidermidis	Vancomycin[b]	

[a] Cefotaxime or ceftriaxone.
[b] Addition of rifampin may be considered. See text for indications.
[c] Value of these antimicrobial agents has not been established.
[d] Superiority of a third-generation cephalosporin over penicillin has not been established.
[e] Addition of an aminoglycoside should be considered.

of ≥2.0 μg/mL) (4–6). The first clinical pneumococcal isolate resistant to penicillin (MIC = 0.6 μg/mL) was reported in 1967 from Australia in a patient with hypogammaglobulinemia and bronchiectasis (7). The first highly resistant strains (MICs of 4 to 8 μg/mL) were described in 1977 in South Africa, followed in the next year by description of multidrug resistant *S. pneumoniae*. Since that time, the frequency of isolation of antimicrobial-resistant pneumococci has increased throughout the world (8–17). In some areas of the United States, 25% to 30% of invasive pneumococcal isolates were found to have either intermediate or high-level resistance to penicillin (8,9).

TABLE 8.2. *Minimal inhibitory concentration breakpoints for antimicrobial agents used to treat* Streptococcus pneumoniae *infections (μg/mL)*

Antimicrobial agent	Susceptible	Nonsusceptible	
		Intermediate	Resistant
Penicillin	≤0.06	0.1–1.0	≥2.0
Ceftriaxone	≤0.5	1.0	≥2.0
Cefotaxime	≤0.5	1.0	≥2.0
Cefepime	≤0.5	1.0	≥2.0
Vancomycin	≤1.0	—	—
Rifampin	≤1.0	2.0	≥4.0
Chloramphenicol	≤4.0	—	≥8.0
Imipenem	≤0.12	0.25–0.5	≥1.0
Meropenem[a]	≤0.12	≥0.25	—

Data from National Committee for Clinical Laboratory Standards. *Methods for dilution antimicrobial susceptibility tests for bacteria that grow aerobically: approved standard,* 4th ed., NCCLS Document M7-A4. Wayne, PA: National Committee for Clinical Laboratory Standards, 1997, with permission.

[a] Susceptibility interpretive criteria have not yet been established by the NCCLS.

A recent survey (1997 to 1998) involving 163 institutions in 43 states of the United States revealed that 35% of respiratory tract pneumococcal isolates were not susceptible to penicillin and 13% of strains were highly resistant (10). In another survey from the Centers for Disease Control and Prevention (CDC) performed in seven different United States regions in 1997, 25% of 3,237 pneumococcal isolates from sterile body sites were not susceptible to penicillin (11); 13.6% were highly resistant. Geographic variability in the incidence of penicillin resistance was also reported; up to 38.8% of isolates in Tennessee were not susceptible to penicillin, whereas the overall incidence was only 15.3% in Maryland. In addition, the incidence varied from different hospitals in the same region, with an incidence ranging from 0 to 39.1% in 22 hospitals in Connecticut. Age may also be a factor in acquisition of drug-resistant pneumococci; in some areas of North America, nearly 40% of pneumococcal isolates from blood or cerebrospinal fluid (CSF) from persons 65 years of age or more had reduced susceptibility to penicillin (18). The problem of penicillin resistance in pneumococci is even greater in other countries of the world. In South Africa, Spain, and Hungary, rates of penicillin nonsusceptibility among pneumococci range from 40% to 70% (14), with high rates also noted in Thailand (57.9%), Vietnam (60.8%), Japan (65.3%), and Korea (79.7%) (15). In Taiwan, the rate of resistance was recently reported to be 56.4% (19). Penicillin resistance has also been found to be a marker for resistance to other β-lactam and non-β-lactam antimicrobial agents, although not for resistance to vancomycin or the fluoroquinolones (7,10,12,15).

Factors reported to predispose to penicillin resistance in pneumococci include patient age (especially less than 6 years or more than 50 years of age), immunosuppression, prolonged hospital stay, children in day care settings, infection by serotypes

14 and 23, and frequent, prolonged, or prophylactic use of antimicrobial therapy (7,13,14,20–22). Children less than 2 years of age (especially if attending day care centers) have the highest risk of being colonized and infected with resistant pneumococci (14,23). However, most studies have identified previous β-lactam therapy as among the most important predictors of the presence of penicillin-nonsusceptible *S. pneumoniae* (13,24); non-β-lactam antimicrobial agents are also capable of selecting for penicillin-nonsusceptible *S. pneumoniae* (24). The risk for selection is greatest in the presence of low antimicrobial concentrations, when agents with poor *in vitro* activity are used, and following prolonged courses of antimicrobial therapy.

The mechanism of penicillin resistance in pneumococci is due to alterations in the structure and molecular size of penicillin-binding proteins (PBPs) (17). It has been suggested that acquisition of penicillin resistance in pneumococci may involve integration of free DNA molecules from the environment, such that a susceptible pneumococcus can incorporate DNA carrying PBP genes of reduced penicillin affinity from nonpneumococcal bacteria, giving rise to a clone of bacteria with low levels of penicillin resistance (25). Under the right selective pressures, this clone may then proliferate via cell division until one of its members undergoes a second recombination, leading to increased antimicrobial resistance in the new clone. Each further recombination will increase the level of resistance. This concept has been supported by genetic and epidemiologic studies. Most areas of the world documented the appearance of low levels of penicillin resistance in pneumococci before highly resistant strains were identified. Resistance has been reported in several different pneumococcal serotypes, although the overwhelming majority of resistant strains are serotypes 6, 14, 19, and 23. Most of the multiresistant strains isolated in the United States disseminated from a multiresistant serotype 23F clone of *S. pneumoniae* that was isolated in Spain as early as 1978 (26).

The antimicrobial therapy of pneumococcal meningitis has been significantly influenced by the emergence of penicillin resistance, such that penicillin is no longer acceptable as empiric therapy when the diagnosis of pneumococcal meningitis is suspected or proven (1,2). The reason for this recommendation is based on failure to achieve adequate CSF concentrations of penicillin to be effective against strains of *S. pneumoniae* that are of intermediate or high-level resistance to penicillin. Serum concentrations of penicillin up to 20 μg/mL can be attained with high-dose intravenous penicillin G (24 million units/day), leading to initial CSF concentrations of approximately 1 μg/mL. Since CSF concentrations of β-lactam antimicrobial agents are needed to be at least 10-fold greater than the minimal bactericidal concentration (MBC) to obtain a bactericidal effect (see Chapter 7), high-dose intravenous penicillin will be inadequate against strains of *S. pneumoniae* with either intermediate or high-level resistance to penicillin. Indeed, early reports documented clinical failure in the majority of patients with penicillin-nonsusceptible *S. pneumoniae* who were treated with penicillin (6,27).

Several alternative agents for the treatment of meningitis caused by penicillin-resistant pneumococci have been evaluated by *in vitro* susceptibility testing, in animal models, and in patients (1,2,27,28). Chloramphenicol is one agent that has been studied in pneumococcal meningitis. It has excellent CSF penetration and is active *in vitro* against most penicillin-resistant pneumococcal strains. However, clinical failures with chloramphenicol have been reported in patients with meningitis caused by penicillin-resistant isolates, likely a result of the poor bactericidal activity of chloramphenicol against these strains (6). In one study, 20 of 25 children with penicillin-resistant isolates had an unsatisfactory outcome (i.e., death, serious neurologic deficit, poor clinical response) when treated with chloramphenicol (29). Despite susceptibility on disc testing, the chloramphenicol MBCs of the penicillin-resistant pneumococcal isolates were significantly higher (>4 μg/mL) than for the penicillin-sensitive isolates, resulting in subtherapeutic bactericidal activity and treatment failure.

The third-generation cephalosporins have been considered the antimicrobial agents of choice in patients with pneumococcal meningitis caused by isolates with intermediate resistance to penicillin (1,2,28). Cefotaxime and ceftriaxone are the third-generation agents of choice; ceftizoxime is not recommended because its MICs to resistant pneumococci tend to be higher than those of either cefotaxime or ceftriaxone (30,31). However, there are reports of meningitis treatment failure with the third-generation cephalosporins in patients with penicillin- and cephalosporin-resistant pneumococcal meningitis, and pneumococcal strains have emerged that are resistant to these agents (MIC ≥ 2 μg/mL) (32–39). One study revealed the incidence of CSF pneumococcal isolates with cefotaxime and ceftriaxone MICs ≥ 0.5 μg/mL to be 16.4% (40). For the third-generation cephalosporins, pneumococcal strains with MICs ≤ 0.5 μg/mL are defined as susceptible, 1.0 μg/mL as intermediate, and ≥ 2.0 μg/mL as resistant. However, when the MIC to the third-generation cephalosporin is ≤ 1 μg/mL, some patients have been treated successfully with either high-dose cefotaxime or ceftriaxone alone (35,41), although one study found that high-dose cefotaxime did not have reliably sufficient CSF bactericidal activity against cephalosporin-resistant pneumococci (42). A recent study in the experimental rabbit model demonstrated that high doses of ceftriaxone were efficacious in meningitis caused by cephalosporin-resistant *S. pneumoniae* (MIC $= 2.0$ μg/mL), although coadministration of dexamethasone significantly increased the rate of therapeutic failure (from 0% to 28%) (43). Cefepime, a fourth-generation cephalosporin, was recently shown to have superior bactericidal efficacy compared with ceftriaxone in an experimental rabbit model of penicillin-resistant pneumococcal meningitis (44), indicating the need to evaluate this agent in the therapy of patients with pneumococcal meningitis.

Vancomycin has been evaluated in the therapy of meningitis caused by penicillin-resistant *S. pneumoniae* (45,46). In one study in 11 adult patients with meningitis caused by intermediate penicillin-resistant pneumococcal strains (45), vancomycin therapy was associated with clinical failure in four patients. There were no failures in 14 subsequent patients treated with ceftriaxone. In two of the failures, CSF vancomycin concentrations were undetectable at 48 hours, and in a third patient, symptoms recurred on the eighth day of antimicrobial therapy. The concomitant administration of dexamethasone and the subsequent decreased inflammation and poor entry of vancomycin into CSF may have contributed to this negative outcome; this explanation has been supported in an experimental rabbit model of pneumococcal meningitis (47,48). In noninflamed meninges, CSF penetration of vancomycin becomes erratic, requiring very high serum concentrations. Since dexamethasone limits the inflammatory process in the meninges, the CSF vancomycin penetration is diminished. These data support the concept that vancomycin should not be used alone for the therapy of pneumococcal meningitis. Of additional concern is the recent description of *S. pneumoniae* strains that are tolerant to vancomycin (49,50). Tolerance is defined as the ability of bacteria to survive in the presence of an antimicrobial agent, neither growing nor undergoing lysis, and is not detected by conventional *in vitro* susceptibility testing. A vancomycin- and cephalosporin-tolerant strain of *S. pneumoniae* was recently isolated from the CSF of a patient with meningitis who then developed recrudescence of meningitis despite therapy with vancomycin plus a third-generation cephalosporin (51). Because tolerance is a precursor phenotype to the development of resistance, these data have important implications in the use of vancomycin for pneumococcal meningitis and indicate the need for continued surveillance for vancomycin-tolerant pneumococci.

Based on the preceding data, as an empiric regimen, the combination of vancomycin plus a third-generation cephalosporin (either cefotaxime or ceftriaxone) is recommended for patients with suspected or proven pneumococcal meningitis (1,2). This combination was synergistic in a rabbit model of penicillin-resistant pneumococcal meningitis (52) and was synergistic, or at least additive, in the CSF of children with meningitis (53,54). The addition of rifampin to vancomycin and/or the third-generation cephalosporin has been recommended by some authorities, although clinical data are lacking. In a mouse model of pneumococcal meningitis that compared rifampin with ceftriaxone (55), there were 11 deaths (26%) in the rifampin group and 21 deaths (49%) in the ceftriaxone group by day 6 of therapy. However, the rapid development of resistance prohibits use of rifampin as monotherapy in pneumococcal meningitis. In contrast, in an *in vitro* study using amoxicillin-resistant *S. pneumoniae* (MIC ≥ 4.0 μg/mL), the addition of rifampin to a third-generation cephalosporin led to a 10-fold decrease in killing of ceftriaxone-susceptible strains (56). In the absence of clinical data, rifampin should be added only if the organism is demonstrated to be susceptible and there is a delay in the expected clinical or bacteriologic response (27). In patients with pneumococcal meningitis who are not responding, intrathecal or intraventricular vancomycin also remains a reasonable option (46). Once susceptibility studies of the isolated pneumococccus are performed, antimicrobial therapy can be modified for optimal treatment (Table 8.1). In addition, a repeat lumbar puncture should be considered after 24 to 48 hours to evaluate therapy if the pneumococcus is penicillin and/or cephalosporin resistant and the patient's clinical condition has not improved or worsened, or if the patient has received adjunctive dexamethasone that might interfere with the ability to interpret the clinical response (27,28). However, some experts believe that a second lumbar puncture is not necessary if therapy was initiated with vancomycin plus either cefotaxime or ceftriaxone, and the clinical response has been good, particularly if dexamethasone was not used (28).

Few studies have addressed whether clinical outcome is worse in patients with pneumococcal meningitis caused by penicillin- and/or cephalosporin-resistant strains. In one retrospective analysis of 55 cases of community-acquired meningitis caused by *S. pneumoniae* (57), the case-fatality rates among adults were lower if treatment included chloramphenicol or a third-generation cephalosporin, although the number of patients receiving differing antimicrobial regimens was very small to make meaningful conclusions. In a multicenter, retrospective study of 180 episodes of pneumococcal meningitis in children (58), mortality and frequency of neurologic sequelae were not influenced by susceptibility of the pneumococcal isolate to penicillin or ceftriaxone. Similar results, with no differences in mortality, were obtained in another analysis of 109 cases of pneumococcal meningitis caused by cefotaxime-nonsusceptible isolates (59). Empiric use of vancomycin, the current prevalence of drug-resistant *S. pneumoniae,* and the degree of nonsusceptibility to cefotaxime may have influenced these findings. These studies indicate the need for continued surveillance of resistance characteristics among *S. pneumoniae,* and the need to correlate resistance to clinical outcome.

With continued emergence of penicillin- and cephalosporin-resistant strains of *S. pneumoniae,* other antimicrobial agents have been evaluated for their efficacy in pneumococcal meningitis. Imipenem has been used successfully in two patients with penicillin- and cephalosporin-resistant pneumococcal meningitis (60,61), although a high incidence of drug-related seizure activity (33% in one study) limits its usefulness in patients with bacterial meningitis (62). Meropenem, a carbapenem with a broad spectrum of *in vitro* activity, including penicillin-resistant pneumococci and far less seizure proclivity than imipenem (63), has recently been approved by the Food and Drug Administration for treatment of bacterial meningitis in children 3 months of age and older. In one study comparing the *in vitro* killing activities of meropenem and other antimicrobial agents at clinically achievable CSF concentrations against highly penicillin-resistant *S. pneumoniae* isolates from children with meningitis (40), no significant difference in the activity of meropenem was observed compared with the combination of vancomycin plus ceftriaxone. Meropenem has been studied for the treatment of meningitis in both adults and children in several clinical trials (64,65), with microbiologic and clinical outcomes similar to those of patients treated with either cefotaxime or ceftriaxone. In one prospective study of 258 children with bacterial meningitis, patients were randomized to receive either meropenem or cefotaxime. There were no significant differences in outcome, with clinical cure (with or without sequelae) seen in 97% and 96% of patients treated with meropenem and cefotaxime, respectively (66). At 5 to 7 weeks, 54% of the meropenem-treated patients and 58% of the cefotaxime-treated patients were cured with no sequelae. Meropenem was also used successfully in one patient with multiply drug-resistant pneumococcal meningitis (67) and in another patient with pneumococcal meningitis in whom the organism had a cefotaxime MIC of 2.0 μg/mL (66). These studies provide excellent documentation of the efficacy of meropenem in the treatment of bacterial meningitis (68). However, further studies are needed to determine the efficacy of meropenem in pneumococcal meningitis caused by penicillin- and cephalosporin-resistant strains before its routine use can be recommended.

The fluoroquinolones have generally lacked sufficient *in vitro* activity against *S. pneumoniae* to warrant their investigation in the therapy of central nervous system infections. However, newer agents have shown excellent *in vitro* activity and have been evaluated in experimental animal models of pneumococcal meningitis. Trovafloxacin has excellent CSF penetration (69) and has been shown to have bactericidal activity in an experimental rabbit model of penicillin-resistant pneumococcal meningitis (70), an effect that was not affected by the coadministration of dexamethasone. The combination of trovafloxacin and vancomycin was found to significantly increase the killing rate in an experimental rabbit model of penicillin-resistant pneumococcal meningitis greater than when each agent was used alone (71). However, concerns about liver toxicity related to trovafloxacin preclude its continued use in the treatment of resistant pneumococcal infections. Another agent, moxifloxacin, has excellent *in vitro* activity against pneumococci isolated from meningitis patients (including penicillin-resistant strains) (72) and was shown to be as effective as ceftriaxone in the rabbit model of meningitis caused by a penicillin-sensitive pneumococcal strain (73). CSF penetration was only slightly reduced by the coadministration of dexamethasone. Moxifloxacin has also shown efficacy in the therapy of penicillin-resistant pneumococcal meningitis in rabbits (74). Similar *in vitro* and animal model results have been demonstrated with gatifloxacin (75,76) and gemifloxacin (77,78). However, clinical trials are needed to determine the usefulness of these agents in patients with bacterial meningitis. Of concern is the recent report of decreased pneumococcal susceptibility to the fluoroquinolones (79) as well as a case of fatal meningitis caused by a levofloxacin-resistant strain of *S. pneumoniae* (80), indicating the need to monitor pneumococcal *in vitro* susceptibility to these agents.

Neisseria meningitidis

Penicillin G and ampicillin have been the antimicrobial agents of choice for meningitis caused by *N. meningitidis*. However, these recommendations may need to be modified in the future based on trends in antimicrobial susceptibility of meningococci. Meningococcal strains have been reported from several areas (particularly Spain) that are relatively resistant to penicillin G with a MIC range of 0.1 to 1.0 μg/mL (81,82). Of 3,264 strains of *N. meningitidis* isolated from blood and CSF from Spain during the period of 1978 to 1985, only one resistant isolate was observed (83). However, nine of 168 (5%) invasive isolates relatively resistant to penicillin G were found in the first 6 months of 1986, which reached a frequency of 20% in 1989. Subsequently, the prevalence of isolates with increased resistance to penicillin and ampicillin were 48.4% and 55.6%, respectively, in one hospital in Spain (84). Penicillin resistance in meningococci is mediated by a reduced affinity of the antibiotic for penicillin-binding proteins 2 or 3 (83,85,86). Decreased meningococcal susceptibility to penicillin has also been reported from Greece, Switzerland, Romania, France, Belgium, the United Kingdom, Malawi, South Africa, and Canada (87). In the United States, meningococcal strains relatively resistant to penicillin have also been described (88–90). In one population-based surveillance study for invasive meningococcal disease in selected areas of the United States, three of 100 isolates had penicillin MICs of 0.125 μg/mL (88). In another active, population-based surveillance in seven geographically dispersed areas of the United States during 1997 (91), three of 90 (3%) isolates were intermediately resistant to penicillin (MIC 0.12 μg/mL), whereas 49 of the remaining 87 isolates had MICs of 0.06 μg/mL.

High-level penicillin resistance as a result of β-lactamase production has also been reported, and the MICs for these strains may be as high as 256 μg/mL (86); β-lactamase-production has not been reported in meningococcal isolates in the United States (88,91).

The clinical significance of these isolates is unclear at present because many patients with meningococcal meningitis caused by strains with intermediate resistance to penicillin have recovered with standard penicillin therapy. However, isolated reports of treatment failure have been described (92,93). Furthermore, in a study from Spain in which reduced susceptibility of *N. meningitidis* to penicillin was seen in 34% of 213 children with meningococcal meningitis (94), reduced penicillin susceptibility was more frequent among strains responsible for death or sequelae (60% versus 32%; $P = 0.04$). These findings should be interpreted with caution, however, because of the low numbers of patients reported.

Based on these data, some authorities would treat patients with meningococcal meningitis with a third-generation cephalosporin (either cefotaxime or ceftriaxone), pending results of *in vitro* susceptibility testing. However, in areas of the world with a low prevalence of resistant isolates, routine *in vitro* susceptibility testing of all meningococcal isolates is probably not warranted (91). Susceptibility testing of the isolate should be performed in patients who fail to appropriately respond to standard therapy.

Other antimicrobial agents have been utilized in patients with meningococcal meningitis. Chloramphenicol is the standard treatment for meningococcal meningitis in developing countries because of its ease of administration (intramuscularly in oil) and low cost (95). However, high-level chloramphenicol resistance (MIC $\geq$ 64 μg/mL) has recently been described (96), because of the presence of the *catP* gene on a truncated transposon that has lost mobility because of internal deletions; transmission of genetic material between strains of *N. meningitidis* probably played an important role in the dissemination of this gene. These data indicate the importance of continued surveillance for these resistant strains. Trovafloxacin was found to be equivalent to ceftriaxone in children with meningococcal meningitis in one report (97), although further studies are needed before any of the fluoroquinolones can be routinely recommended for the therapy of meningococcal meningitis. Meropenem also has excellent *in vitro* activity against meningococcal isolates (98,99) and may prove to be highly effective in the therapy of meningococcal meningitis.

Streptococcus agalactiae

Standard therapy for neonatal meningitis caused by the group B streptococcus is either ampicillin or penicillin G, with a short initial empiric course of an aminoglycoside recommended because of documented *in vitro* synergy and reports detailing the presence of penicillin-tolerant strains (100). Ampicillin or penicillin is also recommended for adult patients with meningitis caused by this organism. In two case series and literature reviews in adult patients with group B streptococcal meningitis (101,102), the case fatality rates were significantly lower for patients treated with penicillin than for patients treated with other antimicrobial agents. However, there were higher proportions of comorbidity and complications on admission in patients not treated with penicillin, such that these patients were treated with antimicrobial agents with a broader spectrum of *in vitro* activity. Alternative agents for therapy of *S. agalactiae* meningitis are the third-generation cephalosporins; vancomycin is reserved for patients who are allergic to β-lactam drugs.

Listeria monocytogenes

For patients with *Listeria* meningitis, recommended therapy is either ampicillin or penicillin G (103–107). The addition of an aminoglycoside should be strongly considered in proven infection due to documented *in vitro* synergy and enhanced killing *in vivo* as documented in a variety of animal models of *Listeria* infection. Although a prospective, randomized clinical trial comparing ampicillin to ampicillin plus gentamicin has never been performed in patients with *Listeria* meningitis, the available experimental data and clinical experience suggest that the addition of an aminoglycoside may improve the efficacy of ampicillin or penicillin (107). Of concern is a recent case report of a neonate with meningitis caused by *L. monocytogenes* with reduced *in vitro* susceptibility to the aminoglycosides (108), indicating the need for continued surveillance of these isolates.

An alternative agent for the treatment of *Listeria* meningitis in the patient who is allergic to or intolerant of penicillins is trimethoprim-sulfamethoxazole (103–107,109–111), which is bactericidal against *Listeria in vitro*. Clinical outcomes in patients treated with trimethoprim-sulfamethoxazole appear at least comparable to the combination of ampicillin and gentamicin, although poor outcomes have been reported (112). Furthermore, in a preliminary study in patients with severe listerial meningoencephalitis, the combination of ampicillin plus trimethoprim-sulfamethoxazole was associated with a much lower rate of treatment failure and with fewer neurologic sequelae than the combination of ampicillin plus an aminoglycoside (113).

Other antimicrobial agents have been examined for their efficacy in *L. monocytogenes* infections. Although chloramphenicol has varying activity against *Listeria in vitro*, its use has been associated with unacceptably high failure and relapse rates in patients with *Listeria* meningitis (114,115). Vancomycin is also unsatisfactory for *Listeria* meningitis, despite favorable *in vitro* susceptibility results and positive results in anecdotal case reports in patients with listeriosis (105,116,117). *Listeria* meningitis has even been reported in a patient receiving vancomycin therapy (118). However, intraventricular administration of vancomycin was successful in one case of recurrent *L. monocytogenes* meningitis (119). Rifampin is bacteriostatic against *L. monocytogenes in vitro* and was no better than penicillin or ampicillin alone when evaluated in the experimental rabbit model of *Listeria* meningitis (120). Meropenem is active *in vitro* and was found to be efficacious in an experimental animal model of *L. monocytogenes* meningitis (121); meropenem was also successfully used in a pediatric renal transplant patient with *Listeria* meningitis (122). Further studies are needed to determine whether meropenem will be clinically efficacious in patients with *Listeria* meningitis. *In vitro* studies suggest that the newer fluoroquinolones may be effective against *Listeria* (123). In one study in an experimental rat model of meningoencephalitis caused by *L. monocytogenes,* trovafloxacin was more active than trimethoprim-sulfamethoxazole (124), suggesting that the newer fluoroquinolones may offer an effective alternative to trimethoprim-sulfamethoxazole in the therapy of *Listeria* meningitis in patients allergic to β-lactam agents; further studies with these drugs in *Listeria* meningitis are needed, however. Despite their broad range of *in vitro* activity, the third-generation cephalosporins are inactive in meningitis caused by *L. monocytogenes* (106,107).

Haemophilus influenzae

Therapy of meningitis caused by *H. influenzae* type b has been markedly altered by the emergence of β-lactamase-producing strains. In a surveillance study of all cases of bacterial meningitis in 27 states of the United States from 1978 through 1981, β-lactamase-producing strains accounted for approximately 24% of all CSF isolates (125). The incidence was 32% in a subsequent surveillance study of five states and Los Angeles County in 1986 (126). Resistance of *H. influenzae* to chloramphenicol has also been described, although more commonly from areas such as Spain than from the United States (50% versus <1% of isolates, respectively) (127–129). Even in patients with chloramphenicol-sensitive isolates, a prospective study of 220 consecutive cases of bacterial meningitis in children older than 3 months of age found chloramphenicol to be bacteriologically and clinically inferior to ampicillin, ceftriaxone, or cefotaxime in the therapy of childhood bacterial meningitis caused predominantly by *H. influenzae* type b (130). Furthermore, the use of chloramphenicol can be problematic because of its unpredictable metabolism in young infants and its pharmacologic interactions with other concomitantly administered drugs (e.g., phenobarbital, rifampin, phenytoin, acetaminophen) that increase the likelihood of toxicity (131).

Based on these concerns, other antimicrobial agents were evaluated for their efficacy in patients with *H. influenzae* meningitis. Initial studies documented that cefuroxime, a second-generation cephalosporin, was as efficacious as the combination of ampicillin and chloramphenicol for childhood bacterial meningitis (132). Other studies have also documented similar efficacy of the third-generation cephalosporins (particularly cefotaxime or ceftriaxone) to the combination of ampicillin plus chloramphenicol for bacterial meningitis (133,134). However, subsequent trials and case reports questioned the efficacy of cefuroxime in *H. influenzae* meningitis. In one report reviewing four prospective trials comparing cefuroxime with ceftriaxone in infants and children with bacterial meningitis, both regimens had comparable efficacy, although some patients did not respond as satisfactorily to cefuroxime with slower rates of CSF sterilization (0% vs. 9% of CSF cultures positive at 24 hours in patients treated with cefuroxime; $P < 0.001$) and a higher incidence of hearing impairment (18% vs. 11%) (135). Another prospective randomized study comparing ceftriaxone with cefuroxime for the treatment of childhood bacterial meningitis documented a more rapid CSF sterilization (2% vs. 12% of CSF cultures positive at 18 to 36 hours; $P = 0.11$) and a lower incidence of hearing impairment (4% vs. 17%; $P = 0.05$) in the patients receiving ceftriaxone (136). Furthermore, there have been reports of treatment failure (137,138) and delayed CSF sterilization in patients receiving cefuroxime for *H. influenzae* meningitis (132), as well as the development of *H. influenzae* meningitis in patients receiving cefuroxime for nonmeningeal *H. influenzae* disease (139). However, cefuroxime continues to be as safe and effective as chloramphenicol or cefotaxime for the treatment of non–central nervous system infections caused by ampicillin-resistant *H. influenzae* type b (140).

Based on these findings, the American Academy of Pediatrics has recommended use of a third-generation cephalosporin as empiric antimicrobial therapy for children with bacterial meningitis (141). Although there have been single case reports of delayed CSF sterilization in patients with *H. influenzae* meningitis treated with ceftizoxime or ceftazidime (142), *in vitro* resistance of *H. influenzae* to the third-generation cephalosporins and fluoroquinolones has not been described to date (143).

Recently, cefepime has been studied in the therapy of bacterial meningitis. Compared with cefotaxime and ceftriaxone, cefepime has similar *in vitro* activity against *H. influenzae, N. meningitidis,* and *S. pneumoniae,* and greater *in vitro* activity against *Enterobacter* species and *Pseudomonas aeruginosa.* In a prospective randomized comparison of cefepime to cefotaxime for treatment of bacterial meningitis in infants and children, cefepime was found to be safe and therapeutically equivalent to cefotaxime (144), and can be considered a suitable therapeutic alternative for treatment of patients with this disease.

Aerobic Gram-Negative Bacilli

The treatment of bacterial meningitis caused by aerobic gram-negative bacilli has been revolutionized by the availability of the third-generation cephalosporins (145–148). Previous mortality rates with standard regimens (usually an aminoglycoside with or without chloramphenicol) ranged from 40% to 90% compared with cure rates of 78% to 94% with the third-generation cephalosporins. Cefotaxime is preferred over ceftriaxone as the third-generation cephalosporin for use in neonates because it has been used more extensively and is not excreted in the bile, which may have an inhibitory effect on the bacterial flora of the intestinal tract (149). Ceftriaxone also has increased protein binding. One particular cephalosporin, ceftazidime, has enhanced *in vitro* activity against *P. aeruginosa* and its use resulted in the cure of 19 of 24 patients in one study of *P. aeruginosa* meningitis when administered alone or in combination with an aminoglycoside (150). In another study of 10 pediatric patients with *Pseudomonas* meningitis, seven patients were cured clinically and nine were cured bacteriologically when treated with ceftazidime-containing regimens (151). Concomitant intrathecal or intraventricular aminoglycoside therapy should be considered in patients with gram-negative meningitis who are not responding to conventional parenteral therapy. However, this mode of administration is rarely needed at present and was associated with a higher mortality rate than systemic therapy alone in infants with gram-negative meningitis and ventriculitis (152).

Based on the emergence of resistance of aerobic gram-negative bacilli to the third-generation cephalosporins (153) and the demonstration of these resistant organisms causing meningitis (154), several other antimicrobial agents have been studied for their efficacy in patients with gram-negative bacillary meningitis. Aztreonam attains excellent CSF concentrations and has been shown to be efficacious in the therapy of gram-negative meningitis (155). Imipenem was found to be efficacious in one case of *Acinetobacter* meningitis (156), although its potential for association with seizure activity limits its usefulness in the therapy of bacterial meningitis. High-dose meropenem (2 g every 8 hours) given for 18 weeks was successful in a lymphoma patient with *P. aeruginosa* meningitis who had failed therapy with ceftazidime plus gentamicin (157), and in a patient with posttraumatic meningitis caused by *P. aeruginosa* (158). More recently, intravenous meropenem was also successfully used in combination with intraventricular polymyxin B in a patient with ventriculoperitoneal shunt-associated ventriculitis caused by a ceftazidime-resistant *Klebsiella pneumoniae* (159). However, development of resistance to meropenem has been described during treatment of a patient with *Acinetobacter* meningitis (160), indicating the need to consider the emergence of resistance in patients who fail to respond.

The fluoroquinolones (e.g., ciprofloxacin, pefloxacin) have been used successfully in some patients with gram-negative meningitis (161–165). In a recent case series of 12 neonates and infants with nosocomial meningitis (in which six cases were attributable to gram-negative bacilli), 10 patients were cured, and in seven children, no neurologic sequelae appeared after a 2- to 4-year follow-up (166). However, the limited published literature on the use of the fluoroquinolones in bacterial meningitis suggests that the primary area of usefulness of these agents is for therapy of multidrug-resistant gram-negative organisms (e.g., meningitis caused by *P. aeruginosa*) or when the response to conventional β-lactam therapy is slow (e.g., meningitis caused by *Salmonella* species). The choice of appropriate antimicrobial therapy is critical in patients with gram-negative bacillary meningitis; in one study of 77 patients with gram-negative bacillary meningitis (167), the overall mortality rate was higher in patients who received inappropriate antimicrobial therapy (100% vs. 28%; $P < 0.001$).

Staphylococci

Staphylococcus aureus meningitis should be treated with nafcillin or oxacillin (168–170), with vancomycin reserved for patients allergic to penicillin or when methicillin-resistant organisms are suspected or isolated. The addition of rifampin should be considered in patients not responding to therapy. Meningitis caused by coagulase-negative staphylococci, the most commonly encountered organisms in CSF shunt infections, is treated with vancomycin (171); rifampin should be added if the patient fails to improve. The intraventricular route of administration may be considered if the infection was difficult to eradicate after antimicrobial administration by the parenteral route (171). Intraventricular teicoplanin, in conjunction with shunt removal, was shown to be efficacious in staphylococcal neurosurgical shunt infections (172), although further studies with this agent are needed before it can be recommended as a first-line agent for these infections.

Duration of Therapy

The duration of therapy for bacterial meningitis has been based more on tradition than on scientific evidence, although some general recommendations can be made (Table 8.3) (173,174). Ten to 14 days of antimicrobial therapy are generally recommended for patients with pneumococcal meningitis. Meningococcal meningitis can be treated for 7 days with intravenous penicillin or ampicillin, and some authors have suggested that 4 days of therapy are adequate (175). This study requires confirmation, however, as only 50 patients were studied and no control group was included. A single dose, or even two to three doses, of long-acting penicillin or chloramphenicol has also been used successfully in developing countries to treat meningococcal meningitis (176,177), although this is not considered standard therapy. Meningitis caused by the group B streptococcus should be treated for 14 to 21 days. Patients with meningitis caused by *L. monocytogenes* should be treated for at least 21 days (106,107), based on failures observed in patients treated for 14 days or less and the presence of microabscesses demonstrated in autopsy studies of patients with focal neurologic findings. In patients with meningitis caused by aerobic gram-negative bacilli, treatment regimens should be continued for 3 weeks due to the high rate of relapse in patients treated with shorter courses of therapy

In infants and children with meningitis caused predominantly by *H. influenzae* type b, several studies have compared 7 with 10 days of treatment, and demonstrated that 7 days of therapy are safe and effective (130,132,178,179). However, chloramphenicol

TABLE 8.3. *Duration of antimicrobial therapy in patients with bacterial meningitis*

Microorganism	Duration of therapy (d)
Streptococcus pneumoniae	10–14
Neisseria meningitidis	7
Streptococcus agalactiae	14–21
Listeria monocytogenes	≥21
Haemophilus influenzae	7
Aerobic gram-negative bacilli	21

Recommendations for therapy are general guidelines; duration of therapy may need to be individualized based upon clinical response.

(when used alone) should be administered for 10 days in patients with *H. influenzae* meningitis, given its inferiority to ampicillin, cefotaxime, and ceftriaxone (130). Recent studies have suggested that even shorter courses of antimicrobial therapy may be efficacious in infants and children with bacterial meningitis. In one randomized trial of 4 versus 7 days of ceftriaxone therapy in children with bacterial meningitis who had a rapid initial recovery (180), no significant differences in outcome were observed between the two groups at completion of therapy or at follow-up 1 to 3 months after discharge. However, duration of therapy for bacterial meningitis must be individualized; based on clinical response, some patients may require longer courses of antimicrobial therapy.

Outpatient Therapy

Patients with acute bacterial meningitis have traditionally remained hospitalized for the duration of parenteral antimicrobial therapy. However, some recent studies have suggested that outpatient parenteral antimicrobial therapy is appropriate for selected patients with bacterial meningitis (181,182). The advantages of outpatient therapy include decreased costs of hospitalization, decreased risk of development of nosocomial infections, and benefits in terms of quality of life (i.e., the psychologic, physical, and nutritional needs of the patient). Concerns have included the potential risk of serious complications (e.g., seizures, focal neurologic findings, secondary fevers, drug reactions) at the end of antimicrobial therapy. However, complications from bacterial meningitis most frequently occur within the first 2 to 3 days, and serious adverse consequences are exceedingly rare after 3 or 4 days of appropriate antimicrobial therapy. Furthermore, secondary fevers are most commonly a result of nosocomial infection, and drug reactions can be easily evaluated in the physicians' office or in an emergency room.

Several studies have examined the use of outpatient parenteral antimicrobial therapy for bacterial meningitis. In one study of 54 children with bacterial meningitis treated with ceftriaxone (183), the mean duration of outpatient therapy was 4.6 days, and no patient developed neurologic dysfunction, cardiovascular instability, or relapse. In addition, no child required readmission to the hospital. In this study, all patients receiving outpatient parenteral antimicrobial therapy required daily physician visits, absence of fever for at least 24 to 48 hours before initiation of home therapy, no neurologic dysfunction except for hearing or vestibular dysfunction, and resolution of any inappropriate secretion of antidiuretic hormone. In another study of outpatient parenteral antimicrobial therapy in 68 patients with central nervous system infections (including 29 patients with meningitis), all infections were cured and no deaths occurred during therapy (184). Careful patient selection for outpatient therapy and close medical follow-up were essential for inclusion in the study.

Based on these reports, selected patients with bacterial meningitis can receive outpatient parenteral antimicrobial therapy. Criteria that may be used to guide outpatient antimicrobial therapy for bacterial meningitis include the following (182,184): (a) inpatient therapy for at least 6 days; (b) no fever for at least 24 to 48 hours before initiation of outpatient therapy; (c) no significant neurologic dysfunction, focal findings, or seizure activity; (d) clinically stable or improving condition; (e) intake of all fluids by mouth; (f) first dose of the outpatient antimicrobial agent given under medical supervision and without reaction; (g) access to home health nursing for administration of the antimicrobial; (h) reliable intravenous line and infusion device, if needed; (i) daily examination by a physician, and established plan for physician visits, nurse visits, laboratory monitoring, and emergencies; (j) patient and/or family compliance with the program; and (k) a safe environment with access to a telephone, utilities, food, and a refrigerator. It must be emphasized, however, that the patient selection process must be carefully performed and that close medical follow-up is essential whenever outpatient parenteral antimicrobial therapy is considered for any patient with bacterial meningitis. In addition, completion of antimicrobial therapy in a skilled nursing facility may be appropriate for selected patients who need continued care but do not require acute hospitalization.

OUTCOME

Mortality

Bacterial meningitis was almost invariably a fatal disease in the preantibiotic era. However, the mortality rate in patients with bacterial meningitis continues to be high, even with the availability of effective antimicrobial agents. Surveillance data collected by the Centers for Disease Control and Prevention reported the case fatality rates in the United States based upon the microorganism isolated (Table 8.4) (125,126,185). In adult patients with bacterial meningitis, high mortality rates have also been reported (Table 8.5) (186,187). In one study of 493 episodes of acute bacterial meningitis in patients 16 years of age or more from 1962 through 1988, the overall case fatality

TABLE 8.4. *Case fatality rates in patients with bacterial meningitis in the United States based on isolated microorganism*

Microorganism	1978–1981	1986	1995
Streptococcus pneumoniae	26%	19%	21%
Neisseria meningitidis	10%	13%	3%
Streptococcus agalactiae	23%	12%	7%
Listeria monocytogenes	29%	22%	15%
Haemophilus influenzae	6%	3%	6%

Data from Schlech WF III, Ward JI, Band JD, et al. Bacterial meningitis in the United States, 1978 through 1981: the national bacterial meningitis surveillance study. *JAMA* 1985;253:1749–1754; Wenger JD, Hightower AW, Facklam RR, et al. Bacterial meningitis in the United States, 1986: report of a multistate surveillance study. *J Infect Dis* 1990;162:1316–1323; and Schuchat A, Robinson K, Wenger JD, et al. Bacterial meningitis in the United States in 1995. *N Engl J Med* 1997;337:970–976, with permission.

TABLE 8.5. *Mortality rates according to microorganism isolated in adults with bacterial meningitis*

Microorganism	Massachusetts General Hospital (1962–1988)	University of Iceland (1975–1994)
Streptococcus pneumoniae	28%	26%
Neisseria meningitidis	10%	16%
Listeria monocytogenes	32%	38%
Haemophilus influenzae	11%	17%
Gram-negative bacilli	36%	—
Staphylococcus aureus	39%	—
Coagulase-negative staphylococci	0%	—
Culture negative	10%	9%

Data from Durand ML, Calderwood SB, Weber DJ, et al. Acute bacterial meningitis in adults: a review of 493 episodes. *N Engl J Med* 1993;328:21–28; and Sigurdardottir B, Bjornsson OM, Jonsdottir KE, et al. Acute bacterial meningitis in adults: a 20-year overview. *Arch Intern Med* 1997;157:425–430, with permission.

rate was 25% and did not vary over the 27-year period of the study (186). For patients with single episodes of community-acquired meningitis, the case fatality rate was 25% compared with a 35% case fatality rate for single episodes of nosocomial meningitis. Furthermore, mortality rates from bacterial meningitis are quite significant in the developing world. In one study of 4,100 cases of bacterial meningitis in northeastern Brazil (188), the overall case fatality rate was 33%, with 50% of deaths occurring within 48 hours of hospitalization; mortality by causative microorganism is shown in Table 8.6.

Specific factors present on admission or during hospitalization have been associated with an increased mortality rate in patients with bacterial meningitis (189). In one

TABLE 8.6. *Number of cases and case fatality rates of 3,973 cases of bacterial meningitis in northeastern Brazil, 1973–1982*

Microorganism	Total cases (% fatality)
Streptococcus pneumoniae	670 (59)
Neisseria meningitidis	881 (14)
Haemophilus influenzae	898 (38)
Enterobacteriaceae	136 (86)
Streptococcus or *Staphylococcus* species	61 (48)
Pseudomonas species	13 (85)
Gram-negative bacilli	141 (39)
Gram-negative diplococci	416 (14)
Gram-positive cocci	24 (30)
Culture and gram stain negative	733 (19)

Data modified from Bryan JP, de Silva HR, Tavares A, et al. Etiology and mortality of bacterial meningitis in northeastern Brazil. *Rev Infect Dis* 1990;12:128–135, with permission.

study of 493 episodes of acute bacterial meningitis in patients 16 years of age or more, risk factors for death among those with single episodes of bacterial meningitis were age 60 years or greater, obtunded mental state on admission, and onset of seizures within 24 hours of admission (186). In another study of pneumococcal meningitis in children, increased mortality was associated with a comatose state, respiratory distress, shock, a peripheral white blood cell count of less than 5,000/mm^3, a serum sodium of less than 135 mEq/L, and a CSF protein concentration of 250 mg/dL or greater (190). There was also a trend to increased mortality in children whose CSF white blood cell counts were less than 1,000/mm^3 compared with those with counts of 1,000/mm^3 or greater (25% versus 9%; $P < 0.06$). The presence of coma and shock was also associated with increased mortality in another study of pneumococcal meningitis in children (58). In patients with meningococcal meningitis, a lowered level of consciousness, history of seizures, hemoglobin of less than 11 g/dL, platelet count of less than 100,000/mm^3, and a coagulation index of less than 0.5 were all associated with increased mortality (191). Hemorrhagic diathesis, focal neurologic signs, and age of 60 years or greater were independent predictors of death in patients with meningococcal disease in another study (192), whereas receipt of adequate antimicrobial therapy was associated with a more favorable prognosis. Increased mortality in patients with listeriosis has been associated with the presence of an underlying disease that predisposes to infection with this organism (193).

Morbidity

Even in patients who survive their episode of acute bacterial meningitis, significant complications may ensue. These complications may result from direct involvement of the central nervous system or may be related to the systemic manifestations of infection (Table 8.7). In one prospective study of 50 infants and children recovering from *H. influenzae* type b meningitis (194), 50% were entirely normal, 9% were normal except for behavioral problems, and 28% had significant handicaps (e.g., hearing

TABLE 8.7. *Complications of bacterial meningitis*

Central nervous system	Systemic
Hearing loss	Septic shock
Language disorders	Adult respiratory distress syndrome
Mental retardation	Disseminated intravascular coagulation
Motor abnormalities	Arthritis
Seizures	Inappropriate secretion of antidiuretic hormone
Subdural effusions	Side effects of therapy
Brain or spinal cord infarction	
Cerebral edema	
Hydrocephalus	
Intracerebral hemorrhage	
Ataxia	
Visual disturbances	
Behavioral problems	
Septic intracranial thrombophlebitis	
Brain abscess	

loss, 20%; language disorders or delayed development of language, 15%; mental retardation, 11%; motor abnormalities, 7%; and seizures, 5%). Subsequent studies have noted similar results. In one prospective review of 185 infants and children followed for a mean duration of 8.9 years (195), 37% of children had neurologic abnormalities 1 month after meningitis. Many of these abnormalities resolved within a year, leaving only 14% of children with persistent defects (10% had only sensorineural hearing loss and 4% had multiple neurologic defects); only the children with permanent neurologic deficits were at risk for seizures. In a retrospective review of 97 children with *H. influenzae* type b meningitis, only 14% had persistent neurologic sequelae (196). No differences in intelligence quotient were found in the patients compared with a control group consisting of their age- and sex-matched siblings.

Of all the neurologic complications reported in infants and children with bacterial meningitis, hearing impairment is an important public health problem; early identification is necessary to ensure proper rehabilitation. In a prospective evaluation of hearing impairment in children with acute bacterial meningitis, 10.3% of patients had persistent bilateral or unilateral sensorineural hearing loss (197). This is consistent with reviews of recent literature, in which the incidence for permanent sensorineural hearing impairment of any degree among survivors of bacterial meningitis was 9.6% (198), leading to recommendations that all children recovering from bacterial meningitis be referred for audiologic assessment (149). Furthermore, fleeting hearing loss caused by reversible cochlear dysfunction may also occur in children with bacterial meningitis, noted in 10% of patients in one study (199).

Significant complications of bacterial meningitis have also been reported in adults. In one prospective clinical study of 86 consecutive adult patients with bacterial meningitis, complications developed in 43 patients (200). The major complications in the central nervous system included angiographically documented cerebrovascular involvement (15.1%), brain swelling (14.0%), hydrocephalus (11.6%), and intracerebral hemorrhage (2.3%). Systemic complications included septic shock (11.6%), adult respiratory distress syndrome (3.5%), and disseminated intravascular coagulation (8.1%). The prognosis for adult patients with cerebrovascular complications is unfavorable, associated with significant morbidity and mortality (201).

ADJUNCTIVE THERAPY

Despite the heightened level of suspicion and early recognition of the acute meningitis syndrome, and the availability of effective bactericidal antimicrobial agents, the morbidity and mortality from bacterial meningitis remain unacceptably high (see earlier). These complications may result from the infectious process itself or from the pathophysiologic consequences of bacterial meningitis (e.g., cerebral edema, increased intracranial pressure, altered cerebral blood flow, neuronal injury), which are caused by the subarachnoid space inflammatory response (see Chapter 3). As a consequence of these factors, various adjunctive treatment strategies have been employed in the hope of improving outcome from this disorder (see later). In addition, intensive care monitoring may be required for certain patients with acute bacterial meningitis, as recently recommended by the British Infection Society Working Party (202): those with (a) cardiovascular instability with hypotension not responding promptly to fluid challenges, oliguria persisting for more than 2 or 3 hours, or increasing metabolic acidosis; (b) respiratory instability with an unprotected airway, dyspnea/tachypnea, or hypoxemia; (c) neurologic impairment and/or seizures; and (d) central nervous system depression sufficient to prejudice the airway and its protective reflexes.

Corticosteroids

Adjunctive dexamethasone has been extensively studied in the treatment of patients with bacterial meningitis (1,2). The value of this agent lies in its ability to attenuate the subarachnoid space inflammatory response that results from antimicrobial-induced lysis of meningeal pathogens, thereby reducing many of the pathophysiologic consequences of bacterial meningitis (see Chapter 3). In a recently published meta-analysis of clinical studies published from 1988 to 1996, adjunctive dexamethasone (0.15 mg/kg every 6 hours for 2 to 4 days) was found to be beneficial for *H. influenzae* type b meningitis and, if commenced with or before parenteral antimicrobial therapy, suggested benefit for pneumococcal meningitis in childhood (203). Evidence of clinical benefit was strongest for hearing outcomes. When using dexamethasone, the timing of administration is crucial; administration before or concomitant with the first dose of an antimicrobial agent is optimal for maximal attenuation of the subarachnoid space inflammatory response. The routine use of adjunctive dexamethasone is not recommended in neonates or adults, pending results of ongoing studies. A complete description of the experimental and clinical studies detailing the use of adjunctive corticosteroids is found in Chapter 7.

Reduction of Intracranial Pressure

There is no evidence that intracranial pressure monitoring is necessary in the routine management of patients with bacterial meningitis. However, patients who present with signs of increased intracranial pressure (e.g., altered level of consciousness ranging from drowsiness to coma, dilated poorly reactive or nonreactive pupils, ocular movement disorders, and/or bradycardia and hypertension) and who are stuporous or comatose may benefit from insertion of an intracranial pressure monitoring device (204–206). Intracranial pressures of more than 20 mm Hg are abnormal and should be treated. Furthermore, there is rationale for treating smaller pressure elevations (i.e., above 15 mm Hg) to avoid larger elevations, so-called plateau waves, which are sustained elevations in intracranial pressure that may occur spontaneously or as the result of small increases in cerebral blood volume (i.e., from hypoxia, fever, or intratracheal suctioning); plateau waves can lead to cerebral herniation and irreversible brain stem injury.

Several methods are available to reduce intracranial pressure (204–206). Some simple methods include the following: (a) elevation of the head of the bed to 30° to maximize venous drainage with minimal compromise of cerebral perfusion;

(b) avoidance of turning the head to the side and hyperextending the neck, as these maneuvers may increase jugular venous pressure and block efflux of CSF through the foramen magnum; and (c) avoidance of intratracheal suctioning or endotracheal intubation. The increased intracranial pressure associated with these maneuvers may be reduced by the intravenous injection of lidocaine (1.5 mg/kg).

Hyperventilation (to maintain the $PaCO_2$ between 27 and 30 mm Hg), which causes cerebral vasoconstriction and reduction in cerebral blood volume, may be employed to reduce intracranial pressure (204–206). However, some experts have questioned the routine use of hyperventilation to reduce intracranial pressure in patients with bacterial meningitis (207,208). In infants and children with bacterial meningitis who have initially normal computed tomographic (CT) scans of the head, hyperventilation can safely reduce elevated intracranial pressure because it is unlikely that cerebral blood flow would be reduced to ischemic thresholds. However, in children with cerebral edema on head CT, cerebral blood flow is more likely to be normal or reduced. Although hyperventilation might decrease intracranial pressure, it would do so at the expense of a significant reduction in cerebral blood flow, possibly approaching ischemic thresholds.

Hyperosmolar agents (e.g., mannitol) decrease intracranial pressure by making the intravascular space hyperosmolar to the brain, permitting movement of water from brain tissue into the intravascular compartment. Mannitol has been reported to be effective in reducing intracranial pressure in patients with bacterial meningitis (209). Mannitol can be given as either a bolus injection (1 g/kg over 10 to 15 minutes) or in small, frequent doses (0.25 g/kg every 2 to 3 hours) followed by repeat injections at 3- to 4-hour intervals to maintain the serum osmolality between 315 and 320 mOsm/L (206). Mannitol can induce a rebound increase in intracranial pressure (204,205), although this is an unusual event and should not prevent use of mannitol in the appropriate circumstances. Glycerol, another osmotic dehydrating agent that can be given orally, has been evaluated in a trial of 122 infants and children with bacterial meningitis (210). Patients in this study were randomized to receive adjunctive intravenous dexamethasone, oral glycerol (4.5 g/kg daily; maximum, 180 g/day), dexamethasone plus glycerol, or neither; 7% of the glycerol-treated patients and 19% of those not given glycerol had audiologic or neurologic sequelae ($P = 0.052$). However, further placebo-controlled, blinded studies are required before glycerol can be recommended routinely in patients with bacterial meningitis.

Patients who continue to have elevated intracranial pressures, despite the preceding measures, may be treated with high-dose barbiturate therapy, which decreases cerebral metabolic demands and cerebral blood flow (204–206). Barbiturates can also cause vasoconstriction in normal tissue, thereby shunting blood to ischemic tissue and protecting the brain from ischemic insult. Pentobarbital is administered in an initial dose of 5 to 10 mg/kg at a rate of 1 mg/kg/min, followed by a dose of 1 to 3 mg/kg/hr. During administration of pentobarbital, the patient is monitored to measure decreases in intracranial pressure (to <20 mm Hg), or the dose can be titrated to development of a burst-suppression pattern on the electroencephalogram. These are the initial goals of therapy rather than measurement of specific drug concentrations, which are often unreliable indicators of effectiveness or toxicity. Cardiac parameters also need to be monitored (by placement of a Swan-Ganz catheter) because of the risk of cardiac toxicity (e.g., decreased cardiac output, decreased contractile force, arrhythmias) with high-dose barbiturate therapy. This mode of treatment for meningitis and elevated intracranial pressure is of unproven benefit, however, and must be considered experimental. Furthermore, some experts have suggested that barbiturate coma should not be used routinely in children in the management of comatose children, irrespective of the etiology (211).

Anticonvulsants

Seizures occur in approximately 30% to 40% of children and 20% to 30% of adults with acute bacterial meningitis (206,208,209). Seizures must be managed quickly and aggressively to avoid permanent anoxic ischemic changes. Status epilepticus that is continuous for 90 minutes or more can cause permanent neurologic injury. For early termination of seizure activity, a short-acting anticonvulsant with a rapid onset of action is recommended (e.g., lorazepam given intravenously at a dose of 1 to 4 mg in adults and as an initial dose of 0.05 mg/kg in children; or diazepam at a dose of 0.25 to 0.4 mg/kg at a rate of 1 to 2 mg/min, maximum dose of 10 mg). This is followed by administration of a long-acting anticonvulsant such as phenytoin. If phenytoin fails to control the seizure activity, the patient should be intubated, mechanically ventilated, and treated with phenobarbital.

Fluid Management

The initial fluid management in patients with acute bacterial meningitis is directed toward treatment of dehydration and volume depletion, which occur as a result of decreased oral intake, vomiting, and/or diarrhea (208). Increased fluids are necessary to restore systemic and cerebral perfusion. Patients should be kept euvolemic and not fluid restricted in an attempt to reduce cerebral edema (202). In one prospective, randomized trial of fluid restriction versus maintenance fluids in acute meningitis (212), children who had a reduction in extracellular water of more than 10% induced by fluid restriction for the first 48 hours had a higher mortality rate than those who received normal maintenance fluids ($P < 0.05$).

More than 50% of children with bacterial meningitis are hyponatremic (serum sodium <135 mEq/L) early in the course of illness, which may be attributed to the syndrome of inappropriate secretion of antidiuretic hormone (SIADH) (206,209,213). Estimates of the frequency of SIADH as the etiology of the hyponatremia range from 7% to 88%. This discrepancy partly reflects differences in the definition of SIADH. The degree of hyponatremia correlates with the presence of seizures, severity of acute disease, and neurodevelopmental outcomes. These findings have also been linked to the high incidence of cerebral edema in patients who die from bacterial meningitis; SIADH leads to water retention, which exacerbates cerebral swelling. Restriction of fluids to correct the hyponatremia is important, although rigid adherence to fluid restriction in children with bacterial meningitis is no longer recommended because of the adverse effects of hypovolemia on cerebral perfusion pressure (see earlier). In hyponatremic patients with no evidence of dehydration or shock, fluid administration should be limited to about 800 to 1,000 mL/m^2/day with a solution containing one-fourth to one-half normal saline and potassium (20 to 40 mEq/L) in 5% dextrose. Once the serum sodium is greater than 135 mEq/L, the fluid can be liberalized gradually over 36 to 48 hours to maintenance rates (1,500 to 1,700 mL/m^2/day).

Surgery

Surgical intervention may be required in some patients with bacterial meningitis. Patients who have suffered a basilar skull fracture with CSF leak may have persistent dural defects that can lead to recurrent episodes of bacterial meningitis (214). Many leaks will cease spontaneously, but surgery is indicated for leaks that persist for several weeks or in patients who present with delayed or recurrent infection. Surgery is not indicated in the acute phase (before 7 days) of leakage. There is no difference in outcome when patients with acutely repaired leaks are compared with those whose leaks stop spontaneously within 7 days. Surgical intervention may also be required in patients who develop recurrent meningitis from congenital or acquired cranial defects and dermal sinuses (215).

Patients with subdural effusions may also require further evaluation (208,216). Although the majority of patients with subdural effusions require no specific treatment because spontaneous resolution will occur, some subdural effusions may enlarge dramatically or become infected, causing local cerebral symptoms. In these patients, fluid should be obtained for analysis (including Gram stain and culture), and temporary drainage should be considered.

Cerebrospinal Fluid Shunt Infections

Numerous methods of treating CSF shunt infections have been reported, although no randomized, prospective studies have been performed (171,215). After obtaining CSF for analysis, antimicrobial therapy should be initiated prior to culture results if meningeal inflammation is present (see Chapter 7). Therapy can then be modified based on culture results (Table 8.1). Occasionally, direct instillation of antimicrobial agents into the ventricles (i.e., through an external ventriculostomy or shunt reservoir) is necessary in patients with infections that are difficult to eradicate or when the patient is unable to undergo the surgical components of therapy (see later). Vancomycin has been directly instilled into the ventricles to overcome the relatively meager CSF penetration after intravenous administration; daily dosages have ranged from 4 to 10 mg. Gentamicin (1 to 2 mg daily for infants and children, and 4 to 8 mg daily for adults) can be utilized, always in combination with a parenteral agent (e.g., a β-lactam), for infections caused by susceptible gram-negative organisms. Empiric dosing should initially be used, with subsequent dosage adjustments based on CSF antimicrobial concentrations.

In addition, patients with CSF shunt infections should undergo removal of all components of the infected shunt at the beginning of antimicrobial therapy, with an external ventriculostomy placed to clear the ventriculitis and monitor CSF findings (171). The ability of many organisms to adhere to the prostheses and survive antimicrobial therapy precludes optimal treatment *in situ*. Furthermore, the propensity for the entire shunt to become contaminated when one portion becomes infected argues against partial revisions. With externalization, treatment success is usually greater than 90%, compared with only 75% when antimicrobial therapy is combined with shunt removal and immediate shunt replacement. Following an antimicrobial hiatus (e.g., approximately 3 days) to verify clearance of the infection, a new shunt can be placed (171).

REFERENCES

1. Tunkel AR, Scheld WM. Acute bacterial meningitis. *Lancet* 1995;346:1675–1680.
2. Tunkel AR, Scheld WM. Acute meningitis. In: Mandell GL, Bennett JE, Dolin R, eds. *Principles and practice of infectious diseases*, 5th ed. Philadelphia: Churchill-Livingstone, 1999:959–997.
3. National Committee for Clinical Laboratory Standards. *Methods for dilution antimicrobial susceptibility tests for bacteria that grow aerobically: approved standard,* 4th ed. NCCLS Document M7-A4. Wayne, PA: National Committee for Clinical Laboratory Standards, 1997.
4. Appelbaum PC. Antimicrobial resistance in *Streptococcus pneumoniae*: an overview. *Clin Infect Dis* 1992;15:77–83.
5. Austrian R. Confronting drug-resistant pneumococci. *Ann Intern Med* 1994;121:807–809.
6. Paris MM, Ramilo O, McCracken GH Jr. Management of meningitis caused by penicillin-resistant *Streptococcus pneumoniae*. *Antimicrob Agents Chemother* 1995;39:2171–2175.
7. Campbell GD, Silberman R. Drug-resistant *Streptococcus pneumoniae*. *Clin Infect Dis* 1998;26: 1188–1195.
8. Hofmann J, Cetron MS, Farley MM, et al. The prevalence of drug-resistant *Streptococcus pneumoniae* in Atlanta. *N Engl J Med* 1995;333:481–486.
9. Jernigan DB, Cetron MS, Breiman RF. Minimizing the impact of drug-resistant *Streptococcus pneumoniae* (DRSP). A strategy from the DRSP working group. *JAMA* 1996;275:206–209.
10. Thornsberry C, Hickey ML, Kahn J, et al. Surveillance of antimicrobial resistance among respiratory tract pathogens in the United States, 1997–1998. *Drugs* 1999;58[Suppl 2]:361–363.
11. Centers for Disease Control and Prevention. Geographic variation in penicillin resistance in *Streptococcus pneumoniae*—selected sites, United States, 1997. *MMWR* 1997;48:656–661.
12. Zhanel GG, Karlowsky JA, Palatnick L, et al. Prevalence of antimicrobial resistance in respiratory tract isolates of *Streptococcus pneumoniae*: results of a Canadian national surveillance study. *Antimicrob Agents Chemother* 1999;43:2504–2509.
13. Ball P. Therapy for pneumococcal infections at the millennium: doubts and certainties. *Am J Med* 1999;28:77S–85S.
14. Jacobs MR. Drug-resistant *Streptococcus pneumoniae*: rational antibiotic choices. *Am J Med* 1999;106:19S–25S.
15. Song J, Lee NY, Ichiyama S, et al. Spread of *Streptococcus pneumoniae* in Asian countries: Asian Network for Surveillance of Resistant Pathogens (ANSORP) Study. *Clin Infect Dis* 1999;28: 1206–1211.
16. Invasive Bacterial Infection Surveillance (IBIS) Group, International Clinical Epidemiology Network (INCLEN). Prospective multicentre hospital surveillance of *Streptococcus pneumoniae* in India. *Lancet* 1999;353:1216–1221.
17. Rocha P, Baleeiro C, Tunkel AR. Impact of antimicrobial resistance on the treatment of invasive pneumococcal infections. *Clin Infect Dis Rep* 2000;2:399–408.
18. Butler JC, Cetron MS. Pneumococcal drug resistance: the new "special enemy of old age." *Clin Infect Dis* 1999;28:730–735.
19. Fung CP, Hu BS, Lee SC, et al. Antimicrobial resistance of *Streptococcus pneumoniae* isolated in Taiwan: an island-wide surveillance study between 1996 and 1997. *J Antimicrob Chemother* 2000;45:49–55.

20. Clavo-Sanchez AJ, Giron-Gonzalez JA, Lopez-Prieto D, et al. Multivariate analysis of risk factors for infection due to penicillin-resistant and multidrug-resistant *Streptococcus pneumoniae*: a multicenter study. *Clin Infect Dis* 1997;24:1052–1059.
21. Yagupsky P, Porat N, Fraser D, et al. Acquisition, carriage, and transmission of pneumococci with decreased antibiotic susceptibility in young children attending a day care facility in southern Israel. *J Infect Dis* 1998;177:1003–1012.
22. Guillemot D, Carbon C, Balkau B, et al. Low dosage and long treatment duration of β-lactam: risk factors for carriage of penicillin-resistant *Streptococcus pneumoniae*. *JAMA* 1998;279:365–370.
23. Ko AI, Reis JN, Coppola SJ, et al. Clonally related penicillin–nonsusceptible *Streptococcus pneumoniae* serotype 14 from cases of meningitis in Salvador, Brazil. *Clin Infect Dis* 2000;30:78–86.
24. Goldstein FW. Penicillin-resistant *Streptococcus pneumoniae*: selection by both β-lactam and non-β-lactam antibiotics. *J Antimicrob Chemother* 1999;44:141–144.
25. Tomasz A. New faces of an old pathogen: emergence and spread of multidrug-resistant *Streptococcus pneumoniae*. *Am J Med* 1999;107:55S–62S.
26. McDougal LK, Facklam R, Reeves M, et al. Analysis of multiply antimicrobial-resistant isolates of *Streptococcus pneumoniae* from the United States. *Antimicrob Agents Chemother* 1992;36: 2176–2184.
27. Kaplan SL, Mason EO. Management of infections due to antibiotic-resistant *Streptococcus pneumoniae*. *Clin Microbiol Rev* 1998;11:628–644.
28. American Academy of Pediatrics, Committee on Infectious Diseases. Therapy for children with invasive pneumococcal infections. *Pediatrics* 1997;99:289–299.
29. Friedland IR, Klugman KP. Failure of chloramphenicol therapy in penicillin-resistant pneumococcal meningitis. *Lancet* 1992;339:405–408.
30. Haas DW, Stratton CW, Griffin JP, et al. Diminished activity of ceftizoxime in comparison to cefotaxime and ceftriaxone against *Streptococcus pneumoniae*. *Clin Infect Dis* 1995;20:671–676.
31. Waites KB, Rivers T. Bactericidal activities of ceftizoxime and cefotaxime against *Streptococcus pneumoniae*. *Antimicrob Agents Chemother* 1998;42:1869–1870.
32. Sloas MM, Barrett FF, Chesney PJ, et al. Cephalosporin treatment failure in penicillin- and cephalosporin-resistant *Streptococcus pneumoniae* meningitis. *Pediatr Infect Dis J* 1992;11:622–626.
33. John CC. Treatment failure with use of a third-generation cephalosporin for penicillin-resistant pneumococcal meningitis: case report and review. *Clin Infect Dis* 1994;18:188–193.
34. Catalan MJ, Fernandez JM, Vazquez A, et al. Failure of cefotaxime in the treatment of meningitis due to relatively resistant *Streptococcus pneumoniae*. *Clin Infect Dis* 1994;18:766–769.
35. Tan TQ, Schutze GE, Mason EO Jr, et al. Antibiotic therapy and acute outcome of meningitis due to *Streptococcus pneumoniae* considered intermediately susceptible to broad-spectrum cephalosporins. *Antimicrob Agents Chemother* 1994;38:918–923.
36. Guibert M, Chahime H, Petit J, et al. Failure of cefotaxime treatment in two children with meningitis caused by highly penicillin-resistant *Streptococcus pneumoniae*. *Acta Paediatr* 1995;84:831–833.
37. Ruiz-Irastorza GR, Garea C, Alonso JJ, et al. Failure of cefotaxime treatment in a patient with penicillin-resistant pneumococcal meningitis and confirmation of nosocomial spread by random amplified polymorphic DNA analysis. *Clin Infect Dis* 1995;21:234–235.
38. Florez C, Silva G, Martin E. Cefotaxime failure in pneumococcal meningitis caused by a susceptible isolate. *Pediatr Infect Dis J* 1996;15:723–724.
39. Pacheco TR, Cooper CK, Hardy DJ, et al. Failure of cefotaxime in an adult with *Streptococcus pneumoniae* meningitis. *Am J Med* 1997;102:303–305.
40. Fitoussi F, Doit C, Benali K, et al. Comparative *in vitro* killing activities of meropenem, imipenem, ceftriaxone and ceftriaxone plus vancomycin at clinically achievable cerebrospinal fluid concentrations against penicillin-resistant *Streptococcus pneumoniae* isolates from children with meningitis. *Antimicrob Agents Chemother* 1998;42:942–944.
41. Viladrich PF, Cabellos C, Pallares R, et al. High doses of cefotaxime in treatment of adult meningitis due to *Streptococcus pneumoniae* with decreased susceptibilities to broad-spectrum cephalosporins. *Antimicrob Agents Chemother* 1996;40:218–220.
42. Friedland IR, Klugman KP. Cerebrospinal fluid bactericidal activity against cephalosporin-resistant *Streptococcus pneumoniae* in children with meningitis treated with high-dose cefotaxime. *Antimicrob Agents Chemother* 1997;41:1888–1891.
43. Cabellos C, Martinez-Lacasa J, Tubau F, et al. Evaluation of combined ceftriaxone and dexamethasone therapy in experimental cephalosporin-resistant pneumococcal meningitis. *J Antimicrob Chemother* 2000;45:315–320.

44. Gerber CM, Cottagnoud M, Neftel K, et al. Evaluation of cefepime alone and in combination with vancomycin against penicillin-resistant pneumococci in the rabbit meningitis model and *in vitro*. *J Antimicrob Chemother* 2000;45:63–68.
45. Viladrich PF, Gudiol F, Linares J, et al. Evaluation of vancomycin for therapy of adult pneumococcal meningitis. *Antimicrob Agents Chemother* 1991;35:2467–2472.
46. Ahmed A. A critical evaluation of vancomycin for treatment of bacterial meningitis. *Pediatr Infect Dis J* 1997;16:895–903.
47. Paris MM, Hickey SM, Uscher MI, et al. Effect of dexamethasone on therapy of experimental penicillin- and cephalosporin-resistant pneumococcal meningitis. *Antimicrob Agents Chemother* 1994;38:1320–1324.
48. Cabellos C, Martinez-Lacasa J, Martos A, et al. Influence of dexamethasone on efficacy of ceftriaxone and vancomycin therapy in experimental pneumococcal meningitis. *Antimicrob Agents Chemother* 1995;39:2158–2160.
49. Novak R, Henriques B, Charpentier E, et al. Emergence of vancomycin tolerance in *Streptococcus pneumoniae*. *Nature* 1999;399:590–593.
50. Gilmore MS, Hoch JA. A vancomycin surprise. *Nature* 1999;399:524–527.
51. McCullers JA, English BK, Novak R. Isolation and characterization of vancomycin-tolerant *Streptococcus pneumoniae* from the cerebrospinal fluid of a patient who developed recrudescent meningitis. *J Infect Dis* 2000;181:369–373.
52. Friedland IR, Paris M, Ehrett S, et al. Evaluation of antimicrobial regimens for treatment of experimental penicillin- and cephalosporin-resistant pneumococcal meningitis. *Antimicrob Agents Chemother* 1993;37:1630–1636.
53. Klugman KP, Friedland IR, Bradley JS. Bactericidal activity against cephalosporin-resistant *Streptococcus pneumoniae* in cerebrospinal fluid of children with acute bacterial meningitis. *Antimicrob Agents Chemother* 1995;39:1988–1992.
54. Doit C, Barre J, Cohen R, et al. Bactericidal activity against intermediately cephalosporin-resistant *Streptococcus pneumoniae* in cerebrospinal fluid of children with bacterial meningitis treated with high doses of cefotaxime and vancomycin. *Antimicrob Agents Chemother* 1997;41:2050–2052.
55. Nau R, Wellmer A, Soto A, et al. Rifampin reduces early mortality in experimental *Streptococcus pneumoniae* meningitis. *J Infect Dis* 1999;179:1557–1560.
56. Fitoussi F, Doit C, Geslin P, et al. Killing activities of trovafloxacin alone and in combination with β-lactam agents, rifampin, or vancomycin against *Streptococcus pneumoniae* isolates with various susceptibilities to extended-spectrum cephalosporins at concentrations clinically achievable in cerebrospinal fluid. *Antimicrob Agents Chemother* 1999;43:2372–2375.
57. Stanek RJ, Mufson MA. A 20-year epidemiological study of pneumococcal meningitis. *Clin Infect Dis* 1999;28:1265–1272.
58. Arditi M, Mason EO Jr, Bradley JS, et al. Three-year multicenter surveillance of pneumococcal meningitis in children: clinical characteristics, and outcome related to penicillin susceptibility and dexamethasone use. *Pediatrics* 1998;102:1087–1097.
59. Fiore AE, Moroney JF, Farley MM, et al. Clinical outcomes of meningitis caused by *Streptococcus pneumoniae* in the era of antibiotic resistance. *Clin Infect Dis* 2000;30:71–77.
60. Aseni F, Otero MC, Perez-Tamarit D, et al. Risk/benefit in the treatment of children with imipenem-cilastatin for meningitis caused by penicillin-resistant pneumococcus. *J Chemother* 1993;5:133–134.
61. Aseni F, Perez-Tamarit D, Otero MC, et al. Imipenem-cilastatin therapy in a child with meningitis caused by a multiply resistant pneumococcus. *Pediatr Infect Dis J* 1989;8:895.
62. Wong VK, Wright HT Jr, Ross LA, et al. Imipenem/cilastatin treatment of bacterial meningitis in children. *Pediatr Infect Dis J* 1991;10:122–125.
63. Bradley JS. Meropenem: a new, extremely broad spectrum beta-lactam antibiotic for serious infections in pediatrics. *Pediatr Infect Dis J* 1997;16:263–268.
64. Schmutzhard E, Williams KJ, Vukmirovits G, et al. A randomised comparison of meropenem with cefotaxime or ceftriaxone for the treatment of bacterial meningitis in adults. *J Antimicrob Chemother* 1995;36:85–97.
65. Bradley JS, Scheld WM. The challenge of penicillin-resistant *Streptococcus pneumoniae* meningitis: current antibiotic therapy in the 1990s. *Clin Infect Dis* 1997;24[Suppl 2]:S213–S221.
66. Odio CM, Puig JR, Feris JM, et al. Prospective, randomized, investigator-blinded study of the efficacy and safety of meropenem vs. cefotaxime therapy in bacterial meningitis in children. *Pediatr Infect Dis J* 1999;18:581–590.

67. John CC, Aouad G, Berman B, et al. Successful meropenem treatment of multiply resistant pneumococcal meningitis. *Pediatr Infect Dis J* 1997;16:1009–1011.
68. Norrby AR. Neurotoxicity of carbapenem antibiotics: consequences for their use in bacterial meningitis. *J Antimicrob Chemother* 2000;45:5–7.
69. Cutler NR, Vincent J, Jhee SS, et al. Penetration of trovafloxacin into cerebrospinal fluid in humans following intravenous infusion of alatrofloxacin. *Antimicrob Agents Chemother* 1997;41:1298–1300.
70. Kim YS, Liu Q, Chow LL, et al. Trovafloxacin in treatment of rabbits with experimental meningitis caused by high-level penicillin-resistant *Streptococcus pneumoniae*. *Antimicrob Agents Chemother* 1997;41:1186–1189.
71. Rodoni D, Hanni F, Gerber CM, et al. Trovafloxacin in combination with vancomycin against penicillin-resistant pneumococci in the rabbit meningitis model. *Antimicrob Agents Chemother* 1999;43:963–965.
72. Tarasi A, Capone A, Tarasi D, et al. Comparative *in vitro* activity of moxifloxacin, penicillin, ceftriaxone and ciprofloxacin against pneumococci isolated from meningitis. *J Antimicrob Chemother* 1999;43:833–835.
73. Schmidt H, Dalhoff A, Stuertz K, et al. Moxifloxacin in the therapy of experimental pneumococcal meningitis. *Antimicrob Agents Chemother* 1998;42:1397–1401.
74. Ostergaard C, Sorensen TK, Knudsen JD, et al. Evaluation of moxifloxacin, a new 8-methoxyquinolone, for treatment of meningitis caused by a penicillin-resistant *Pneumococcus* in rabbits. *Antimicrob Agents Chemother* 1998;42:1706–1712.
75. Odland BA, Jones RN, Verhoef J, et al. Antimicrobial activity of gatifloxacin (AM-1155, CG5501), and four other fluoroquinolones tested against 2,284 recent clinical strains of *Streptococcus pneumoniae* from Europe, Latin America, Canada, and the United States. *Diag Microbiol Infect Dis* 1999;34:315–320.
76. Lustar I, Friedland IR, Wubbel L, et al. Pharmacodynamics of gatifloxacin in cerebrospinal fluid in experimental cephalosporin-resistant pneumococcal meningitis. *Antimicrob Agents Chemother* 1998;42:2650–2655.
77. Heaton VJ, Goldsmith CE, Ambler JE, et al. Activity of gemifloxacin against penicillin- and ciprofloxacin-resistant *Streptococcus pneumoniae* displaying topoisomerase- and efflux-mediated resistance mechanisms. *Antimicrob Agents Chemother* 1999;43:2998–3000.
78. Smirnov A, Wellmer A, Gerber J, et al. Gemifloxacin is effective in experimental pneumococcal meningitis. *Antimicrob Agents Chemother* 2000;44:767–770.
79. Chen DK, McGeer A, de Azavedo JC, et al. Decreased susceptibility of *Streptococcus pneumoniae* to fluoroquinolones in Canada. *N Engl J Med* 1999;341:233–239.
80. Wortmann GW, Bennett SP. Fatal meningitis due to levofloxacin-resistant *Streptococcus pneumoniae*. *Clin Infect Dis* 1999;29:1599–1600.
81. Campos J, Mendelman PN, Sako MU, et al. Detection of relatively penicillin G-resistant *Neisseria meningitidis* by disk susceptibility testing. *Antimicrob Agents Chemother* 1987;31:1478–1482.
82. van Esso D, Fontanals D, Uriz S, et al. *Neisseria meningitidis* with decreased susceptibility to penicillin. *Pediatr Infect Dis* 1987;6:438–439.
83. Saez-Nieto JA, Lujan R, Berron S, et al. Epidemiology and molecular basis of penicillin-resistant *Neisseria meningitidis* in Spain: a 5-year history (1985–1989). *Clin Infect Dis* 1992;14:394–402.
84. Campos J, Trujillo G, Seuba T, et al. Discriminative criteria for *Neisseria meningitidis* isolates that are moderately susceptible to penicillin and ampicillin. *Antimicrob Agents Chemother* 1992;36:1028–1031.
85. Mendelman PM, Campos J, Chaffin DO, et al. Relatively penicillin G resistance in *Neisseria meningitidis* and reduced affinity of penicillin-binding protein 3. *Antimicrob Agents Chemother* 1988;32:706–709.
86. Oppenheim BA. Antibiotic resistance in *Neisseria meningitidis*. *Clin Infect Dis* 1997;24[Suppl 1]:S98–S101.
87. van Deuren M, Brandtzaeg P, van der Meer JWM. Update on meningococcal disease with emphasis on pathogenesis and clinical management. *Clin Microbiol Rev* 2000;13:144–166.
88. Jackson LA, Tenover FC, Baker C, et al. Prevalence of *Neisseria meningitidis* relatively resistant to penicillin in the United States, 1991. *J Infect Dis* 1994;169:438–441.
89. Buck GE, Adams M. Meningococcus with reduced susceptibility to penicillin isolated in the United States. *Pediatr Infect Dis J* 1994;13:156–157.
90. Woods CR, Smith AL, Wasilauskas BL, et al. Invasive disease caused by *Neisseria meningitidis* relatively resistant to penicillin in North Carolina. *J Infect Dis* 1994;170:453–456.

91. Rosenstein NE, Stocker SA, Popovic T, et al. Antimicrobial resistance of *Neisseria meningitidis* in the United States, 1997. *Clin Infect Dis* 2000;30:212–213.
92. Casado-Flores J, Osona B, Comingo P, et al. Meningococcal meningitis during penicillin therapy for meningococcemia. *Clin Infect Dis* 1997;25:1479.
93. Goldani LZ. Inducement of *Neisseria meningitidis* resistance to ampicillin and penicillin in a patient with meningococcemia treated with high doses of ampicillin. *Clin Infect Dis* 1998;26:772.
94. Cubells CL, Garcia JJG, Martinez JR, et al. Clinical data in children with meningococcal meningitis in a Spanish hospital. *Acta Paediatr* 1997;86:26–29.
95. Shaw WV. Chloramphenicol resistance in meningococci. *N Engl J Med* 1998;339:917–918.
96. Galimand M, Gerbaud G, Guibourdenche M, et al. High-level chloramphenicol resistance in *Neisseria meningitidis*. *N Engl J Med* 1998;339:868–874.
97. Hopkins S, Williams D, Dunne M, et al. A randomized, controlled trial of oral or IV trovafloxacin vs. ceftriaxone in the treatment of epidemic meningococcal meningitis. In: *Program and abstracts of the 36th Interscience Conference on Antimicrobial Agents and Chemotherapy*. Washington, DC: American Society for Microbiology, 1996.
98. Van de Beek D, Hensen EF, Spanjaard L, et al. Meropenem susceptibility of *Neisseria meningitidis* and *Streptococcus pneumoniae* from meningitis patients in The Netherlands. *J Antimicrob Chemother* 1997;40:895–897.
99. Abadi FJ, Yakuby DE, Pennington TH. *In vitro* activities of meropenem and other antimicrobial agents against British meningococcal isolates. *Chemotherapy* 1999;45:253–257.
100. Saez-Llorens X, McCracken GH Jr. Antimicrobial and anti-inflammatory treatment of bacterial meningitis. *Infect Dis Clin North Am* 1999;13:619–636.
101. Dunne DW, Quagliarello V. Group B streptococcal meningitis in adults. *Medicine (Baltimore)* 1993;72:1–10.
102. Domingo P, Barquet N, Alvarez M, et al. Group B streptococcal meningitis in adults: report of twelve cases and review. *Clin Infect Dis* 1997;25:1180–1187.
103. Gellin BG, Broome CV. Listeriosis. *JAMA* 1989;261:1313–1320.
104. Berenguer J, Solera J, Dolores-Diaz M, et al. Listeriosis in patients infected with human immunodeficiency virus. *Rev Infect Dis* 1991;13:115–119.
105. Cherubin CE, Appleman MD, Heseltime PNR, et al. Epidemiological spectrum and current treatment of listeriosis. *Rev Infect Dis* 1991;13:1108–1114.
106. Lorber B. Listeriosis. *Clin Infect Dis* 1997;24:1–11.
107. Myolanakis E, Hohmann EL, Calderwood SB. Central nervous system infection with *Listeria monocytogenes*. 33 years' experience at a general hospital and review of 776 episodes from the literature. *Medicine (Baltimore)* 1998;77:313–336.
108. Tsakris A, Papa A, Douboyas J, et al. Neonatal meningitis due to multi-resistant *Listeria monocytogenes*. *J Antimicrob Chemother* 1997;39:553–554.
109. Levitz RE, Quintiliani R. Trimethoprim-sulfamethoxazole for bacterial meningitis. *Ann Intern Med* 1984;100:881–890.
110. Spitzer PG, Hammer SM, Karchmer AW. Treatment of *Listeria monocytogenes* infection with trimethoprim-sulfamethoxazole: case report and review of the literature. *Rev Infect Dis* 1986;8:427–430.
111. Friedrich LV, White RL, Reboli AC. Pharmacodynamics of trimethoprim-sulfamethoxazole in *Listeria* meningitis: a case report. *Pharmacotherapy* 1990;10:301–304.
112. Hof M, Nichterlein T, Kretschmar M. Management of listeriosis. *Clin Microbiol Rev* 1997;10:345–357.
113. Merle-Melet M, Dossou-Gbete L, Maurer P, et al. Is amoxicillin-cotrimoxazole the most appropriate antibiotic regimen for *Listeria* meningoencephalitis? Review of 22 cases and the literature. *J Infect* 1996;33:79–85.
114. Cherubin CE, Marr JS, Sierra MF, et al. *Listeria* and gram-negative bacillary meningitis in New York City, 1972–1979: frequent causes of meningitis in adults. *Am J Med* 1981;71:199–209.
115. Stamm AM, Dismukes WE, Simmons BP, et al. Listeriosis in renal transplant recipients: report of an outbreak and review of 102 cases. *Rev Infect Dis* 1982;4:665–682.
116. Yu V, Miller WP, Wing EJ, et al. Disseminated listeriosis presenting as acute hepatitis: case reports and review of hepatic involvement in listeriosis. *Am J Med* 1982;262:1026–1028.
117. Blatt SP, Zajac RA. Treatment of *Listeria* bacteremia with vancomycin. *Rev Infect Dis* 1991;13:181–182.
118. Baldassarre JS, Ingerman MJ, Nansteel J, et al. Development of *Listeria* meningitis during vancomycin therapy: a case report. *J Infect Dis* 1991;164:221–222.

119. Richards SJ, Lambert CM, Scott AC. Recurrent *Listeria monocytogenes* meningitis treated with intraventricular vancomycin. *J Antimicrob Chemother* 1992;29:351–353.
120. Scheld WM. Evaluation of rifampin and other antibiotics against *Listeria monocytogenes in vitro* and *in vivo*. *Rev Infect Dis* 1983;5:S593–S599.
121. Nairn K, Shepard G, Edwards JR. Evidence of meropenem in experimental meningitis. *J Antimicrob Chemother* 1995;36:73–84.
122. Weston VC, Punt J, Vloebeghs M, et al. *Listeria monocytogenes* meningitis in a penicillin-allergic paediatric renal transplant patient. *J Infect* 1998;37:77–78.
123. Facinelli B, Magi G, Prenna M, et al. *In vitro* extracellular and intracellular activity of two newer and two earlier fluoroquinolones against *Listeria monocytogenes*. *Eur J Clin Microbiol Infect Dis* 1997;16:827–833.
124. Michelet C, Leib SL, Bentue-Ferrer D, et al. Comparative efficacies of antibiotics in a rat model of meningoencephalitis due to *Listeria monocytogenes*. *Antimicrob Agents Chemother* 1999;43:1651–1656.
125. Schlech WF III, Ward JI, Band JD, et al. Bacterial meningitis in the United States,1978 through 1981. The national bacterial meningitis surveillance study. *JAMA* 1985;253:1749–1754.
126. Wenger JD, Hightower AW, Facklam RR, et al. Bacterial meningitis in the United States, 1986: report of a multistate surveillance study. *J Infect Dis* 1990;162:1316–1323.
127. Campos J, Garcia-Tornel S, Sanfeliu I. Susceptibility studies of multiply resistant *Haemophilus influenzae* isolated from pediatric patients and contacts. *Antimicrob Agents Chemother* 1984;25: 706–709.
128. Campos J, Garcia-Tornel S, Gairi JM, et al. Multiply resistant *Haemophilus influenzae* type b causing meningitis: comparative clinical and laboratory study. *J Pediatr* 1986;108:897–902.
129. Givner LB, Abramson JS, Wasilauskas B. Meningitis due to *Haemophilus influenzae* type b resistant to ampicillin and chloramphenicol. *Rev Infect Dis* 1989;11:329–334.
130. Peltola J, Anttila M, Renkonen OV, et al. Randomised comparison of chloramphenicol, ampicillin, cefotaxime, and ceftriaxone for childhood bacterial meningitis. *Lancet* 1989;1:1281–1287.
131. McCracken GH Jr. Current management of bacterial meningitis in infants and children. *Pediatr Infect Dis J* 1992;11:169–174.
132. Marks WA, Stutman HR, Marks MI, et al. Cefuroxime versus ampicillin plus chloramphenicol in childhood bacterial meningitis: a multicenter randomized controlled trial. *J Pediatr* 1986;109: 123–130.
133. Del Rio M, Chrane D, Shelton S, et al. Ceftriaxone versus ampicillin and chloramphenicol for treatment of bacterial meningitis in children. *Lancet* 1983;1:1241–1244.
134. Jacobs RF, Wells TG, Steele RW, et al. A prospective randomized comparison of cefotaxime vs. ampicillin and chloramphenicol for bacterial meningitis in children. *J Pediatr* 1985;107: 129–133.
135. Lebel MH, Hoyt MJ, McCracken GH Jr. Comparative efficacy of ceftriaxone and cefuroxime for treatment of bacterial meningitis. *J Pediatr* 1989;114:1049–1054.
136. Schaad UB, Suter S, Gianella-Borradori A, et al. A comparison of ceftriaxone and cefuroxime for the treatment of bacterial meningitis in children. *N Engl J Med* 1990;322:141–147.
137. Arditi M, Herold BC, Yogev R. Cefuroxime treatment failure and *Haemophilus influenzae* meningitis: case report and review of the literature. *Pediatrics* 1989;84:132–135.
138. Mendelman PM, Chaffin DO, Krilov LR, et al. Cefuroxime treatment failure of nontypable *Haemophilus influenzae* meningitis associated with alteration of penicillin-binding proteins. *J Infect Dis* 1990;162:1118–1123.
139. Foweraker JE, Millar MR, Smith I. Meningitis caused by *Haemophilus influenzae* type b infection after epiglottitis. *Br Med J* 1989;298:1003–1004.
140. Vallejo JG, Kaplan SL, Mason EO Jr. Treatment of meningitis and other infections due to ampicillin-resistant *Haemophilus influenzae* type b in children. *Rev Infect Dis* 1991;13:197–200.
141. American Academy of Pediatrics, Committee on Infectious Diseases. Treatment of bacterial meningitis. *Pediatrics* 1988;81:904–907.
142. Hatch DL, Overturf GD. Delayed cerebrospinal fluid sterilization in infants with *Haemophilus influenzae* type b meningitis. *J Infect Dis* 1989;160:711–715.
143. Jorgensen JH. Update on mechanisms and prevalence of antimicrobial resistance in *Haemophilus influenzae*. *Clin Infect Dis* 1992;14:1119–1123.
144. Saez-Llorens X, Castano E, Garcia R, et al. Prospective randomized comparison of cefepime and cefotaxime for treatment of bacterial meningitis in infants and children. *Antimicrob Agents Chemother* 1995;39:937–940.

145. Cherubin CE, Eng RHK, Norrby R, et al. Penetration of newer cephalosporins into cerebrospinal fluid. *Rev Infect Dis* 1989;11:526–548.
146. Kaplan SL, Patrick CC. Cefotaxime and aminoglycoside treatment of meningitis caused by gram-negative enteric organisms. *Pediatr Infect Dis J* 1990;9:810–814.
147. Cherubin CE, Corrado ML, Nair SR, et al. Treatment of gram-negative bacillary meningitis: role of the new cephalosporin antibiotics. *Rev Infect Dis* 1982;4:S453–S464.
148. Landesman SH, Corrado ML, Shah PM, et al. Past and current roles of cephalosporin antibiotics in treatment of meningitis: Emphasis on use in gram-negative bacillary meningitis. *Am J Med* 1981;71:693–703.
149. Feigin RD, McCracken GH Jr, Klein JO. Diagnosis and management of meningitis. *Pediatr Infect Dis J* 1992;11:785–814.
150. Fong IW, Tomkins KB. Review of *Pseudomonas aeruginosa* meningitis with special emphasis on treatment with ceftazidime. *Rev Infect Dis* 1985;7:604–612.
151. Rodriguez WJ, Khan WN, Cocchetto DM, et al. Treatment of *Pseudomonas* meningitis with ceftazidime with or without concurrent therapy. *Pediatr Infect Dis J* 1990;9:83–87.
152. McCracken GH Jr, Mize SG, Threlkeld N. Intraventricular gentamicin therapy in gram-negative bacillary meningitis of infancy: report of the second neonatal meningitis cooperative study group. *Lancet* 1980;1:787–791.
153. Kaye KS, Fraimow HS, Abrutyn E. Pathogens resistant to antimicrobial agents: epidemiology, molecular mechanisms, and clinical management. *Infect Dis Clin North Am* 2000;14:293–319.
154. Lu CH, Chang WN, Chuang YC. Resistance to third-generation cephalosporins in adult gram-negative bacillary meningitis. *Infection* 1999;27:208–211.
155. Kilpatrick M, Girgis N, Farid Z, et al. Aztreonam for treating meningitis caused by gram-negative rods. *Scand J Infect Dis* 1991;23:125–6.
156. Rodriguez K, Dickinson GM, Greenman RL. Successful treatment of gram-negative bacillary meningitis with imipenem/cilastatin. *South Med J* 1985;78:732–733.
157. Donnelly JP, Horrevorts AM, Sauerwein RW, et al. High-dose meropenem in meningitis due to *Pseudomonas aeruginosa*. *Lancet* 1992;339:1117.
158. Chmelik V, Gutvirth J. Meropenem treatment of post-traumatic meningitis due to *Pseudomonas aeruginosa*. *J Antimicrob Chemother* 1993;32:922–923.
159. Segal-Maurer S, Mariano N, Qavi A, et al. Successful treatment of ceftazidime-resistant *Klebsiella pneumoniae* ventriculitis with intravenous meropenem and intraventricular polymyxin B: case report and review. *Clin Infect Dis* 1999;28:1134–138.
160. Nunez ML, Martinez-Toldos C, Bru M, et al. Appearance of resistance to meropenem during the treatment of a patient with meningitis by *Acinetobacter*. *Scand J Infect Dis* 1998;30:421–423.
161. Segev S, Barzilai A, Rosen N, et al. Pefloxacin treatment of meningitis caused by gram-negative bacteria. *Arch Intern Med* 1989;149:1314–1316.
162. Schonwald S, Beus I, Lisic M, et al. Ciprofloxacin in the treatment of gram-negative bacillary meningitis. *Am J Med* 1989;87:248S–249S.
163. Tunkel AR, Scheld WM. Treatment of bacterial meningitis. In: Wolfson JS, Hooper DC, eds. *Quinolone antimicrobial agents*. Washington, DC: American Society for Microbiology, 1993: 481–495.
164. Wong-Beringer A, Beringer P, Lovett MA. Successful treatment of multidrug-resistant *Pseudomonas aeruginosa* meningitis with high-dose ciprofloxacin. *Clin Infect Dis* 1997;25:936–937.
165. D'Antuono VS, Brown I. Successful treatment of *Enterobacter* meningitis with ciprofloxacin. *Clin Infect Dis* 1998;26:206–207.
166. Kremery V Jr, Filka J, Uher J, et al. Ciprofloxacin in treatment of nosocomial meningitis in neonates and in infants: report of 12 cases and review. *Diag Microbiol Infect Dis* 1999;35:75–80.
167. Lu CH, Chang WN, Chuang YC, et al. The prognostic factors of adult gram-negative bacillary meningitis. *J Hosp Infect* 1998;40:27–34.
168. Schlesinger LS, Ross SC, Schaberg DR. *Staphylococcus aureus* meningitis: a broad-based epidemiologic study. *Medicine (Baltimore)* 1987;66:148–156.
169. Kim JH, van der Horst C, Mulrow CD, et al. *Staphylococcus aureus* meningitis: review of 28 cases. *Rev Infect Dis* 1989;11:698–706.
170. Jensen AG, Espersen F, Skinhoj P, et al. *Staphylococcus aureus* meningitis: a review of 104 nationwide, consecutive cases. *Arch Intern Med* 1993;153:1902–1908.
171. Kaufman BA. Infections of cerebrospinal fluid shunts. In: Scheld WM, Whitley RJ, Durack DT, eds. *Infections of the central nervous system*, 2nd ed. Philadelphia: Lippincott-Raven, 1997:555–577.

172. Cruciani M, Navarra A, Di Perri G, et al. Evaluation of intraventricular teicoplanin for the treatment of neurosurgical shunt infections. *Clin Infect Dis* 1992;15:285–289.
173. Radetsky M. Duration of treatment in bacterial meningitis: a historical inquiry. *Pediatr Infect Dis J* 1990;9:2–9.
174. O'Neill P. How long to treat bacterial meningitis. *Lancet* 1993;341:530.
175. Viladrich PF, Pallares R, Ariza J, et al. Four days of penicillin therapy for meningococcal meningitis. *Arch Intern Med* 1986;146:2380–2382.
176. Macfarlane JT, Anjorin FI, Cleland PG, et al. Single injection treatment of meningococcal meningitis. 1. Long-acting penicillin. *Trans R Soc Trop Med Hyg* 1979;73:693–697.
177. Wali SS, Macfarlane JT, Weir WRC, et al. Single injection treatment of meningococcal meningitis. 2. Long-acting chloramphenicol. *Trans R Soc Trop Med Hyg* 1979;73:698–702.
178. Jadavji T, Biggar WD, Gold R, et al. Sequelae of acute bacterial meningitis in children treated for seven days. *Pediatrics* 1985;78:21–25.
179. Lin TY, Chrane DF, Nelson JD, et al. Seven days of ceftriaxone therapy is as effective as ten days' treatment for bacterial meningitis. *JAMA* 1985;253:3559–3563.
180. Roine I, Ledermann W, Foncea LM, et al. Randomized trial of four vs. seven days of ceftriaxone treatment for bacterial meningitis in children with rapid initial recovery. *Pediatr Infect Dis J* 2000;19:219–222.
181. Steele R, Marcy S. Outpatient management of bacterial meningitis. *Pediatr Infect Dis J* 1989;8:258–260.
182. Waler JA, Rathore MH. Outpatient management of pediatric bacterial meningitis. *Pediatr Infect Dis J* 1995;14:89–92.
183. Bradley J, Ching D, Phillips S. Outpatient therapy of serious pediatric infections with ceftriaxone. *Pediatr Infect Dis J* 1988;7:160–164.
184. Tice AD, Strait K, Ramey R, et al. Outpatient parenteral antimicrobial therapy for central nervous system infections. *Clin Infect Dis* 1999;29:1394–1399.
185. Schuchat A, Robinson K, Wenger JD, et al. Bacterial meningitis in the United States in 1995. *N Engl J Med* 1997;337:970–976.
186. Durand ML, Calderwood SB, Weber DJ, et al. Acute bacterial meningitis in adults. A review of 493 episodes. *N Engl J Med* 1993;328:21–28.
187. Sigurdardottir B, Bjornsson OM, Jonsdottir KE, et al. Acute bacterial meningitis in adults: a 20-year overview. *Arch Intern Med* 1997;157:425–430.
188. Bryan JP, de Silva HR, Tavares A, et al. Etiology and mortality of bacterial meningitis in northeastern Brazil. *Rev Infect Dis* 1990;12:128–135.
189. Kaplan SL. Clinical presentations, diagnosis, and prognostic factors of bacterial meningitis. *Infect Dis Clin North Am* 1999;13:579–594.
190. Kornelisse RF, Westerbeek CML, Spoor AB, et al. Pneumococcal meningitis in children: prognostic indicators and outcome. *Clin Infect Dis* 1995;21:1390–1397.
191. Andersen J, Backer V, Voldsgaard P, et al. Acute meningococcal meningitis: analysis of features of the disease according to the age of 255 patients. *J Infect* 1997;34:227–235.
192. Barquet N, Domingo P, Cayla JA, et al. Prognostic factors in meningococcal disease: development of a bedside predictive model and scoring system. *JAMA* 1997;278:491–496.
193. Skogberg K, Syrjänen J, Jahkola M, et al. Clinical presentation and outcome of listeriosis in patients with and without immunosuppressive therapy. *Clin Infect Dis* 1992;14:815–821.
194. Sell SHW. Long-term sequelae of bacterial meningitis in children. *Pediatr Infect Dis* 1983;2:90–93.
195. Pomeroy SL, Holmes SJ, Dodge PR, et al. Seizures and other neurologic sequelae of bacterial meningitis in children. *N Engl J Med* 1990;323:1651–1657.
196. Taylor HG, Mills EL, Ciampi A, et al. The sequelae of *Haemophilus influenzae* meningitis in school-age children. *N Engl J Med* 1990;323:1657–1663.
197. Dodge PR, Davis H, Feigin RD, et al. Prospective evaluation of hearing impairment as a sequela of acute bacterial meningitis. *N Engl J Med* 1984;311:869–874.
198. Fortnum HM. Hearing impairment after bacterial meningitis: a review. *Arch Dis Child* 1992;67:1128–1133.
199. Richardson MP, Reid A, Tarlow MJ, et al. Hearing loss during bacterial meningitis. *Arch Dis Child* 1997;76:134–138.
200. Pfister HW, Feiden W, Einhäupl KM. Spectrum of complications during bacterial meningitis in adults: results of a prospective clinical study. *Arch Neurol* 1993;50:575–581.

201. Pfister HW, Borasio GD, Dirnagl U, et al. Cerebrovascular complications of bacterial meningitis in adults. *Neurology* 1992;42:1497–1504.
202. Begg N, Cartwright KAV, Cohen J, et al. Consensus statement on diagnosis, investigation, treatment and prevention of acute bacterial meningitis in immunocompetent adults. *J Infect* 1999;39:1–15.
203. McIntyre PB, Berkey CS, King SM, et al. Dexamethasone as adjunctive therapy in bacterial meningitis: a meta-analysis of randomized clinical trials since 1988. *JAMA* 1997;278:925–931.
204. Ropper AH. Raised intracranial pressure in neurologic disease. *Semin Neurol* 1984;4:397–407.
205. Lyons MK, Meyer FB. Cerebrospinal fluid physiology and the management of increased intracranial pressure. *Mayo Clin Proc* 1990;65:684–707.
206. Ross KL, Tunkel AR, Scheld WM. Acute bacterial meningitis in children and adults. In: Scheld WM, Whitley RJ, Durack DT, eds. *Infections of the central nervous system,* 2nd ed. Philadelphia: Lippincott-Raven, 1997:335–401.
207. Ashwal S, Stringer W, Tomasi L, et al. Cerebral blood flow and carbon dioxide reactivity in children with bacterial meningitis. *J Pediatr* 1990;117:523–530.
208. Ashwal S. Neurologic evaluation of the patient with acute bacterial meningitis. *Neurol Clin* 1995;13:549–577.
209. Kaplan SL, Fishman MA. Supportive therapy for bacterial meningitis. *Pediatr Infect Dis J* 1987;6:670–677.
210. Kilpi T, Peltola H, Jauhiainen T, et al. Oral glycerol and intravenous dexamethasone in preventing neurologic and audiologic sequelae of childhood bacterial meningitis. *Pediatr Infect Dis J* 1995;14:270–278.
211. Trauner DA. Barbiturate therapy in acute brain injury. *J Pediatr* 1986;109:742–746.
212. Singhi SC, Singhi PD, Srinivas B, et al. Fluid restriction does not improve the outcome of acute meningitis. *Pediatr Infect Dis J* 1995;14:495–503.
213. Duke T. Fluid management of bacterial meningitis in developing countries. *Arch Dis Child* 1998;79:181–185.
214. Tunkel AR, Scheld WM. Acute infectious complications of head injury. In: Braakman R, ed. *Handbook of clinical neurology,* vol. 57: *Head injury.* Amsterdam: Elsevier Science Publishing, 1990:317–326.
215. Kaufman BA, Tunkel AR, Pryor J, et al. Meningitis in the neurosurgical patient. *Infect Dis Clin North Am* 1990;4:677–701.
216. Snedeker JD, Kaplan SL, Dodge PR, et al. Subdural effusion and its relationship with neurologic sequelae of bacterial meningitis in infancy: a prospective study. *Pediatrics* 1990;86:163–170.

9

Prevention

Bacterial meningitis continues to be an important cause of morbidity and mortality in both industrialized and developing countries throughout the world, despite the availability of effective bactericidal antimicrobial agents. Until recently, three species of bacteria (*Haemophilus influenzae, Neisseria meningitidis,* and *Streptococcus pneumoniae*) were responsible for more than 80% of all cases of bacterial meningitis (see Chapter 2). The spread of meningitis caused by these microorganisms may be interrupted by the following means: (a) reduction of the pool of infection among asymptomatic nasopharyngeal carriers by antimicrobial therapy or vaccination; (b) amelioration of adverse environmental conditions that favor the spread of respiratory infections; and (c) protection of susceptible new hosts by chemoprophylaxis (1). The latter approach has received the most attention and has been effective in control of outbreaks in selected patients at risk for development of invasive disease caused by specific meningeal pathogens. Furthermore, recent declines in the incidence of bacterial meningitis have been the result of successful use of conjugate vaccines. This chapter will review the rationale and recommendations for the use of chemoprophylaxis to prevent secondary cases of bacterial meningitis and the efficacy of vaccines as primary prevention in decreasing the incidence of this devastating infection.

CHEMOPROPHYLAXIS

It has become clear in recent years that the spread of several types of bacterial meningitis can be prevented by chemoprophylaxis with antimicrobial agents of contacts of meningitis cases. Chemoprophylaxis is utilized to eliminate the nasopharyngeal carriage in contacts and patients, prevent contacts from developing the disease, and perhaps treat infection in those incubating the disease (2). However, chemoprophylaxis will likely not prevent incubating disease and should never be considered a substitute for close surveillance of contacts, who need to be monitored for development of symptoms and signs of illness within the first week or so following onset of symptoms in the index case. There is always much concern regarding who should receive chemoprophylaxis after an index case of bacterial meningitis is identified, and many persons deem themselves to have been "close contacts" of the index patient.

Generally, close contacts are described as persons who frequently sleep and eat in the same dwelling or who have intimate contact with an index case (3). Here I will discuss the epidemiology of microorganism acquisition and review specific recommendations for chemoprophylaxis based on the microorganism isolated in the index patient.

Haemophilus influenzae Type B

Invasive disease may occur in nonvaccinated household contacts of patients with *H. influenzae* type b meningitis (4,5). The risk is markedly age dependent (4), reported highest for children under 2 years of age (4.4%) in one study (4). The attack rate decreased progressively in children between the ages of 2 and 4 years (1.2%) and in those between the ages of 4 and 6 years (0.06%). No secondary cases were reported in contacts who were 6 years of age and older. Most secondary cases (75%) occur within 6 days of onset of disease in the index case; although untreated household contacts remain at increased risk for *H. influenzae* type b disease for at least 1 month after onset in the index case, the risk diminishes over time. Studies in the United States have established that the secondary attack rate in children in households with children under 5 years of age is 500 to 800 times higher during the month after exposure (6,7). Day care outside of the home is considered another risk factor for transmission. Several reports have shown at least a 1% risk of secondary disease in day care contacts (8), which is 25 times greater than the expected rate of primary *H. influenzae* type b disease in this age group (9). The children in day care facilities in whom secondary disease is most likely to develop include those who are under 24 months of age, have been exposed in the classroom setting to a person with invasive *H. influenzae* type b disease, and have not received rifampin (10). The risk is also related to the size of the day care center, with the risk higher in centers with more than four children (11). There is controversy, however, as to the magnitude of the risk to children in day care settings. Two prospective studies reported that the risk of subsequent *H. influenzae* type b disease in children attending day care facilities was substantially lower than previously reported among household contacts of patients with the disease (12,13). Further studies are needed to clarify these issues.

The rationale for the use of chemoprophylaxis for prevention of secondary disease is eradication of nasopharyngeal colonization of *H. influenzae* type b, thereby preventing transmission to young, susceptible contacts and to prevent the development of invasive disease in those already colonized. Early reports examined the effectiveness of a number of antimicrobial agents in the elimination rate of nasopharyngeal carriage of *H. influenzae* type b (Table 9.1) (4). Rifampin has been shown to be the most effective antimicrobial agent for elimination of nasopharyngeal carriage because of its ability to achieve high concentrations in respiratory secretions (14). In one randomized, blinded trial of rifampin versus placebo for chemoprophylaxis, four cases of secondary invasive disease caused by *H. influenzae* type b developed among 765 placebo-treated controls compared with no cases among 1,112 rifampin recipients (15), suggesting the efficacy of rifampin in the prevention of secondary *H. influenzae* type b disease. However, failures have occurred with rifampin and

TABLE 9.1. *Elimination rate of nasopharyngeal carriage of* Haemophilus influenzae *type b after treatment with various antimicrobial agents*

Regimen	Elimination rate
No therapy or placebo	26%
Cefaclor	18%
Erythromycin-sulfasoxazole	20%
Trimethoprim-sulfamethoxazole	58%
Ampicillin	70%
Rifampin (10 mg/kg dose)	71%
Rifampin (20 mg/kg dose)	96%

Data modified from Band JD. Chemoprophylaxis of *Haemophilus influenzae* type b disease: a strategy for preventing secondary cases. In: Sell SH, Wright PF, eds. Haemophilus influenzae: *epidemiology, immunology, and prevention of disease.* New York: Elsevier Science, 1982: 309–315, with permission.

rifampin-resistant strains of *H. influenzae* type b exist. The current recommendation for chemoprophylaxis is rifampin (20 mg/kg daily for 4 days; 600 mg maximum per dose) for all individuals, including adults, in households with at least one child younger than 48 months of age whose immunization status with the *H. influenzae* type b conjugate vaccine is incomplete (16,17). Complete immunization is defined as having had at least one dose of conjugate vaccine at 15 months of age or older, two doses between 12 and 14 months, or a two- or three-dose primary series when younger than 12 months of age with a booster/reinforcing dose at 12 months of age or older. A contact is defined as a child who either is a household member or has spent 4 or more hours each day with the index case for at least 5 of the 7 days preceding the day the index case was hospitalized. As a result of the efficacy of the *H. influenzae* type b conjugate vaccines (see later), chemoprophylaxis is not recommended when all household contacts younger than 48 months of age have completed their immunization series unless the vaccinated child is immunocompromised, because the immunization series may have been ineffective in this patient group. The index patient may also need to receive rifampin prophylaxis because some antimicrobial agents (i.e., ampicillin, chloramphenicol) given for invasive *H. influenzae* type b disease do not necessarily eliminate nasopharyngeal colonization. One study suggested that 2 days of rifampin therapy were equally efficacious to 4 days' treatment (18), although this requires further confirmation before a recommendation to shorten duration of chemoprophylaxis can be made. Rifampin is not recommended for pregnant women who are contacts of infected infants, since the risk of rifampin to the fetus has not been established. Ceftriaxone may be utilized in this setting, although the efficacy of ceftriaxone for *H. influenzae* type b chemoprophylaxis has not been proven.

Recommendations for chemoprophylaxis of contacts in day care centers are not as clearly defined. Chemoprophylaxis is not currently recommended for day care contacts 2 years of age or older unless two or more cases occur in the day care center within a 60-day period and the day care center has unvaccinated or incompletely vaccinated children (17). Administration of rifampin to all attendees and supervisory personnel is indicated as recommended for household contacts. For unvaccinated or incompletely vaccinated children younger than 2 years of age in this setting, the question of whether to administer chemoprophylaxis needs to be individualized and should be considered more strongly in day care centers that resemble households where children have prolonged contact (i.e., for at least 25 hours) with the index case in the week before the index case was hospitalized.

Neisseria meningitidis

Chemoprophylaxis is also necessary for contacts of patients with invasive meningo-coccal disease; up to 10% of meningococcal meningitis cases have had contact with another known case (2). The estimated prevalence of meningococcal carriage in the United States is 5% to 10% under nonepidemic conditions (19), although carriage rates are less than 1% in children under 4 years of age (20). Up to 30% of teenagers and 10% of adults carry meningococci in the upper respiratory tract at any point in time (21). Carriage rates are highest among close contacts of an index case. The transmission of meningococci is facilitated by crowding, close contact, low socioeco-nomic conditions, climactic factors such as temperature and humidity, concomitant viral infections, and smoking, and in those who are nonsecretors of the Lewis blood group (2). These factors often lead to higher carriage rates among close contacts of index cases and in populations living in close or poor environments. In closed popu-lations, such as military recruits, carriage rates can reach levels of 50% or more (22). In one report, 5% to 15% of military recruits became carriers of new meningococcal strains each month (23). Carriage may last a long time (at least months) in about 25% of carriers, is intermittent in one-third, and is transient or infrequent in the remain-ing 40% (24). However, overall carriage rates have not been especially useful in the prediction of outbreaks of meningococcal disease, and carriage rates determined by swab cultures are underestimates of transmission and acquisition (25).

Household contacts exposed to a patient with meningococcal disease have an in-creased risk of developing invasive disease that is from 500 to 4,000 times higher than the risk of those who are not exposed (26). The risk is more than 100-fold in day care children compared with the age-adjusted risk for the general population (3), and dormitory living has been found to increase the risk 11-fold. Transmission of N. meningitidis leading to development of invasive disease has also been documented in a campus bar, dance club, and sports club (27–29). Secondary systemic meningo-coccal disease most often develops within 7 days of recognition of the index case, with 70% to 80% of secondary cases occurring within 14 days of the primary case. In one report, 57% of secondary cases occurred within the first week, 18% during the second week, 9% during the third week, and 16% during the fourth to sixth weeks (30). In contrast, another study found that nine (53%) of 17 secondary cases occurred 5 to 39 weeks after the primary case (31).

Chemoprophylaxis to prevent invasive meningococcal disease is recommended for close contacts of the index case, defined as household contacts, day care center members, and anyone directly exposed to the patient's oral secretions (e.g., through kissing, mouth-to-mouth resuscitation, endotracheal intubation, or endotracheal tube management) (32). Chemoprophylaxis may also need to be administered to the index case prior to hospital discharge because certain antimicrobial agents (e.g., high-dose penicillin or chloramphenicol) do not reliably eradicate meningococci from the nasopharynx of colonized patients. Chemoprophylaxis should be administered as soon as possible (ideally within 24 hours) after the case is identified. Administration 14 days or more after onset of illness in the index patient is probably of limited value. Chemoprophylaxis is not recommended for those contacts at low risk for developing invasive meningococcal disease (17). These are casual contacts (e.g., a school or work mate who has no history of direct exposure to the patient's oral secretions), indirect contacts (i.e., contact is only with a high-risk contact and not with the index patient), and medical personnel who have no direct exposure to the patient's oral secretions.

The optimal chemoprophylactic agent of choice to prevent invasive meningococcal disease is controversial. The sulfonamides were the first antimicrobial agents utilized to provide mass chemoprophylaxis during World War II, although resistance to these agents among meningococci is now widespread; sulfonamides should only be used if the *in vitro* susceptibility of *N. meningitidis* to these agents has been established (2). Minocycline has shown efficacy in eradicating meningococcal carriage, although its use has been compromised by an unacceptably high incidence of adverse effects. Several other antimicrobial regimens have been recommended as chemoprophylaxis against development of meningococcal disease (Table 9.2). The Centers for Disease Control and Prevention currently recommends administration of rifampin at 12-hour intervals for 2 days (32), which generally has an efficacy of more than 90%. However, rifampin has several shortcomings, including nasopharyngeal eradication rates of only about 70% to 80% in some studies, adverse events, necessity for multiple doses over 2 days, and emergence of resistant organisms (up to 10% to 27% of isolates) that may then cause invasive disease. In addition, rifampin is not recommended for pregnant women because the drug is teratogenic in laboratory animals. In the search for alternative agents, ceftriaxone (intramuscular administration of 250 mg in adults and 125 mg in children) eliminated the serogroup A carrier state in 97% of patients for up to 2 weeks in one study (33), although parenteral administration is required. In another report, ceftriaxone was equivalent to rifampin (98.2% versus 97.6%, respectively) in eliminating nasopharyngeal carriage of serogroup B *N. meningitidis* (34). Additional studies have demonstrated a single dose of oral ciprofloxacin (500 mg in adults) to be more than 90% effective in elimination of nasopharyngeal carriage of *N. meningitidis* (35–37). Ciprofloxacin concentrations in nasal secretions have been shown to exceed the MIC_{90} for meningococci (38), and ciprofloxacin may well supplant rifampin for chemoprophylaxis in adults. Ciprofloxacin is not generally recommended for use in children because of concerns regarding cartilage damage, although a recent consensus report concluded that ciprofloxacin can be used for chemoprophylaxis in children when no acceptable alternative agent is available (39). Azithromycin (500 mg orally once) was also shown to be as effective as a four-dose regimen of rifampin in the eradication of meningococci from the nasopharynx (40). In pregnant patients,

TABLE 9.2. *Schedule for administration of antimicrobial agents for chemoprophylaxis against invasive meningococcal disease*

Antimicrobial agent	Age group	Dosage, route, and duration of administration
Rifampin	Children <1 mo	5 mg/kg orally every 12 h for 2 d
Rifampin	Children ≥1 mo	10 mg/kg orally every 12 h for 2 d
Rifampin	Adults	600 mg orally every 12 h for 2 d
Ceftriaxone	Children <15 yr	125 mg intramuscular single dose
Ceftriaxone	Adults	250 mg intramuscular single dose
Ciprofloxacin	Adults	500 mg orally single dose
Azithromycin	Adults	500 mg orally single dose

Data from Centers for Disease Control and Prevention. Control and prevention of meningococcal disease and control and prevention of serogroup C meningococcal disease: evaluation and management of suspected outbreaks. *MMWR* 1997;46:1–11; and Girgis N, Sultan Y, Frenck RW Jr, et al. Azithromycin compared with rifampin for eradication of nasopharyngeal colonization by *Neisseria meningitidis. Pediatr Infect Dis J* 1998;17:816–819, with permission.

ceftriaxone is probably the safest alternative agent for chemoprophylaxis. Widespread chemoprophylaxis to low-risk contacts (see later) should be discouraged because of the concerns of emergence of resistant organisms and the possible future limitations of this approach.

Streptococcus pneumoniae

The risk of secondary pneumococcal disease in contacts of infected patients has not been defined, although outbreaks have been described in closed populations such as gold miners, military recruits, and jail inmates (16). In one outbreak in a day care center (41), treatment of 97% of the day care center children and staff with rifampin (10 mg/kg twice daily for 2 days) resulted in a 70% reduction (i.e., only partial eradication) of positive nasopharyngeal cultures for *S. pneumoniae,* but did not prevent new acquisition of this microorganism by three children and one family member. At present, the need for or benefit of prophylactic administration of antimicrobial agents to contacts of a person with pneumococcal disease has not been demonstrated. Therefore chemoprophylaxis is not recommended (17). However, daily antimicrobial prophylaxis is recommended for children with functional or anatomic asplenia, irrespective of their immunization status, for the prevention of pneumococcal disease. Therapy with oral penicillin (125 mg twice daily) in infants and children with sickle cell disease reduces the incidence of pneumococcal infections by 84% (42). The Centers for Disease Control and Prevention have recommended daily penicillin prophylaxis for children with sickle cell hemoglobinopathy beginning before 4 months of age (43), although there is no consensus as to the age when prophylaxis should be discontinued. One study demonstrated that children with sickle cell anemia who were receiving regular medical attention and who did not have a prior severe pneumococcal infection or a surgical splenectomy could safely discontinue prophylactic penicillin at approximately 5 years of age (44). Further studies are needed to define the age at which antimicrobial prophylaxis may be discontinued in these high-risk patients.

Streptococcus agalactiae

Group B streptococci are frequently harbored in the genitourinary and lower gastrointestinal tracts of adults, and cultures of both lower vaginal and anorectal sites isolate these microorganisms in 15% to 35% of asymptomatic pregnant women (45,46). Vertical transmission of group B streptococci to neonates occurs in 40% to 73% of culture-positive women, although only 1% to 2% of infants develop early-onset disease caused by this microorganism. A number of factors have been identified that have been associated with an increased risk of early-onset group B streptococcal disease (Table 9.3) (47). Several studies have demonstrated that the intravenous or intramuscular administration of antimicrobial agents after the onset of labor or rupture of the membranes is highly effective in reducing neonatal colonization with group B streptococci. One meta-analysis of seven trials (including studies of carriers with and without risk factors) estimated a 30-fold reduction in early-onset neonatal group B streptococcal disease with intrapartum antimicrobial chemoprophylaxis (48), although because of the heterogeneity of the therapeutic interventions and flaws in trial methods, the combination of results in these trials may not have been appropriate (49).

During the 1990s, however, the incidence of disease caused by mother-to-child transmission of the group B streptococcus fell from 1.7 to 0.6 cases per 1,000 live births (50), likely a result of the increased use of penicillin during labor in women at high risk of transmitting the infection to their newborns. The Centers for Disease Control and Prevention have established guidelines for prevention of group B streptococcal infection by intrapartum chemoprophylaxis (51,52). One of two strategies was recommended: (a) a screening-based approach (Fig. 9.1) in which vaginal/rectal

TABLE 9.3. *Factors associated with an increased risk of early-onset group B streptococcal disease*

Premature delivery
Low birth weight
Increased interval between membrane rupture and delivery
Rupture of membranes before onset of labor
Amnionitis
Intrapartum fever
Maternal vaginal or rectal colonization with group B streptococcus
Heavy (dense) colonization with group B streptococcus
African American race
Maternal age <20 yr
Group B streptococcal bacteriuria during current pregnancy
Low concentrations of antibody to type-specific capsular polysaccharide of the group B
    streptococcus
Previous stillbirth or spontaneous abortion
Multiple gestation/sibling of affected twin
Previous delivery of an infant with group B streptococcal disease
Cesarean section
Urinary tract infection during pregnancy
Prolonged duration of intrauterine monitoring

Data adapted from Allen UD, Navas L, King SM. Effectiveness of intrapartum penicillin prophylaxis in preventing early-onset group B streptococcal infection: results of a meta-analysis. *Can Med Assoc J* 1993;149:1659–1665, with permission.

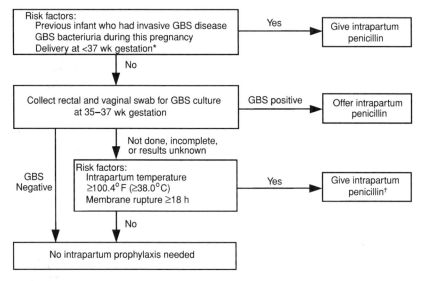

FIG. 9.1. Algorithm for prevention of early-onset group B streptococcal disease in neonates, using prenatal screening at 35–37 wk gestation. *If membranes ruptured at <37 wk gestation, and the mother has not begun labor, collect group B streptococcal culture and either (a) administer antibiotics until cultures are completed and the results are negative or (b) begin antibiotics only when positive cultures are available. No prophylaxis is needed if culture obtained at 35–37 wk gestation was negative. †Broader spectrum antibiotics may be considered at the physician's discretion, based on clinical indications. (From Centers for Disease Control and Prevention. Adoption of hospital policies for prevention of perinatal group B streptococcal disease—United States, 1997. *MMWR* 1998;47:65–70, with permission.)

swabs are collected at 35 to 37 weeks' gestation for culture in selective broth medium, and carriers and those women delivering before 37 weeks with unknown carrier status are then offered intrapartum antimicrobial prophylaxis; and (b) a risk-based strategy (Fig. 9.2) in which women of unknown carrier status receive intrapartum chemoprophylaxis based on threatened delivery at less than 37 weeks' gestation, rupture of the membranes of 18 hours or more, or intrapartum fever of 38°C or more. Based on these strategies, a review of early-onset group B streptococcal infections during 1995 in four areas of North America suggested that risk-based and screening-based strategies would reduce early-onset disease by 41% and 78%, respectively (53). Substantial decreases in early-onset group B streptococcal disease were also reported in individual hospitals and larger geographic areas where these policies were implemented. Surveillance data from the Centers for Disease Control and Prevention indicated that early-onset disease declined by 53% between 1993 and 1997 (51), an effect accompanied by a significant increase in the proportion of hospitals adopting preventive policies (54). In one institution where superb compliance with screening was achieved, the rate fell from 11.6 to 1.4 cases per 10, 000 live births (55).

Chemoprophylaxis should consist of intrapartum intravenous ampicillin (2 g initially, then 1 to 2 g every 4 hours) or penicillin G (5 million units initially, then 2.5 million units every 4 hours) until delivery (52). In the penicillin-allergic patient,

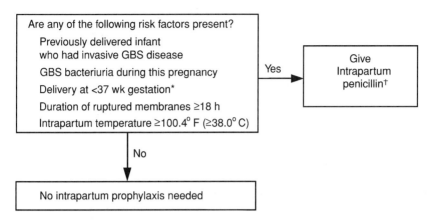

FIG. 9.2. Algorithm for prevention of early-onset of group B streptococcal disease in neonates, using risk factors. *If membranes ruptured at <37 wk gestation, and the mother has not begun labor, collect group B streptococcal culture and either (a) administer antibiotics until cultures are completed and the results are negative or (b) begin antibiotics only when positive cultures are available. †Broader spectrum antibiotics may be considered at the physician's discretion, based on clinical indications. (From Centers for Disease Control and Prevention. Adoption of hospital policies for prevention of perinatal group B streptococcal disease–United States, 1997. *MMWR* 1998;47: 65–70, with permission.)

intravenous clindamycin (900 mg every 8 hours until delivery) is recommended; intravenous erythromycin (500 mg every 6 hours until delivery) is the suggested alternative agent. Concerns regarding the use of intrapartum chemoprophylaxis include the possibility of an unacceptably high number of adverse reactions from administration of the antimicrobial agent and the risk for emergence of antimicrobial-resistant microorganisms (51,52). Although group B streptococci continue to be susceptible to penicillin, resistance to erythromycin and clindamycin have been reported in 7.4% and 3.4%, respectively, of invasive group B streptococcal isolates (56). In another laboratory surveillance study of invasive disease caused by group B streptococci in adults (57), resistance to erythromycin was 6.7% and to clindamycin was 4.4%, although all isolates were susceptible to penicillin, ampicillin, and vancomycin. Other alternatives (e.g., the cephalosporins) may need to be considered for intrapartum chemoprophylaxis in penicillin-allergic women. Continued surveillance studies are also needed to monitor the possible adverse effects of intrapartum chemoprophylaxis with antimicrobial agents (58). Recently, polymerase chain reaction (PCR) has been evaluated for rapid detection of group B streptococci in pregnant women at delivery and was found to have a sensitivity of 97% and specificity of 100% (59); validation of this technique in routine clinical practice might obviate the need for prenatal screening and reduce the use of antimicrobial prophylaxis in women who are not colonized (60).

Basilar Skull Fracture

The incidence of bacterial meningitis following basilar skull fracture ranges from 0.2% to 17.8%, with an incidence of up to 50% in patients with a cerebrospinal fluid (CSF) leak (61). A number of studies have reported on the use of prophylactic antimicrobial agents in patients with basilar skull fractures and CSF leak, based on the premise that in patients with a dural defect, the CSF is exposed to pathogenic microorganisms from the nasopharynx, nasal or mastoid sinuses, or external auditory canal. The use of antimicrobial chemoprophylaxis in this setting remains controversial. Some experts recommend against the use of antimicrobial chemoprophylaxis whereas others recommend routine chemoprophylaxis for a period ranging from 3 to 14 days or until 1 week after CSF leakage has resolved. However, the interpretation and comparison of the various studies examining this question are confounded by multiple variables, including the use of retrospective data, small sample size, patient selection, choice of antimicrobial agents, and definition of infection. In one review of articles published between 1970 and 1989 of 848 cases of basilar skull fracture (62), 19 (4%) of 519 patients who received prophylactic antimicrobial therapy developed meningitis versus 10 (3%) of the 329 patients not receiving prophylaxis. In addition, a recent meta-analysis of 1,241 patients (719 of whom received antimicrobial prophylaxis) among 12 published trials suggested that antimicrobial prophylaxis did not decrease the risk of bacterial meningitis (63). The common odds ratio of 1.15, although indicating an increased meningitis risk among patients not treated with antimicrobial therapy, did not reach statistical significance. Patients with basilar skull fracture associated with CSF leak were analyzed separately and, again, there was no significant effect of prophylactic administration of antimicrobial agents. There have been two prospective, randomized, controlled trials that examined prophylactic use of antimicrobial agents after basilar skull fracture (64,65). In one study of 157 patients with skull fractures (43 of whom had basilar skull fractures) (65), the only patient who developed meningitis had a basilar skull fracture and CSF otorrhea and did not receive antimicrobial prophylaxis.

Based on the available data, the prophylactic use of antimicrobial therapy in patients with basilar skull fracture does not appear to reduce the risk of bacterial meningitis and is not recommended. Furthermore, use of prophylactic antimicrobial agents may result in selection and growth of resistant organisms and development of more serious infections that may be difficult to eradicate. Patients with a basilar skull fracture should be monitored carefully. If symptoms or signs of bacterial meningitis develop, an aggressive diagnostic and therapeutic approach should be initiated.

Cerebrospinal Fluid Shunts

Placement of CSF shunts is complicated by infection in 2% to 40% of cases (66). Although many trials have examined the use of prophylactic antimicrobial therapy in the prevention of CSF shunt infections, these studies are conflicting and inconclusive, and the practice of administration of antimicrobial prophylaxis remains controversial. Therefore the technique of meta-analysis has been applied to the various studies of use of prophylactic antimicrobial agents in CSF shunt surgery. In one meta-analysis (67), 12 of 37 trials met the selection criteria and were included in the analysis. In the aggregate, the use of prophylactic antimicrobial therapy was associated with a significant reduction in subsequent CSF shunt infection (risk ratio of 0.52, with an approximate risk reduction of 50%). However, the infection rate in the treatment groups in these trials averaged 6.8% (range from 1.9% to 17%), an unacceptably high clean wound infection rate. In addition, only one of the 12 trials achieved statistical significance favoring the use of antimicrobial prophylaxis (68). Positive results favoring prophylaxis were also confirmed in another meta-analysis of antimicrobial prophylaxis for CSF shunts (69). The beneficial effect of prophylaxis was strongly related to the baseline infection rate and disappeared when the baseline infection rate was 5% or less. Therefore the aggregate data suggest that prophylactic antimicrobial therapy does reduce the risk of infection in CSF shunt surgery (66). The greatest risk reduction occurs in those groups with a relatively high baseline rate of infection, perhaps more than 12%. One expert recommends the use of an antistaphylococcal antimicrobial agent given intravenously just after induction of anesthesia and before incision, with the agent continued only intraoperatively (66). In the absence of definitive prospective data, this approach is recommended in patients undergoing CSF shunt surgery.

VACCINATION

Vaccination to prevent infection with specific meningeal pathogens is a very useful measure for decreasing the incidence of bacterial meningitis. Strategies for vaccination have focused on prevention of invasive disease caused by *H. influenzae* type b, *N. meningitidis, S. pneumoniae,* and *S. agalactiae.* The efficacy of currently available vaccines is discussed in detail in the following sections.

Haemophilus influenzae Type B

The use of vaccination to prevent invasive disease caused by *H. influenzae* type b began in the 1970s with the use of capsular polysaccharide vaccines consisting of the polyribosylribitol phosphate (PRP) of the outermost layer of *H. influenzae* type b (70). The response to vaccination was age dependent, with serum antibody concentrations of 0.15 μg/mL or more providing short-term protection and concentrations 1.0 μg/mL or more indicative of long-term protection (71). However, this vaccine was not effective among children less than 18 months of age, the time when many infants develop invasive disease caused by this microorganism. In the late 1980s, the *H. influenzae* type b conjugate vaccines became available. Each conjugate vaccine consisted of a carrier protein covalently conjugated to PRP or parts of the PRP with or without a linker; the process of conjugation changed the polysaccharide from a T-cell-independent to a T-cell-dependent antigen, and greatly improved immunogenicity (72,73). In addition, repeat doses of *H. influenzae* type b conjugate vaccines elicited booster responses and allowed maturation of class-specific immunity with the predominance of IgG antibody. The first *H. influenzae* type b conjugate vaccine (PRP-D) was licensed for use in December 1987 but was not consistently immunogenic in children less than 18 months of age and is therefore not recommended for use in infants. There are currently three chemically and immunologically distinct *H. influenzae* type b conjugate vaccines licensed for use in infants as young as 6 weeks of age. All are highly immunogenic and

TABLE 9.4. *Incidence of* Haemophilus influenzae *type b meningitis before and after vaccination with conjugate vaccines in children aged 0–4 yr in selected areas of the world*

Geographic area (yr of comparison)	Incidence before vaccination[a]	Incidence after vaccination[a]
United States (1987 vs 1995)	54	<1
Canada (1985 vs 1994)	~44	<1
Brazil (1988–1996 vs 1997)	22	10
Chile (1995 vs 1998)	40	<2
Uruguay (1992–1993 vs 1995)	17–22	1
Scandinavia (1970s vs 1995)	31	<1
Austria (1991 vs 1993–1996)	11	<1
The Netherlands (1970s vs 1993–1994)	22–40	0.3
Spain (1993–1995 vs 1997)	14	~0
Switzerland (1976–1990 vs 1991–1993)	26	8
United Kingdom, England and Wales (1991–1992 vs 1993–1994)	15	0.6
Israel (1989–1992 vs 1995)	18	<1
Australia, Sydney region (1991–1992 vs 1993–1994)	21	6

Adapted from Peltola H. Worldwide *Haemophilus influenzae* type b disease at the beginning of the 21st century: global analysis of the disease burden 25 years after the use of the polysaccharide vaccine and a decade after the advent of conjugates. *Clin Microbiol Rev* 2000;13:302–317, with permission.
[a] Incidence per 100,000 per yr.

more than 95% of infants develop protective antibody concentrations after a primary series of two or three doses. Comparative clinical trials of the efficacy of conjugate vaccines in industrialized nations have revealed that these vaccines have decreased the number of cases of *H. influenzae* type b meningitis by more than 90% (74–77). The conjugate vaccines have also been quite efficacious in decreasing the incidence of *H. influenzae* type b meningitis throughout the world (Table 9.4) (73).

The American Academy of Pediatrics recommends that all infants, including those born prematurely, should receive a primary series of *H. influenzae* type b conjugate vaccine beginning at 2 months of age (17,78). The number of doses in the primary series depends upon the type of vaccine utilized (Table 9.5). A primary series of PRP-OMP vaccine is two doses, and HbOC and PRP-T require a three-dose primary series. A booster dose is also recommended at 12 to 15 months of age regardless of which vaccine is used in the primary series. All three of the vaccines are interchangeable. Vaccine should not be given to a child younger than 6 weeks of age because it may induce tolerance to additional doses of the *H. influenzae* type b conjugate vaccine. Unvaccinated children more than 7 months of age may not require a full series of vaccine doses (Table 9.5). Children older than 59 months of age do not need vaccination with *H. influenzae* type b conjugate vaccine because the majority of these children are immune, probably from asymptomatic infection as infants. However, children and adults at high risk for invasive *H. influenzae* type b disease (i.e., those with functional or anatomic asplenia, immunodeficiency—especially IgG2 subclass deficiency, immunosuppression from cancer chemotherapy, and infection with human immunodeficiency virus) should be given at least one dose of any of the licensed *H. influenzae* type b conjugate vaccines.

TABLE 9.5. *Recommended routine vaccination schedule for the* Haemophilus influenzae *type b conjugate vaccines*

Vaccine	Age at first dose (mo)	Primary series	Booster
HbOC or PRP-T	2–6	3 doses, 2 mo apart	12–15 mo
PRP-OMP	2–6	2 doses, 2 mo apart	12–15 mo
HbOC, PRP-T, or PRP-OMP	7–11	2 doses, 2 mo apart	12–18 mo
HbOC, PRP-T, or PRP-OMP	12–14	1 dose	2 mo later
HbOC, PRP-T, PRP-OMP, or PRP-D	15–59	1 dose	—

HbOC, *H. influenzae* type b polysaccharide conjugated to mutant diphtheria toxoid; PRP-D, *H. influenzae* type b polysaccharide conjugated to diphtheria toxoid; PRP-OMP, *H. influenzae* type b polysaccharide conjugated to outer membrane protein of serogroup B meningococcus; PRP-T, *H. influenzae* type b polysaccharide conjugated to tetanus toxoid.

The *H. influenzae* type b conjugate vaccines also reduce oropharyngeal colonization by *H. influenzae* type b, leading to a herd protective effect. Clinical studies in Finland (79), Iceland (80), the United States (81,82), and Gambia (83) have demonstrated that the prevalence of *H. influenzae* type b carriage declined significantly after large-scale vaccination programs. The calculated efficacy of PRP-D vaccine in preventing colonization with *H. influenzae* type b was 64% to 81% (82). However, recent studies of oropharyngeal *H. influenzae* type b carriage in the Netherlands (84) and among Alaska Native children (85) found that vaccination did not reduce or eliminate oropharyngeal carriage. This suggests the importance of monitoring the impact of *H. influenzae* type b conjugate vaccines in different populations in terms of vaccine efficacy and the impact of vaccination on carriage. In contrast, another population-based study of the incidence of invasive *H. influenzae* disease (caused by serotype b, other serotypes, and nontypeable strains) in Alaskan residents 10 years of age and older demonstrated that the overall statewide incidence of invasive *H. influenzae* infections decreased by 33% in this age group after the initiation of an infant *H. influenzae* type b vaccination program (86), perhaps by decreasing *H. influenzae* type b carriage in child reservoirs. Despite reports of lack of herd immunity following vaccination with *H. influenzae* type b conjugate vaccines, the majority of published studies demonstrated a positive effect of the conjugate vaccines on carriage that has furthered the decline in the incidence of invasive *H. influenzae* type b disease in vaccinated populations (72). Further studies should help to clarify this issue.

Recently, it has been suggested that three doses of the *H. influenzae* type b conjugate vaccine may not be imperative in conferring protection against invasive disease (3,72,73). One dose of *H. influenzae* type b conjugate confers protection of about 50% and the second dose increases the degree of protection considerably. However, the third dose adds only approximately 5% to protection. Since there is no need for long-term immunity to *H. influenzae* type b because natural immunity develops during childhood regardless of whether or not the infant was vaccinated, two doses of *H. influenzae* type b should suffice for most children. This is especially important in developing countries, where reducing the number of doses of costly *H. influenzae* type b conjugate vaccines would be one way to facilitate large-scale vaccination in regions with limited resources. Based on this rationale, a policy was adopted in Finland in which only two doses of conjugate vaccine were administered primarily, followed by a booster dose at 14 to 18 months of age (87). The United Kingdom chose another strategy in which three doses of PRP-T were given at 2, 3, and 4 months of age and no booster dose was administered (88). This was based on the finding that adequate concentrations of antibody persisted long after an accelerated vaccination schedule (89). In a subsequent United Kingdom study, 43 vaccine failures were described (31 failures among infants receiving PRP-T), which still gave an overall vaccine efficacy of 98.1% (90). These authors also suggested that priming with tetanus toxoid may lead to a significant level of protection after only one dose of PRP-T in infancy, which, if confirmed, may influence future decisions regarding the order of vaccine administration. Further studies will determine whether reduced frequency of dosing can be employed in the prevention of invasive *H. influenzae* type b disease.

Neisseria meningitidis

Since invasive disease caused by *N. meningitidis* occurs in patients devoid of specific bactericidal or opsonizing antibodies (91), vaccination to induce formation of these antibodies is the best way to prevent disease (3,26,92,93). Serogroup A and C meningococcal polysaccharide vaccines have been shown to be immunogenic and have established clinical efficacy for the control of outbreaks and epidemics of invasive disease caused by these meningococcal serogroups. However, these vaccines are less immunogenic in infants and small children, age groups at significant risk for invasive disease. Serogroup A polysaccharide vaccine appeared to be protective against invasive disease in one trial of infants and children from 3 months to 5 years of age (94), although the small number of infants under 1 year of age in this trial made it difficult to assess efficacy in this age group, and a response comparable to that among adults was not achieved until 4 or 5 years of age. In other studies, antibody responses to the serogroup A polysaccharide vaccine were shown to occur at the ages of 7 and 12 months (95,96). In one study, efficacy was estimated at 87% in the first year and 54% by 3 years after vaccination (97), but there was little protection in children younger than 3 years of age by 2 years after vaccination. In contrast, the serogroup C meningococcal polysaccharide component is poorly immunogenic in recipients less than 2 years of age. In one study in the United States, 60% of children ages 18 to 24 months had low titers of bactericidal antibody in response to vaccination with the serogroup C meningococcal vaccine (98). Furthermore, antibody concentrations to serogroup C polysaccharide fall rapidly after vaccination. In one Canadian study, only 20% of children (ages 2 to 6 years) had detectable bactericidal antibody by 12 months after vaccination (99). After vaccination of adults with serogroup A/C vaccines, total antibody and bactericidal activity peaked at 1 month post vaccination and declined rapidly over the next 2 years, although activity peaked above baseline for 10 years (100).

The serogroup A and C polysaccharide vaccines have demonstrated estimated clinical efficacies of 85% to 100% in older children and adults, and are useful in controlling epidemics caused by these meningococcal serogroups (32). Successful vaccination during serogroup A meningococcal epidemics has been reported throughout the world, and mass vaccination in sub-Saharan Africa and worldwide has resulted in herd immunity to serogroup A meningococcal meningitis (101). Duration of efficacy, however, decreases markedly during the first 3 years following a single dose of vaccine, an effect that occurs more rapidly in infants and children than in adults. Vaccines containing serogroup Y and W135 polysaccharides are also safe and immunogenic in adults and children more than 2 years of age (32). Although vaccination with these polysaccharides induces production of bactericidal antibodies, clinical protection has not been documented. Bactericidal antibody responses are elicited in adults with the licensed quadrivalent vaccine (activity against serogroups A, C, Y, and W135). This vaccine consists of 50 μg of each the respective purified bacterial capsular polysaccharides.

Vaccination with the quadrivalent meningococcal vaccine is currently recommended for persons 2 years of age or more in certain high-risk groups as follows (32): (a) those with terminal complement component or properdin deficiency or dysfunction; (b) anatomic or functional asplenia; (c) those who travel to areas with hyperendemic or epidemic meningococcal disease (e.g., Nigeria); and (d) military recruits. Research, industrial, and clinical laboratory personnel who routinely are exposed to *N. meningitidis* in solutions that may be aerosolized should also be considered for vaccination. Persons who have had their spleens removed as a result of trauma or nonlymphoid tumors and those with inherited complement deficiencies have acceptable antibody responses to vaccination, but the clinical efficacy of vaccination has not been established. Vaccination can be used as an adjunct to chemoprophylaxis, although vaccination does not reduce the transfer of bacteria to nonvaccinated persons, and the nasopharyngeal carrier state is unaffected (92). The vaccine has also been utilized in community outbreak settings, with an efficacy of 85% among 2- to 29-year-olds in one study (102). Vaccination is not recommended for routine use in the United States because of the overall low risk of infection, the inability to protect against serogroup B disease (see later), and the inability to provide lasting immunity to young children. However, because of the recent increase in invasive meningococcal disease in adolescents and young adults of high school and college age in the United States, and studies of meningococcal infection in United States college students, the Advisory Committee on Immunization Practices has recently recommended that college freshman dormitory residents and their parents be provided information about meningococcal infection and the benefits of vaccination, and that other undergraduate students wishing to reduce their risk of meningococcal disease can also choose to be vaccinated (103). Given the devastating nature of invasive meningococcal disease and the availability of a safe and effective vaccine, it is reasonable to promote the use of meningococcal vaccination in college students.

With the success of conjugate polysaccharide vaccines against invasive disease caused by *H. influenzae* type b (see earlier), conjugate vaccines for use against disease caused by serogroups A and C meningococci have been developed (93).

These vaccines contain meningococcal polysaccharide conjugated to a protein such as tetanus toxoid, diphtheria, or CRM_{197} and are immunogenic and induce immunologic memory in young children. They may also provide protection against carriage of meningococci, creating sufficient herd immunity to block transmission and thereby protect age groups that are not vaccinated; however, the effect of vaccination on nasopharyngeal carriage is currently being investigated. In one randomized, controlled trial in 182 healthy infants, meningococcal C conjugate vaccine was well tolerated and children were able to achieve higher meningococcal C IgG concentrations after three doses (at 2, 3, and 4 months of age) than those who received a hepatitis B control vaccine (104). At 12 months, antibody concentrations remained significantly higher in children vaccinated with the meningococcal C conjugate vaccine. Similar results were observed after administration of three doses of a *N. meningitidis* A + C diphtheria toxoid conjugate vaccine (MenD) to infants from Niger (105). This vaccine also demonstrated superior immunogenicity to the A + C meningococcal polysaccharide vaccine.

Based on these data, the United Kingdom has become the world's first country to implement routine immunization with a monovalent serogroup C meningococcal conjugate vaccine (106). Three doses of vaccine are recommended for children aged 2, 3, and 4 months; two doses for children more than 4 months and under 1 year of age; and one dose for all others. This latter group will be vaccinated in a catch-up campaign to immunize all school-aged children and young adults to the age of 20 years. It is predicted that the overall incidence of meningococcal disease after widespread vaccination should decrease by 40%, and deaths by even more, because of the relative severity of serogroup C disease (107). However, although there are excellent immunogenicity and safety data for the serogroup C meningococcal protein-polysaccharide conjugate vaccines, they have not yet been tested in phase III trials or in mass vaccination programs. There is also concern that vaccination may lead to an increase in the carriage of non-serogroup C hypervirulent meningococci (i.e., serogroup B, W135, or Y variants of the ET-37 complex), which might have a substantial effect on disease rates (107). These concerns indicate the need for careful surveillance in those persons with high rates of meningococcal carriage and in those who are to be included in the first round of vaccination. Furthermore, variation in serogroup distribution in various regions of the world (e.g., serogroup A in sub-Saharan Africa, serogroups C and Y in the United States) suggest the need for development and availability of multivalent meningococcal conjugate vaccines (108).

One other major obstacle to the control of invasive meningococcal disease is the lack of a suitable vaccine against serogroup B. The serogroup B capsular polysaccharide is poorly immunogenic (3,92,93), leading to examination of outer membrane proteins as potential immunogens. The immunogenicity and protective efficacy of several outer membrane protein vaccines have been evaluated in Chile, Cuba, Norway, and Brazil, with efficacies ranging from 57% to 83% in older children and adults (109–112), although no efficacy was seen in a study in children 4 years of age or less (113), the group often at highest risk for development of invasive disease. Given the discrepancies between trials studying these outer membrane protein vaccines, a recent prospective, double-blind, randomized controlled immunogenicity study compared the serum bactericidal activity elicited by the Cuban, Norwegian, or a control vaccine (114). The Cuban and Norwegian vaccines feature two different class 1 outer membrane proteins. Children (aged 2 to 4 years) and adult (aged 17 to 30 years) recipients of either meningococcal vaccine were more likely than controls to develop an immune response to the heterologous epidemic strain (i.e., the strain from which the other vaccine was derived). Infants (younger than 1 year of age), however, did not respond. In contrast, against homologous vaccine type strains (i.e., the strain from which the vaccine was derived), the response rate was 67% or higher among children and adults and 90% or higher among infants. These data indicate that vaccines prepared from strains sharing class 1 outer membrane proteins with epidemic strains will be more effective than vaccines prepared from other strains, suggesting that "designer" vaccines could be prepared to fit different epidemic strains as they occur (115). Prospective, randomized, double-blind clinical studies are needed to determine the efficacy of serogroup B meningococcal outer membrane protein vaccines in the prevention of epidemics caused by these microorganisms.

Streptococcus pneumoniae

The use of the current 23-valent pneumococcal vaccine (containing purified capsular polysaccharide antigen of serotypes 1, 2, 3, 4, 5, 6B, 7F, 8, 9N, 9V, 10A, 11A, 12F, 14, 15B, 17F, 18C, 19A, 19F, 20, 22F, 23F, and 33F) is recommended for prevention of bacteremic pneumococcal disease in certain high-risk groups (43): (a) persons 65 years of age and more; and (b) persons 2 to 64 years of age with chronic cardiovascular disease, chronic pulmonary disease, diabetes mellitus, alcoholism, chronic liver disease, CSF leaks, functional or anatomic asplenia, and living in special environments or social settings (including Alaskan natives and certain American Indian populations). Immunocompromised persons 2 years of age or more with human immunodeficiency virus infection, hematologic or generalized malignancies, chronic renal failure, nephrotic syndrome, illness that requires immunosuppressive chemotherapy (including corticosteroids), and organ or bone marrow transplant should also be vaccinated. The efficacy of this vaccine in prevention of pneumococcal meningitis has never been proven, however, although it may be assumed that the overall efficacy of the vaccine is about 50% against pneumococcal meningitis (with a wide 95% confidence interval) (116,117). In immunocompetent patients, the efficacy against pneumococcal meningitis caused by the vaccine strains was 63% compared with an efficacy of only 22% when immunocompromised patients were also included in the analysis.

Since children less than 2 years of age have the highest rate of invasive pneumococcal infection and because the 23-valent pneumococcal vaccine has no proven efficacy in the prevention of invasive pneumococcal infections in this age group, it became important to develop a more efficacious vaccine. Recently, pneumococcal vaccine preparations that conjugate capsular polysaccharide antigens to carrier proteins from a nontoxic variant of diphtheria toxin (CRM_{197}), tetanus toxoid, or a meningococcal outer membrane protein complex have been developed (118). A multivalent vaccine is created by separately conjugating individual capsular polysaccharides to a carrier protein and, in a separate step, combining these polysaccharide conjugates to create the final preparation (119). At present, pneumococcal conjugate formulations under study generally include polysaccharides of seven common invasive pneumococcal serotypes (4, 6B, 9V, 14, 18C, 19F, and 23F), nine serotypes (addition of serotypes 1 and 5), or 11 serotypes (addition of serotypes 3 and 7F). In phase I and phase II studies, these conjugate vaccines were safe and had the ability to induce production of sufficient amounts of specific anticapsular antibodies and induce immunologic memory (118). One recently published multicenter, controlled, double-blind study examined the efficacy of a heptavalent conjugate pneumococcal vaccine (coupled to the protein carrier CRM_{197}) compared with meningococcus type C CRM_{197} conjugate in 37,868 infants and children (120). Vaccine was administered in four doses at 2, 4, 6, and 12 to 15 months of age. Efficacy of the pneumococcal conjugate vaccine was 97.4% ($P < 0.001$) in fully vaccinated children in the prevention of invasive pneumococcal disease caused by the pneumococcal serotypes in the vaccine. The efficacy in the intention-to-treat analysis group was 93.9%. The overall efficacy was 89.1% ($P < 0.001$) against invasive pneumococcal disease regardless of serotype. If these data are confirmed in clinical practice, this vaccine is likely to have a major impact on the epidemiology of pneumococcal infections. In a recent cost-effective analysis of pneumococcal conjugate vaccination of healthy infants and children in a hypothetical United States birth cohort of 3.8 million infants (121), it was estimated that vaccination would prevent more than 12,000 cases of meningitis and bacteremia, and 112 deaths caused by pneumococcal infection for each United States birth cohort.

Based on the preceding information, the American Academy of Pediatrics Committee on Infectious Diseases has recommended vaccination of all infants less than 2 years of age with the currently licensed heptavalent pneumococcal conjugate vaccine (Prevnar) (122). The vaccine is administered in four doses at 2, 4, 6, and 12 to 15 months of age. Children who are unvaccinated and are 7 to 11 months of age should be given a total of three doses (two doses in a primary series 6 to 8 weeks apart and one dose at 12 to 15 months of age), and children who are unvaccinated and are 12 to 23 months of age should be given a total of two doses (6 to 8 weeks apart). Healthy children who are unvaccinated at 24 months of age or older need only one dose of the vaccine. The committee also recommends that the vaccine be given for all children ages 24 to 59 months who are at high risk of invasive pneumococcal infection. These include children with sickle cell disease and other types of functional or anatomic asplenia, human immunodeficiency virus infection or primary immunodeficiency, a condition requiring immunosuppressive therapy or solid organ transplantation, diabetes mellitus, and chronic cardiac, pulmonary, or renal disease.

With the licensure of the pneumococcal conjugate vaccine, continued surveillance for pneumococcal serotypes causing invasive disease is critical and may have implications for the serotype formulation of future conjugate vaccines (123,124). Studies of carriage have suggested a reduction in colonization by vaccine serotypes after immunization (125,126), although in some cases there is an increase in carriage of nonvaccine serotypes (127). The relevance of this finding is unclear, however, since pneumococcal isolates of the nonvaccine serotypes are thought to be much less likely than vaccine serotypes to cause disease. Continued follow-up of invasive pneumococcal disease since licensure of the conjugate vaccine will help to define these important issues.

REFERENCES

1. Greenwood BM. Selective primary health care: strategies for control of disease in the developing world. XIII: acute bacterial meningitis. *Rev Infect Dis* 1984;6:374–389.
2. Cuevas LE, Hart CA. Chemoprophylaxis of bacterial meningitis. *J Antimicrob Chemother* 1993; 31:79–91.
3. Peltola H. Prophylaxis of bacterial meningitis. *Infect Dis Clin North Am* 1999;13:685–710.
4. Band JD. Chemoprophylaxis of *Haemophilus influenzae* type b disease: a strategy for preventing secondary cases. In: Sell SH, Wright PF, eds. Haemophilus influenzae: *epidemiology, immunology, and prevention of disease.* New York: Elsevier Science Publishing, 1982:309–315.
5. Peter G. Treatment and prevention of *Haemophilus influenzae* type b meningitis. *Pediatr Infect Dis J* 1987;6:787–790.
6. Ward JI, Fraser DW, Baraff LJ, et al. *Haemophilus influenzae* meningitis: a national study of secondary spread in household contacts. *N Engl J Med* 1979;301:122–126.
7. Glode MP, Daum RS, Goldmann DA, et al. *Haemophilus influenzae* type b meningitis: a contagious disease of children. *Br Med J* 1980;280:899–901.
8. Broome CV, Mortimer EA, Katz SL, et al. Use of chemoprophylaxis to prevent the spread of *Haemophilus influenzae* b in day-care facilities. *N Engl J Med* 1987;316:1226–1228.
9. Cochi SL, Fleming DW, Hightower AW, et al. Primary invasive *Haemophilus influenzae* type b disease: a population-based assessment of risk factors. *J Pediatr* 1986;108:887–896.
10. Fleming DW, Leibenhaut MH, Albanes D, et al. Secondary *Haemophilus influenzae* type b in day-care facilities: risk factors and prevention. *JAMA* 1985;254:509–514.
11. Istre GR, Conner JS, Broome CV, et al. Risk factors for primary invasive *Haemophilus influenzae* disease: increased risk from day care attendance and school-aged household members. *J Pediatr* 1985;106:190–195.
12. Osterholm MT, Pierson LM, White KE, et al. The risk of subsequent transmission of *Haemophilus influenzae* type b disease among children in day care. *N Engl J Med* 1987;316:1–5.
13. Murphy TV, Clements JF, Breedlove JA, et al. Risk of subsequent disease among day-care contacts of patients with systemic *Haemophilus influenzae* type b disease. *N Engl J Med* 1987;316:5–10.
14. Cox F, Trincher R, Rissing JP, et al. Rifampin prophylaxis for contacts of *Haemophilus influenzae* type b disease. *JAMA* 1981;245:1043–1045.
15. Band JD, Fraser DW, Ajello G, et al. Prevention of *Hemophilus influenzae* type b disease. *JAMA* 1984;251:2381–2386.
16. Lieberman JM, Greenberg DP, Ward JI. Prevention of bacterial meningitis. vaccines and chemoprophylaxis. *Infect Dis Clin North Am* 1990;4:703–729.
17. Peter G, Hall CB, Halsey NA, et al. *Haemophilus influenzae* infections. In: *1997 Red book: report of the Committee on Infectious Diseases,* 24th ed. Elk Grove Village, IL: American Academy of Pediatrics, 1997:222–231.
18. Green M, Li KI, Wald ER, et al. Duration of rifampin chemoprophylaxis for contacts of patients infected with *Haemophilus influenzae* type b. *Antimicrob Agents Chemother* 1992;36: 545–547.
19. Greenfield S, Sheehe PR, Feldman HA. Meningococcal carriage in a population of "normal" families. *J Infect Dis* 1971;123:67–73.
20. Gold R, Goldschneider I, Lepow ML, et al. Carriage of *Neisseria meningitidis* and *Neisseria lactamica* in infants and children. *J Infect Dis* 1978;137:112–121.
21. Caugant DA, Hoiby EA, Magnus P, et al. Asymptomatic carriage of *Neisseria meningitidis* in a randomly sampled population. *J Clin Microbiol* 1994;32:323–330.
22. Fraser PK, Bailey GK, Abbot JD, et al. The meningococcal carrier-state. *Lancet* 1973;1:1235–1237.
23. Anderson J, Berthelsen L, Bech JB, et al. Dynamics of meningococcal carrier state and characterization of the carrier strains: a longitudinal study within three cohorts of military recruits. *Epidemiol Infect* 1998;121:85–94.
24. Stephens DS. Uncloaking the meningococcus: dynamics of carriage and disease. *Lancet* 1999;353:941–942.

25. Jones GR, Christodoulides M, Brooks JL, et al. Dynamics of carriage of *Neisseria meningitidis* in a group of military recruits: subtype stability and specificity of immune response following colonization. *J Infect Dis* 1998;178:451–456.
26. Riedo FX, Plikaytis BD, Broome CV. Epidemiology and prevention of meningococcal disease. *Pediatr Infect Dis J* 1995;14:643–657.
27. Imrey PB, Jackson LA, Ludwinski PH, et al. Meningococcal carriage, alcohol consumption, and campus bar patronage in a serogroup C meningococcal disease outbreak. *Antimicrob Agents Chemother* 1995;33:3133–3137.
28. Cookson ST, Corrales JL, Lotero JO, et al. Disco fever: epidemic meningococcal disease in northeastern Argentina associated with disco patronage. *J Infect Dis* 1998;178:266–269.
29. Koh YM, Barnes GH, Kaczmarski E, et al. Outbreak of meningococcal disease linked to a sports club. *Lancet* 1998;352:706–707.
30. De Wals P, Hertoghe L, Borlee-Grimee I, et al. Meningococcal disease in Belgium: secondary attack rate among household day-care nursery and pre-elementary school contacts. *J Infect* 1981;3[Suppl 1]:53–61.
31. Cooke RPD, Riordan T, Jones DM, et al. Secondary cases of meningococcal infection among close family and household contacts in England and Wales, 1984–1987. *Br Med J* 1989;298:555–558.
32. Centers for Disease Control and Prevention. Control and prevention of meningococcal disease and control and prevention of serogroup C meningococcal disease: evaluation and management of suspected outbreaks. *MMWR* 1997;46:1–11.
33. Schwartz B, Al-Tobaiqi A, Al-Ruwais A, et al. Comparative efficacy of ceftriaxone and rifampicin in eradicating pharyngeal carriage of group A *Neisseria meningitidis*. *Lancet* 1988;1:1239–1242.
34. Simmons G, Jones N, Calder L. Equivalence of ceftriaxone and rifampicin in eliminating nasopharyngeal carriage of serogroup B *Neisseria meningitidis*. *J Antimicrob Chemother* 2000;45:909–911.
35. Dworzack DL, Sanders CC, Horowitz EA, et al. Evaluation of single-dose ciprofloxacin in the eradication of *Neisseria meningitidis* from nasopharyngeal carriers. *Antimicrob Agents Chemother* 1988;32:1740–1741.
36. Gaunt PN, Lambert BE. Single dose ciprofloxacin for the eradication of pharyngeal carriage of *Neisseria meningitidis*. *J Antimicrob Chemother* 1988;21:489–496.
37. Tunkel AR, Scheld WM. Treatment of bacterial meningitis. In: Hooper DC, Wolfson JS, eds. *Quinolone antimicrobial agents,* 2nd ed. Washington, DC: American Society for Microbiology, 1993: 381–395.
38. Darouiche R, Perkins B, Musher D, et al. Levels of rifampin and ciprofloxacin in nasal secretions: correlation with MIC_{90} and eradication of nasopharyngeal carriage of bacteria. *J Infect Dis* 1990;162:1124–1127.
39. Schaad UB, Salam MA, Aujard Y, et al. Use of fluoroquinolones in pediatrics: consensus report of an International Society of Chemotherapy Commission. *Pediatr Infect Dis J* 1995;14:1–9.
40. Girgis N, Sultan Y, French RW Jr, et al. Azithromycin compared with rifampin for eradication of nasopharyngeal colonization by *Neisseria meningitidis*. *Pediatr Infect Dis J* 1998;17:816–819.
41. Rauch AM, O'Ryan M, Van R, et al. Invasive disease due to multiply resistant *Streptococcus pneumoniae* in a Houston, Texas, day-care center. *Am J Dis Child* 1990;144:923–927.
42. Gaston MH, Verter JI, Woods G, et al. Prophylaxis with oral penicillin in children with sickle cell anemia: a randomized trial. *N Engl J Med* 1986;314:1593–1599.
43. Centers for Disease Control and Prevention. Prevention of pneumococcal disease: recommendations of the Advisory Committee on Immunization Practices (ACIP). *MMWR* 1997;46:1–23.
44. Faletta JM, Woods GM, Verter JI, et al. Discontinuing penicillin prophylaxis in children with sickle cell anemia. *J Pediatr* 1995;127:685–690.
45. Zangwill KM, Schuchat A, Wenger JD, et al. Group B streptococcal disease in the United States, 1990: report from a multistate active surveillance system. *MMWR* 1992;41:25–32.
46. Committee on Infectious Diseases and Committee on Fetus and Newborn. Guidelines for prevention of group B streptococcal (GBS) infection by chemoprophylaxis. *Pediatrics* 1992;90:775–778.
47. Schuchat A. Epidemiology of group B streptococcal disease in the United States: shifting paradigms. *Clin Microbiol Rev* 1998;11:497–513.
48. Allen UD, Navas L, King SM. Effectiveness of intrapartum penicillin prophylaxis in preventing early-onset group B streptococcal infection: results of a meta-analysis. *Can Med Assoc J* 1993;149: 1659–1665.
49. Ohlsson A, Myhr TL. Intrapartum chemoprophylaxis of perinatal group B streptococcal infections: a critical review of randomized controlled trials. *Am J Obstet Gynecol* 1994;170:910–917.

50. Schrag SJ, Zywicki S, Farley MM, et al. Group B streptococcal disease in the era of intrapartum antibiotic prophylaxis. *N Engl J Med* 2000;342:15–20.
51. Schuchat A. Group B streptococcus. *Lancet* 1999;353:51–56.
52. Centers for Disease Control and Prevention. Prevention of perinatal group B streptococcal disease: a public health perspective. *MMWR* 1996;45:1–24.
53. Rosenstein N, Schuchat A, Neonatal GBS Disease Study Group. Opportunities for prevention of perinatal group B streptococcal disease: a multistate surveillance analysis. *Obstet Gynecol* 1997;90: 901–906.
54. Centers for Disease Control and Prevention. Adoption of hospital policies for prevention of perinatal group B streptococcal disease—United States, 1997. *MMWR* 1998;47:65–70.
55. Brozanski BS, Jones JG, Krohn MA, et al. Effect of a screening-based prevention policy on prevalence of early-onset group B streptococcal sepsis. *Obstet Gynecol* 2000;95:496–501.
56. Fernandez M, Hickman ME, Baker CJ. Antimicrobial susceptibilities of group B streptococci isolated between 1992 and 1996 from patients with bacteremia or meningitis. *Antimicrob Agents Chemother* 1998;42:1517–1519.
57. Tyrrell GJ, Senzilet LD, Spika JS, et al. Invasive disease due to group B streptococcal infection in adults: results from a Canadian, population-based, active laboratory surveillance study, 1996. *J Infect Dis* 2000;182:168–173.
58. Towers V, Carr MH, Padilla G, et al. Potential consequences of widespread antipartal use of ampicillin. *Am J Obstet Gynecol* 1998;179:879–883.
59. Bergeron MG, Ke D, Menard C, et al. Rapid detection of group B streptococci in pregnant women at delivery. *N Engl J Med* 2000;343:175–179.
60. Schuchat A. Neonatal group B streptococcal disease: screening and prevention. *N Engl J Med* 2000;343:209–210.
61. Tunkel AR, Scheld WM. Acute infectious complications of head trauma. In: Braakman R, ed. *Handbook of clinical neurology, head injury.* Amsterdam: Elsevier Science Publishers, 1990:317–326.
62. Rathore MH. Do prophylactic antibiotics prevent meningitis after basilar skull fracture? *Pediatr Infect Dis J* 1991;10:87–88.
63. Villalobos T, Arango C, Kubilis P, et al. Antibiotic prophylaxis after basilar skull fracture. *Clin Infect Dis* 1998;27:364–369.
64. Klastersky UJ, Sadegli M, Brihaye J. Antimicrobial prophylaxis in patients with rhinorrhea or otorrhea: a double-blind study. *Surg Neurol* 1976;8:111–114.
65. Demetriades D, Charalambides D, Lakhoon I, et al. Role of prophylactic antibiotics in open and basilar skull fractures of the skull: a randomized study. *Injury* 1992;23:377–380.
66. Kaufman BA. Infections of cerebrospinal fluid shunts. In: Scheld WM, Whitley RJ, Durack DT, eds. *Infections of the central nervous system,* 2nd ed. Philadelphia: Lippincott-Raven, 1997:555–577.
67. Langley JM, LeBlanc JC, Drake J, et al. Efficacy of antimicrobial prophylaxis in placement of cerebrospinal fluid shunts: meta-analysis. *Clin Infect Dis* 1993;17:98–103.
68. Blomstedt GC. Results of trimethoprim-sulfamethoxazole prophylaxis in ventriculostomy and shunting procedures: a double-blind randomized trial. *J Neurosurg* 1985;62:694–697.
69. Haines SJ, Walters BC. Antibiotic prophylaxis for cerebrospinal fluid shunts: a meta-analysis. *Neurosurgery* 1994;34:87–92.
70. Peltola H, Käyhty H, Sivonen A, et al. *Haemophilus influenzae* type b capsular polysaccharide vaccine in children: a double-blind field study of 100,000 vaccinees 3 months to 5 years of age in Finland. *Pediatrics* 1977;60:730–737.
71. Käyhty H, Peltola H, Karanko V, et al. The protective level of serum antibodies to the capsular polysaccharide of *Haemophilus influenzae* type b. *J Infect Dis* 1983;147:1100.
72. Peltola H. Vaccines against bacterial meningitis. In: Scheld WM, Whitley RJ, Durack DT, eds. *Infections of the central nervous system,* 2nd ed. Philadelphia: Lippincott-Raven, 1997:1013–1039.
73. Peltola H. Worldwide *Haemophilus influenzae* type b disease at the beginning of the 21st century: global analysis of the disease burden 25 years after the use of the polysaccharide vaccine and a decade after the advent of conjugates. *Clin Microbiol Rev* 2000;13:302–317.
74. Eskola J, Käyhty H, Takala AK, et al. A randomized, prospective field trial of a conjugate vaccine in the protection of infants and children against invasive *Haemophilus influenzae* type b disease. *N Engl J Med* 1990;323:1381–1387
75. Black SB, Shinefield HE, Fireman B, et al. Efficacy in infancy of oligosaccharide conjugate *Haemophilus influenzae* type b (HbOC) vaccine in a United States population of 61,080 children. *Pediatr Infect Dis J* 1991;10:97–104.

76. Santosham M, Wolff M, Reid R, et al. The efficacy in Navajo infants of a conjugate vaccine consisting of *Haemophilus influenzae* type b polysaccharide and *Neisseria meningitidis* outer-membrane protein complex. *N Engl J Med* 1991;324:1767–1772.

77. Booy R, Hodgson S, Carpenter L, et al. Efficacy of *Haemophilus influenzae* type b conjugate vaccine PRP-T. *Lancet* 1994;344:362–366.

78. American Academy of Pediatrics, Committee on Infectious Diseases. Recommended childhood immunization schedule—United States, January–December 2000. *Pediatrics* 2000;105:148–151.

79. Takala AD, Eskola J, Leinonen M, et al. Reduction of oropharyngeal carriage of *Haemophilus influenzae* type b (Hib) in children immunized with an Hib conjugate vaccine. *J Infect Dis* 1991;164:982–986.

80. Jonsdottir K, Steingrimsson O, Olafsson O. Immunization of infants in Iceland against *Haemophilus influenzae* type b. *Lancet* 1992;340:252–253.

81. Mohle-Boetani JC, Ajello G, Breneman E, et al. Carriage of *Haemophilus influenzae* type b in children after widespread vaccination with *Haemophilus influenzae* type b vaccines. *Pediatr Infect Dis J* 1993;12:589–593.

82. Murphy TV, Pastor P, Medley F, et al. Decreased *Haemophilus* colonization in children vaccinated with *Haemophilus influenzae* type b conjugate vaccine. *J Pediatr* 1993;122:517–523.

83. Adegbola RA, Mulholland EK, Secka O, et al. Vaccination with a *Haemophilus influenzae* type b conjugate vaccine reduces oropharyngeal carriage of *H. influenzae* type b among Gambian children. *J Infect Dis* 1998;177:1758–1761.

84. Van Alphen L, Spanjaard L, van der Ende A, et al. Effect of nationwide vaccination of 3-month-old infants in The Netherlands with conjugate *Haemophilus influenzae* type b vaccine: high efficacy and lack of herd immunity. *J Pediatr* 1997;131:869–873.

85. Galil K, Singleton R, Levine OS, et al. Reemergence of invasive *Haemophilus influenzae* type b disease in a well-vaccinated population in remote Alaska. *J Infect Dis* 1999;179:101–106.

86. Perdue DG, Bulkow LR, Gellin BG, et al. Invasive *Haemophilus influenzae* disease in Alaskan residents aged 10 years and older before and after infant vaccination programs. *JAMA* 2000;283:3089–3094.

87. Peltola H, Eskola J, Käyhty H, et al. Clinical comparison of the *Haemophilus influenzae* type b polysaccharide-diphtheria toxoid and the oligosaccharide-CRM$_{197}$ protein vaccines in infancy. *Arch Pediatr Adolesc Med* 1994;148:620–625.

88. Booy R, Hodgson S, Carpenter L, et al. Efficacy of *Haemophilus influenzae* type b conjugate vaccine PRP-T. *Lancet* 1994;344:362–366.

89. Booy R, Taylor SA, Dobson SRM, et al. Immunogenicity and safety of PRP-T conjugate vaccine given according to the British accelerated immunization schedule. *Arch Dis Child* 1992;67:475–478.

90. Booy R, Heath PT, Slack MPE, et al. Vaccine failures after primary immunization with *Haemophilus influenzae* type-b conjugate vaccine without booster. *Lancet* 1997;349:1197–1202.

91. Jones GR, Williams JN, Christodoulides M, et al. Lack of immunity in university students before an outbreak of serogroup C meningococcal infection. *J Infect Dis* 2000;181:1172–1175.

92. Van Deuren M, Brandtzaeg P, van der Meet JWM. Update on meningococcal disease with emphasis on pathogenesis and clinical management. *Clin Microbiol Rev* 2000;13:144–166.

93. Pollard AJ, Levin M. Vaccines for prevention of meningococcal disease. *Pediatr Infect Dis J* 2000;19:333–345.

94. Peltola H, Mäkelä PH, Käyhty H, et al. Clinical efficacy of meningococcus group A capsular polysaccharide vaccine in children three months to five years of age. *N Engl J Med* 1977;297:686–691.

95. Gold R, Lepow ML, Goldschneider I, et al. Immune response of human infants of polysaccharide vaccines of group A and C *Neisseria meningitidis*. *J Infect Dis* 1977;136[Suppl 1]:S31–S35.

96. Goldschneider I, Lepow ML, Gotschlich EC, et al. Immunogenicity of group A and group C meningococcal polysaccharides in human infants. *J Infect Dis* 1973;128:769–776.

97. Reingold AL, Broome CV, Hightower AW, et al. Age-specific differences in duration of clinical protection after vaccination with meningococcal polysaccharide A vaccine. *Lancet* 1985;2:114–118.

98. Lieberman JM, Chiu SS, Wong VK, et al. Safety and immunogenicity of a serogroups A/C *Neisseria meningitidis* oligosaccharide-protein conjugate vaccine in young children: a randomized controlled trial. *JAMA* 1996;275:1499–1503.

99. Mitchell LA, Ochnio JJ, Glover C, et al. Analysis of meningococcal serogroup C-specific antibody levels in British Columbian children and adolescents. *J Infect Dis* 1996;173:1009–1013.

100. Zangwill KM, Stout RW, Carlone GM, et al. Duration of antibody response after meningococcal polysaccharide vaccine in US Air Force personnel. *J Infect Dis* 1994;169:847–852.

101. Robbins JB, Towne DW, Gotschlich EC, et al. "Love's Labours Lost": failure to implement mass vaccination against group A meningococcal meningitis in sub-Saharan Africa. *Lancet* 1997;350:880–882.

102. Rosenstein N, Levine O, Taylor JP, et al. Efficacy of meningococcal vaccine and barriers to vaccination. *JAMA* 1998;279:435–439.
103. Harrison LH. Preventing meningococcal infection in college students. *Clin Infect Dis* 2000;30: 648–651.
104. MacLennan JM, Shackley F, Heath PT, et al. Safety, immunogenicity, and induction of immunologic memory by a serogroup C meningococcal vaccine in infants. *JAMA* 2000;283:2795–2801.
105. Campagne G, Garba A, Fabre P, et al. Safety and immunogenicity of three doses of a *Neisseria meningitidis* A + C diphtheria conjugate vaccine in infants from Niger. *Pediatr Infect Dis J* 2000;19:144–150.
106. Public Health Laboratory Service. Vaccination programme for group C meningococcal infection is launched. *Commun Dis Rep CDR Weekly* 1999;9:261–264.
107. Maiden MCJ, Spratt BG. Meningococcal conjugate vaccine: new opportunities and new challenges. *Lancet* 1999;354:615–616.
108. Perkins BA. New opportunities for prevention of meningococcal disease. *JAMA* 2000;283: 2842–2843.
109. Sierra GVG, Campa HC, Varcacel NM, et al. Vaccine against group B *Neisseria meningitidis*: protection trial and mass vaccination results in Cuba. *NIPH Ann* 1991;14:195–207.
110. Bjune G, Hoiby EA, Gronnesby JK, et al. Effect of outer membrane vesicle vaccine against group B meningococcal disease in Norway. *Lancet* 1991;338:1093–1096.
111. Milagres LG, Ramos SR, Sacchi CT, et al. Immune response of Brazilian children to a *Neisseria meningitidis* serogroup B outer membrane protein vaccine: comparison with efficacy. *Infect Immun* 1994;62:4419–4424.
112. Boslego JB, Garcia J, Cruz C. Efficacy, safety, and immunogenicity of a meningococcal vaccine group B (15:P1.3) outer membrane protein vaccine in Iquique, Chile. *Vaccine* 1995;13:821–829.
113. De Moraes JC, Perkins BA, Camargo MCC, et al. Protective efficacy of a serogroup B meningococcal vaccine in Sao Paulo, Brazil. *Lancet* 1992;340:1074–1078.
114. Tappero JW, Lagos R, Ballesteros AM, et al. Immunogenicity of 2 serogroup B outer-membrane protein meningococcal vaccines: a randomized controlled trial in Chile. *JAMA* 1999;281:1520–1527.
115. Wenger JD. Serogroup B meningococcal disease: new outbreaks, new strategies. *JAMA* 1999;281:1541–1543.
116. Bolan G, Broome CV, Facklam RR, et al. Pneumococcal vaccine efficacy in selected populations in the United States. *Ann Intern Med* 1986;104:1–6.
117. Butler JC, Breiman RF, Campbell JF, et al. Pneumococcal polysaccharide vaccine efficacy: an evaluation of current recommendations. *JAMA* 1993;270:1826–1831.
118. Eskola J, Anttila M. Pneumococcal conjugate vaccines. *Pediatr Infect Dis J* 1999;18:543–551.
119. Watson W. Pneumococcal conjugate vaccines. *Pediatr Infect Dis J* 2000;19:331–332.
120. Black S, Shinefield H, Fireman B, et al. Efficacy, safety and immunogenicity of heptavalent pneumococcal conjugate vaccine in children. *Pediatr Infect Dis J* 2000;19:187–195.
121. Lieu TA, Ray GT, Black SB, et al. Projected cost-effectiveness of pneumococcal conjugate vaccination of healthy infants and young children. *JAMA* 2000;283:1460–1468.
122. American Academy of Pediatrics, Committee on Infectious Diseases. Policy statement: recommendations for the prevention of pneumococcal infections, including use of pneumococcal conjugate vaccine (Prevnar), pneumococcal polysaccharide vaccine, and antibiotic prophylaxis. *Pediatrics* 2000;106:362–366.
123. Hausdorff WP, Bryant J, Paradiso PR, et al. Which pneumococcal serogroups cause the most invasive disease: implications for conjugate vaccine formulation and use, part I. *Clin Infect Dis* 2000;30:100–121.
124. Hausdorff WP, Bryant J, Kloek C, et al. The contribution of specific pneumococcal serogroups to different disease manifestations: implications for conjugate vaccine formulation and use, part II. *Clin Infect Dis* 2000;30:122–140.
125. Dagan R, Melamed R, Muallem M, et al. Reduction of a nasopharyngeal carriage of pneumococci during the second year of life by a heptavalent conjugate pneumococcal vaccine. *J Infect Dis* 1996;174:1271–1278.
126. Dagan R, Muallem M, Leroy O, et al. Reduction of pneumococcal nasopharyngeal carriage in early infancy after immunization with tetravalent pneumococcal vaccines conjugated to either tetanus toxoid or diphtheria toxoid. *Pediatr Infect Dis J* 1997;16:1060–1064.
127. Obaro SK, Adegbola RA, Banya WA, et al. Carriage of pneumococci after pneumococcal vaccination. *Lancet* 1996;348:271–272.

10

The Future

Over the last two centuries, there has been a major evolution in the understanding of the clinical manifestations, diagnostic approach, and management of the patient with bacterial meningitis. Since the first detailed description of "epidemic cerebrospinal fever" (i.e., meningococcal meningitis) in 1805, clinicians have examined various approaches to the therapy of this devastating disorder. With the advent of lumbar puncture in the late nineteenth century, drainage of cerebrospinal fluid (along with irrigation of the subarachnoid space with Ringer's lactate or chemical agents) was employed, although it would be another 15 years before the use of antimeningococcal antiserum was shown to be efficacious in experimental animals with meningococcal infections. The intrathecal administration of antimeningococcal antiserum into patients with meningococcal meningitis was subsequently shown to decrease mortality from as much as 90% to about 30%.

The introduction of antimicrobial agents in the twentieth century (sulfonamides in the late 1930s and penicillin in the 1940s) revolutionized the management of the patient with bacterial meningitis. Whereas the outcome from this disorder was fatal in untreated patients with rare exceptions, the mortality rate was dramatically lowered after treatment with antimicrobial agents. However, despite the availability of effective bactericidal antimicrobial agents, the morbidity and mortality from bacterial meningitis remains unacceptably high. The approach to the patient with bacterial meningitis in the twenty-first century will need to focus on several avenues to further improve the prognosis in patients with this disorder. These are highlighted in the following discussion.

EARLY RECOGNITION OF THE MENINGITIS SYNDROME

Early recognition of the acute meningitis syndrome with rapid initiation of antimicrobial therapy may improve outcome in patients with acute bacterial meningitis. Although this principle of therapy for bacterial meningitis makes intuitive sense, there are no prospective clinical data to support this concept. Especially in the developing world, an inordinate delay from the time of development of symptoms to the initiation of antimicrobial therapy may contribute to the higher mortality rate observed in these countries. Since it cannot be predicted when an individual patient with bacterial meningitis will progress to a high level of clinical severity, the duration of symptoms prior to hospitalization cannot be used as an indicator of when to first administer antimicrobial therapy. Clinicians must have a high level of suspicion in considering this diagnosis and initiate antimicrobial therapy before the patient's condition advances to a high level of clinical severity, at which time antimicrobial agents and other strategies may not be as efficacious in improving outcome.

DEVELOPMENT AND AVAILABILITY OF NEW ANTIMICROBIAL AGENTS

A major issue facing clinicians caring for patients with acute bacterial meningitis is the emergence of microorganisms resistant to standard antimicrobial agents. This is currently most evident in the therapeutic approach to the patient with pneumococcal meningitis. Worldwide increases in the prevalence of resistance of *Streptococcus pneumoniae* to penicillin G have changed the approach to empiric antimicrobial therapy of pneumococcal meningitis, such that the standard is now vancomycin combined with a third-generation cephalosporin, pending *in vitro* susceptibility testing. However, pneumococcal resistance to the third-generation cephalosporins has also emerged, and vancomycin-tolerant pneumococci have recently been described. The new carbapenem, meropenem, has been approved for the treatment of bacterial meningitis, although too few meningitis patients with resistant pneumococcal strains have been treated with this agent to determine its efficacy. The newer fluoroquinolones (e.g., levofloxacin, moxifloxacin, gatifloxacin) have excellent *in vitro* activity against resistant pneumococci, but clinical studies with these agents in pneumococcal meningitis have not been published. Emergence of penicillin resistance in *Neisseria meningitidis* may also require clinicians to alter the therapeutic approach in patients with meningococcal meningitis. Development of newer agents with *in vitro* activity against these resistant microorganisms is urgently needed, so that we will continue to have effective antimicrobial agents to treat these devastating infections.

Of additional concern is the availability of effective antimicrobial therapy in developing countries for patients with bacterial meningitis caused by these resistant microorganisms. Penicillin and chloramphenicol have been used most extensively in the developing world because of ease of administration and low cost. The utilization of newer antimicrobial agents may be limited secondary to expense, even though therapy with agents that cannot reliably and rapidly sterilize the cerebrospinal fluid may be associated with worse outcome. Continued worldwide surveillance for trends in antimicrobial resistance in meningeal pathogens, populations at risk, and morbidity and mortality in response to treatment is critical in order to determine the optimal therapeutic approach for patients with bacterial meningitis.

DEVELOPMENT OF NEW ADJUNCTIVE THERAPIES

Research over the last three decades has elucidated many of the pathogenic and pathophysiologic mechanisms operable in bacterial meningitis. We now have a better understanding of the mechanisms by which meningeal pathogens colonize the host and produce invasive disease, as well as the bacterial and host determinants that cause breakdown of the blood-brain barrier, induce subarachnoid space inflammation, produce cerebral edema, increase intracranial pressure, alter cerebral blood flow, and produce neurologic injury in patients with bacterial meningitis. These studies have led to the recommendation that adjunctive dexamethasone (which attenuates the subarachnoid space inflammatory response after antimicrobial-induced lysis of meningeal pathogens) be routinely used in infants and children with *Haemophilus influenzae* type b meningitis, and considered strongly for children with pneumococcal meningitis if commenced concomitant with or just before the first dose of an antimicrobial agent. This approach has reduced morbidity in infants and children with bacterial meningitis. There is controversy, however, as to whether adjunctive dexamethasone should be routinely used in all patients with bacterial meningitis. Furthermore, use of adjunctive dexamethasone may not be considered until after administration of antimicrobial therapy, at which time dexamethasone is less likely to have a therapeutic benefit.

Therapeutic approaches to adjunctive therapy should target the pathophysiologic consequences of bacterial meningitis, since many of these manifestations are evident once the patient seeks medical attention. Recent studies have elucidated the mechanisms of neuronal injury that occur in patient with bacterial meningitis, highlighting the importance of reactive oxygen and nitrogen intermediates in these processes. Drugs directed against these intermediates might offer important therapeutic advances. Development of adjunctive strategies to target these events might be used after administration of antimicrobial therapy or later in the disease course, resulting in an improvement in outcome.

VACCINATION

With the exception of the development of antimicrobial agents, the most significant advance in the fight against bacterial meningitis has been the virtual elimination of meningitis caused by *H. influenzae* type b in countries where routine immunization with the *H. influenzae* type b conjugate vaccine has been implemented. Even in countries where vaccine use has been moderate, significant reductions in the incidence of invasive *H. influenzae* type b disease have been documented, suggesting that herd immunity (perhaps from the ability of the *H. influenzae* type b conjugate vaccine to reduce nasopharyngeal colonization) is enhanced by vaccination. Recent licensure of the pneumococcal conjugate vaccine in the United States and the serogroup C meningococcal conjugate vaccine in the United Kingdom might also be expected to reduce the incidence of bacterial meningitis caused by these microorganisms; surveillance studies post licensure are needed to determine whether the efficacy of these vaccines is comparable to that observed with the *H. influenzae* type b conjugate vaccine. Effective vaccines against serogroup B meningococcus and group B streptococcus must be developed and will have implications in the control of invasive disease caused by these microorganisms.

Vaccination is the best strategy for the control of bacterial meningitis worldwide. Major epidemics of meningococcal disease still occur regularly in many areas of the world. Mass immunization with meningococcal polysaccharide vaccines can halt epidemics of invasive meningococcal disease. However, in developing countries where the incidence and mortality from bacterial meningitis far exceeds the rates in industrialized nations, the major barrier to immunization has been expense. Future studies may determine the optimal number of dosages of the conjugate vaccines required for significant protection, the effectiveness of these vaccines in prevention of nasopharyngeal colonization and development of herd immunity in reduction of outbreaks, and the ability to use vaccines in combination without affecting immunogenicity. However, it is also critical to produce vaccines at a low cost to improve availability for the populations at greatest need.

Clearly, the continued utilization of effective vaccines against the various meningeal pathogens is critical to prevent the development of invasive disease, which can lead to significant mortality as well as the devastating sequelae that have been associated with bacterial meningitis. Availability and use of these vaccines may eventually make bacterial meningitis a disease of the past.

Subject Index

Note: Page numbers followed by "*f*" indicate figures; those followed by "*t*" indicate tables.

Sulfadiazine
  adjunctive therapy with corticosteroids,
    clinical trial outcome, 182*t*
  early therapeutic use of, 12, 13
Sulfamethoxazole, percent penetration into CSF,
    167*t*
Sulfanilamide, first use of, in treatment of
    meningitis, 11–14
Sulfonamides
  chemoprophylactic use of, for *Neisseria
    meningitidis* meningitis, 231
  development of, 11–14
  therapeutic use of, first, 12–13
Surface components, bacterial, in
    colonization/invasion process, 45–47
Surgery, 217

T
Thalidomide, effect on inflammatory response,
    61
Therapy
  antimicrobial. See Antimicrobial therapy
  antiserum development for, 9–10
  historical perspective on, 9–14
  penicillin development for, 13–14
  secondary infection in, 10
  sulfonamide development for, 11–14
Ticarcillin, percent penetration into CSF,
    167*t*
TNF (tumor necrosis factor)
  in blood-brain barrier permeability, 56
  in neuronal apoptosis, 73
  in subarachnoid space inflammation, 59–60
Tobramycin
  percent penetration into CSF, 167*t*
  recommended dosage, in normal renal and
    hepatic function, 176*t*
Transcytosis, in central nervous system invasion,
    51–52
Trimethoprim, percent penetration into CSF,
    167*t*
Trimethoprim-sulfamethoxazole
  recommended dosage, in normal renal and
    hepatic function, 176*t*
  therapeutic use of
    in aerobic gram-negative bacillary
      meningitis, 196*t*
    in *Listeria monocytogenes* meningitis, 196*t*,
      204
Trovafloxacin
  percent penetration into CSF, 167*t*

therapeutic use of
  in *Listeria monocytogenes* meningitis, 205
  in *Neisseria meningitidis* meningitis, 203
  in *Streptococcus pneumoniae* meningitis,
    202
Tumor necrosis factor (TNF)
  in blood-brain barrier permeability, 56
  in neuronal apoptosis, 73
  in subarachnoid space inflammation, 59–60

V
Vaccines
  future developments in, 252–253
  for *Haemophilus influenzae* type b meningitis
    prevention, 1, 19–21, 19*t*, 30–31
    doses conferring immunity, 239–240
    efficacy of, 229, 237–238
    oropharyngeal colonization reduction, 239
    schedule for, 238–239, 238*t*
  for *Neisseria meningitidis* meningitis
    prevention, 1, 19–20
    conjugate vaccine development, 241–242
    conjugate vaccine implementation, 242
    efficacy of, 240
    recommendations for, 241
    serogroup A and C, 240–241
    serogroup B vaccine development, 242–243
  for pathogenic colonization, 239
  for *Streptococcus pneumoniae* meningitis
    prevention, 1, 19–20
    conjugate vaccine, 244
    efficacy of, 243–244
    recommendations for, 244
Vancomycin
  percent penetration into CSF, 167*t*
  recommended dosage, in normal renal and
    hepatic function, 176*t*
  therapeutic use of
    in *Listeria monocytogenes* meningitis, 204
    in penicillin resistant *Streptococcus
      pneumoniae* meningitis, 196*t*, 199–200
    in staphylococcal meningitis, 196*t*,
      207–208
    in *Streptococcus agalactiae* meningitis,
      196*t*, 204
Virus infection
  in differential diagnosis, 119–134. *See also
    under* Differential diagnosis
  upper respiratory tract, in
    colonization/invasion process, 46
Virulence factors. *See* Bacterial virulence factors